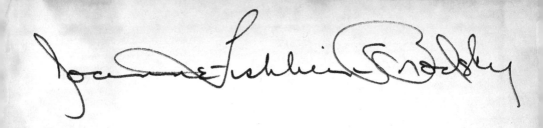

Psychosocial nursing

Psychosocial nursing

Theory and Practice in
Hospital and Community Mental Health

by **Frances Monet Carter Evans**
Professor, School of Nursing
University of San Francisco

The Macmillan Company, New York
Collier-Macmillan Limited, London

The Macmillan Company
866 Third Avenue, New York, New York 10022
Collier-Macmillan Canada, Ltd., Toronto, Ontario

Library of Congress catalog card number: 71-131475

PRINTING   5678910   YEAR   3456789

to **H**enry
and to my brothers
James and Charles

Preface

This book is an effort to look at psychiatric nursing in a new light and to show how it relates to current problems. Emphasis is placed on psychosocial aspects of nurse-patient relationships.

It reflects a basic concern with the role of the psychiatric nurse in the prevention of mental disorders, the promotion of mental health of individuals and families, and the provision of quality nursing care for those patients with incipient and diagnosed mental disorder in diverse settings.

This book has been written for nursing students and is intended to provide some of the basic psychosocial content relevant to the practice of psychiatric nursing.

F. M. C. E.
San Francisco

Acknowledgments

In the writing of this book I wish to acknowledge the inspiration and encouragement of Marion E. Kalkman, who has also aided me in many aspects of my professional education. The late Suzanne Aimée Bernfeld helped me in the clarification of some of the concepts contained in this volume.

I am deeply indebted to my patients, students, colleagues, and teachers without whom this book would not have been written. Appreciation is hereby expressed to my editors T. P. McConahay and Henry Van Swearingen for their valuable assistance. For comments on Chapters 2 and 3, respectively, I wish to extend appreciation to my colleagues Corrine Orsi and Sister Mary Martha Kiening. Thanks are also due the late Jennie Davis and Gloria Stracke, Phyllis Chiara, and Sylvia Douglas for their help in typing the manuscript.

Furthermore, I wish to express my appreciation to the authors and publishers whose works are quoted in this book. All works quoted are credited in footnotes.

All names of patients in the case material in this book are fictitious.

Contents

1 Introduction

In psychiatry, changes in philosophy of treatment and the emphasis upon prevention require a new focus in the education of nurses. The shift from hospital to community-centered care is in process, and psychiatric care within the home community is now a reality in many states. The merging of sociology, anthropology, and the public health point of view with psychiatry gives the profession a new direction. Not only is it necessary to know intrapsychic processes; the dimensions of the ecological units of the home, neighborhood, and community must also receive full attention of the psychiatric nurse.

At the same time, trends in educational programs at a generic level are moving toward the teaching of clinical nursing and away from the specialty areas. Integration of psychiatric-mental health concepts in generic programs has been going on for more than ten years. Integrated programs in nursing include segments of all traditional "specialties"—medical-surgical, community, maternal-child health, and psychiatric mental health nursing—in all courses. This new approach emphasizes the holistic view of man in the provision of nursing care. Professional nursing now includes concern not only for the intrapsychic "wounds" of the patient but for the effect these have upon his total functioning as a human being, as a member of a family, and of the society which has contributed to his condition. Attention is thereby being given to relevant aspects of the sociocultural background of the patient and his family in family-centered nursing.

The psychiatric nurse is concerned with those persons with mental problems and also with helping persons to achieve high level wellness. The ideas presented here are built upon the theoretical framework of man as a continuum of psyche, soma, family, society, and culture—all in reciprocal relationships. These systems are in a constant state of interaction with each other, and there are no fine lines of demarcation among them. A change in one system, however, affects all the others. Stress overload in one system requires overtime from all the others. The nurse can no longer administer to one system and ignore the others if effective care is to be provided for the patient. Therefore, in this book, pertinent mental health concepts related to the psyche, soma, family, society, and culture of persons are presented.

Concepts relating to wellness are emphasized to assist the student in identifying the strengths of patients and families. This text encompasses some discussion of all phases of the life cycle, but emphasizes the middle years and aging. It is written for nursing students who find patients in diverse settings: out-patient departments, homes, convalescent homes, mental hospitals, day treatment centers, and community mental health centers. Knowledge required for prevention and intervention in nursing is presented. Some concepts are part of the life cycle model, others are part of the model of mental disorder. As the nurse does more community work, both models are required for primary preventive action and better care of the patient with diagnosed mental problems. The well part of the patient, his strengths, and his coping deficits are all important considerations in the nurse-patient relationship. Use of the full potential of each individual for a full and happy life is the ultimate aim of psychiatric-mental health work. Therefore, some aspects of human development and crises of life are included in Chapter 2 as knowledge relevant for the nurse to measure the positive mental health of individuals and to provide anticipatory guidance for them. This knowledge of what is in store for each person as he progresses through the expected crises of life provides a yardstick for the nurse in assessment of levels of wellness. Since much of nursing also deals with individuals and families in crisis, there is an emphasis on the early recognition of crises, the immediacy of need, and the opportunity for growth in crisis resolution. In regard to those who are already mentally disordered, it gives an idea of what they must regain to achieve positive mental health.

Although the care of the mentally retarded has traditionally been included in psychiatry, it is now moving into the medical and educational model and is not included in this book (Lemkau, 1968).

As care of certain conditions of patients has moved from psychiatry into general medicine (epilepsy, for example), psychiatry reaches out to other areas; today it is to the promotion of mental health. The idea of anticipatory thinking with regard to the expected crises of life is an important concept in primary prevention and has broad application in nursing. If an individual has a chance to prepare for what is in store for him in life, he will be less vulnerable to mental disorder. The unexpected crises continue to unfold and are rich areas for secondary and tertiary prevention in nursing. The existence of psychiatric symptoms in every pathological process which produces disease has implications for those in the health professions to contribute to the prevention of mental disorder (Lemkau, 1968). The epidemiology of mental disorder receives a new emphasis in the identification of populations at risk through the study of ecology and demography.

Conflict, tension, anxiety, social deprivation, sensory deprivation, and other losses offer opportunities for direct preventive action in nursing, whether it be psychiatric first aid or long-term nursing care.

In recognition of the men in nursing, I have attempted to refer to nurses and to nursing students, where appropriate, without use of the feminine pronoun.

Psychological aspects of human behavior are treated in this book. A basic assumption is that nursing students also learn about biological man and that many other sources are available on that subject. A "close-up" picture of psychosocial aspects of nursing is provided herein.

Preview

Chapter 2 presents some facets of the life cycle model of human development and crisis points with particular stress upon the meaning of life's crises for the middle-aged and aging person. Components of unexpected crises are presented with emphasis upon the responsibility of the nurse to recognize them in patients and families. Much of the material is derived from the work of Havighurst (1953), Erikson (1963), Caplan (1964), and others.

Chapter 3 presents some aspects of the life style and characteristics of the contemporary family, including sources of strain and techniques of equilibrium maintenance. Basic needs and characteristics of positive mental health of individual members are included. Impact of disequilibrium is presented with examples of adequate coping and coping deficits. Different aspects of home visits and family therapy are also considered.

Chapter 4 includes classification and ecology of mental disorder as it relates to epidemiology. Effects of migration, relocation, and poverty are considered. Milieu therapy is discussed in relation to the concept of the therapeutic community, with particular emphasis upon group psychotherapy. Some aspects of T-groups are discussed in terms of their use as learning tools.

Chapter 5 relates to therapeutic communication; cultural components of communication (ethnocentrism, time, waiting, and territoriality) are discussed. Therapeutic interaction as it relates to the helping relationship in nursing is included. Phases of the helping relationship, component parts and concomitant problems, are considered, along with some aspects of therapeutic use of self. A discussion of interviewing as a method of measurement, which in itself receives little attention in nursing, concludes the chapter.

Chapter 6 outlines conflict, tension, and anxiety as these psychodynamics relate to patients under stress. Coping behavior is presented, and defenses against anxiety which are commonly encountered in nursing practice are discussed with therapeutic tasks outlined. Sensory deprivation, confinement, immobilization, social isolation, and psychophysiological problems receive emphasis in this chapter; stress of changes in body image are outlined, examples given, and therapeutic tasks of the nurse delineated. Some of the psychophysiological and psychoneurotic disorders are also discussed.

Chapter 7 presents the problem of loss as it relates to depression, manic depressive illness, the process of grief and mourning and to dying, death, and bereavement. The intellectual and social renaissance in identifying needs of the dying and bereaved receives attention here. Emphasis is upon understanding one's own attitude toward death as fundamental to the helping relationship.

Chapter 8 presents the concept of aggression as it relates to nursing practice. It discusses aggression within the social and ethological contexts and the need for release of aggression. Nursing intervention with suspicious hostile and paranoid patients is outlined.

The suicidal crisis comprises Chapter 9. Epidemiology of suicide and etiological factors make up part of this chapter, with alienation as a focus. Prevention by early recognition of the crisis and preventive intervention by the nurse are emphasized.

Chapter 10 is concerned with the withdrawn and autistic patient. The new focus on preventive intervention in nursing stresses early recognition of this kind of behavior in all age groups. Cultural determinants as they relate to mental disorder are discussed. Characteristics of the withdrawn, autistic patient and the components of therapeutic care are presented, with emphasis given to the termination process of the nurse-patient relationship. Some aspects of treatment and aftercare are discussed.

Chapter 11 concludes the book with presentation of problems related to drug use and drug dependence and their relevance for the nursing student.

References

Caplan, Gerald: *An Approach to Community Mental Health*. New York: Grune & Stratton, 1961.

———— *Principles of Preventive Psychiatry*. New York: Basic Books, 1964.

Erikson, Erik H.: *Childhood and Society*. New York: W. W. Norton, 1963.

Evans, Frances Monet Carter: *The Role of the Nurse in Community Mental Health*. New York: The Macmillan Co., 1968.

Havighurst, Robert J.: *Human Development and Education*. New York: Longmans, Green & Co., 1953.

Lemkau, Paul V.: "Prevention in Psychiatry," *The British Journal of Social Psychiatry*, **2**:2:127–33, Spring, 1968.

Suggested readings

American Public Health Association: *Mental Disorders: A Guide to Control Methods*. New York: American Public Health Association, 1962.

Hadley, Betty Jo: "Evolution of a Conception of Nursing," *Nursing Research*, **18**:5:400–405, September-October, 1969.

Johnson, Dorothy E.: "Theory in Nursing: Borrowed and Unique," *Nursing Research*, **17**:3:206–209, May-June, 1968.

Keller, Marjorie K.: "The Worker, the Work Society and Baccalaureate Education," University of Tennessee, College of Nursing, mimeographed paper, 1969.

Klein, Donald C.: *Community Dynamics and Mental Health*. New York: John Wiley & Sons, 1968.

Leininger, Madeleine M.: "Community Psychiatric Nursing: Trends, Issues and Problems," *Perspectives in Psychiatric Care*, **7**:1:10–20, 1969.

2 Human development and crisis points

The new emphasis upon the nurse's role in prevention of mental disorder, in the maintenance of positive mental health and in the restoration of health requires knowledge of the ingredients of mental health. Considering these aspects of human development and some of the crisis points in the life cycle may stimulate the reader to perceive the role of the nurse in prevention of mental disorder and to be better able to assist individuals in stress. Although much human relations study is currently directed toward the "here and now," what we are today has its roots in our past. Certain characteristics of adulthood can be traced to babyhood. For instance, when an adult gets very thirsty, he may drink with the noises and passion he evidenced when he was a baby. With the collection of many similar observations, the student of human behavior asserts that *the early behavioral patterns are never destroyed, they are modified.*

This chapter emphasizes developmental phases and crises that are pertinent to nursing, with more attention given to later periods of life. These have not previously received as much study as earlier phases.

Structural concept of the mind: id, ego, and superego

In psychoanalytic theory, the id is that part of the mind encompassing biological urges or needs. Corresponding to the unconscious, instinctive desires and strivings of the person—the libido or impulsive energy of man—it is identical with the unconscious (Potter, 1962).

The ego is defined in terms of the control of functions and processes: thinking, perception, motor activity, understanding, communication, and defenses. The ego is the rational aspect of the personality; it helps to maintain biopsychosocial balance. It develops as the child explores his environment, grasps a part of himself, and perceives that it is his body, different from his surroundings. It marks the combination of the eye perceiving an object, the arm reaching for it, the hand grasping it and bringing it back to the mouth. There are observation, perception, execution, and reception of an object. The entire process requires the breaking down of the simply pleasurable rhythmical movements for the accomplishment of something in which several things are combined.

The ego helps the individual delay gratifications. It functions to preserve the sense of reality, to feel the actions of the world, to mediate between the id and the superego, and to keep a person on an even keel (Menninger, 1963). It thereby aids in adaptation, adjustment, and survival.

The superego, developed later in childhood, derives from and centers around moral demands—particularly prohibitions of parents and society. An unconscious force that blocks unacceptable drives, it is concerned with the "do's" and "dont's" given to the child from parents and his culture. Freud (1923) stated that the "ego is first and foremost a bodily ego; it is not merely a surface entity, but is itself the projection of a surface." [1] A footnote, described as authorized by Freud, adds that the "ego is ultimately derived from bodily sensations, chiefly from those springing from the surface of the body. It may thus be regarded as a mental projection of the surface of the body, besides, as we have seen above, representing the superficies of the mental apparatus." [2] Freud's description of the ego encompasses the concept of body image as presented in this book.

Body image

As the child differentiates his own body from his environment, his body image [3] is formed; *tactile, optic, auditory,* and *kinesthetic* impressions aid in its development. One of the earliest controls is that of the image of the body—the libidinal pleasures of sucking, for example. Other special senses— olfactory, gustatory, visceral, and body sensation—also contribute to the development of body image. Gorman (1969) states that all the sensory functions and the development of the ego work together dynamically from birth to form the body image.

---

[1] Freud, Sigmund: *The Ego and the Id.* Standard Edition. London: The Hogarth Press, Vol. 19, 1961, p. 26.
[2] Freud, *ibid.,* p. 26.
[3] The concept of one's body, based on conscious and unconscious aspects of experience.

Life's crises

Two different types of crises occur in human beings, anticipated and un-anticipated. Unanticipated crises refer to emergencies such as the sudden death of a loved one or eviction; anticipated crises are experienced by everyone—the eight stages of man, for example (Erikson, 1963). Primary preventive techniques in psychiatry involve use of anticipatory guidance to educate people as to what to expect in the various stages of life, ways to meet these changes, and, with parents, how to help children surmount crises of human development and of life in general. The concept that there is something in each phase of life for everyone is as important as the idea of losing something as one phases out of one stage to another.

Unexpected crises, as they affect the individual, are those laden with emotion, threatening events and incidents that present themselves to individuals who find that previous problem-solving methods do not work. A crisis poses some of the following points:

1. A threat or danger to life goals
2. Tension and/or anxiety
3. It evokes or awakens unresolved problems in the past
4. It is a turning point in which healthy or unhealthy adaptation can occur

It is more important to view a crisis as a situation in which *growth* is possible; a psychiatric nurse should work toward that growth. Crisis intervention is the action required, and it takes many forms. It may mean conveying a feeling of deep concern to the suicidal person, helping a poverty-stricken family to become self-supporting, or assisting an aging individual to find appropriate living quarters.

A crisis is also a role transition point, i.e., birth, school entrance, adolescence, leaving one's family for college, and marriage. At these points, new relation-ships are formed and old relationships take on new aspects.

In Erikson's developmental life cycle model of man, each phase of life has a crisis introduction and a task to be accomplished. As the crisis is resolved and the task met, the individual is better equipped to move on to the next phase. It is important for the reader to distinguish between the stage-specific crises of Erikson (1963) which have to be met by everyone and those which are unexpected.

Infancy and early childhood

In infancy, the child at first seems to want mostly to rest. The embryonic life has been broken by birth, hunger, cold, and other discomforts, each of which acts as a stimulus. The infant reacts to remove the disturbing stimulus and to return to rest. At this time the general action is one of defense.

Two principal defense reactions occur: (1) destruction (devouring food is an example) and (2) flight (e.g., closing the eyes, turning the head). They comprise the aggression instinct; in adulthood, this may be referred to as hate. The opposite reaction that develops is love. The infant hears and seems to like certain sounds. By rhythmical repetition, he begins to find some actions desirable to which he formerly objected.

The human face and figure combine sound and motion; this combination is one of the most constant aspects of the infant's environment, providing certain satisfactions such as contact comfort, motion stimulation, and food. It is logical, therefore, that the infant's first love object is the mother or the mother substitute. The developing child needs the assistance of another person to whom he may become attached. Following, clinging, and feeling secure in the presence of this person and depending on him all are indications of attachment behavior. Crying in the absence of the person or at intimations of absence occurs readily and ceases when the person returns (Bowlby, 1969).

Love appears later than defense. This progressive tendency Freud called sex, or libido, the impulsive energy of man. It is during this phase of life that developmental aspects of anxiety occur. The smiling response shows the infant's awareness of another human being; it is the beginning of the differentiation of animate from inanimate objects. During the first year of life eighth-month anxiety also develops. Object constancy has developed with the mother or the mother substitute as the major object in his environment. It is here that the child is calm with the mother and uncomfortable with strangers. *Stranger anxiety* may reach its peak at 12 months.

Separation anxiety also develops in the infant phase and continues throughout life to old age. Separation anxiety refers to feelings of abandonment—being alone, unloved by, and alienated from others. It can occur in the normal individual as well as in the most regressed psychotic person. In later life, an extreme degree may result in formation of delusions. The infant may express separation anxiety by crying every time a person enters the house with his coat on. I have observed this phenomenon while visiting a home for children who were abandoned by their mothers. Crying when the mother leaves is another common sign of separation anxiety. The listlessness of babies in a foundling home described by Spitz (1945) and Ribble (1965) and the turning away from food may be other indications. Bowlby's (1952) study of a two-year-old in a hospital documented reactions to separation from family. His earlier monograph (1951) surveyed the literature of separation.

The first feelings of wanting to be like others are developed during the first year. The erotogenic pleasures are mostly derived from this oral phase of development where the mouth is involved. Other areas of the body, the eyes, and the skin also give pleasure. The oral phase involves (1) passive receptivity (Erikson calls it the "getting" phase), (2) incorporative (the child learns that his own activities can destroy, for example, biting). This phase is the period of origin of the concepts of the good and bad mother, the "good me" and the "bad me" derived from the concept of the good and bad mother.

Achievements of the first year of life relate to the pleasures of the erotogenic zones, development of the ego and body image, and the differentiation between the id and the ego, and the formation of defense mechanisms.

DEFENSE MECHANISMS

The defense mechanisms of the early life of the child can be divided into primary process and secondary process. Primary processes are the most rudimentary ways that infantile ego is defended or tension and anxiety handled. Dreams and psychoses also represent primary process thinking. Symbolization, displacement, condensation, and incorporation are examples of primary process defenses.

"*Symbolization* is an unconscious mental process operating by association and based on similarity and abstract representation whereby one object or idea comes to stand for another through some part, quality, or aspect which the two have in common. The symbol carries in more or less disguised form the feelings vested in the initial object or idea." [4] *Incorporation* is a defense mechanism in which the psychic representation of a person or parts of him are figuratively ingested. An example is the infantile fantasy that the mother's breast has been ingested and is part of one's self. *Displacement* is an unconscious defense mechanism, in which an emotion is transferred from its original object to a more acceptable substitute. *Condensation* is a psychological process in which two or more concepts are fused so that a single symbol represents the multiple parts (American Psychiatric Association, 1969).

Secondary process defenses occur when the ego is older and more able to tolerate tension and frustration; they enable the ego to deal with these. The following paragraph describes certain secondary process defenses.

Identification is a defense mechanism operating unconsciously by which an individual attempts to pattern himself after another. It is to be differentiated from imitation, which is a conscious process. *Projection* is a defense mech-

---

[4] American Psychiatric Association: *A Psychiatric Glossary*. Washington, D.C.: American Psychiatric Association, 1969, p. 95.

anism, operating unconsciously, whereby that which is emotionally un-acceptable in the self is rejected and ascribed to others. *Repression* is unconscious forgetting. Many stored and forgotten events are repressed. Repression represents an internal flight of painful material and it is sometimes used to refer to all the defense mechanisms. It is sometimes confused with suppression. *Suppression* is a conscious process of crowding out undesirable material from consciousness, controlling it, and forcing it completely out of memory into the unconscious. *Denial* is a defense mechanism, operating unconsciously, in which conflict and anxiety are resolved by disavowing thoughts, feelings, wishes, needs, or other reality factors that are consciously intolerable.

DEVELOPMENTAL TASKS AND DEVELOPMENTAL STAGES

Developmental tasks, faced by everyone in the course of growth and matura-tion, are things that each person has to accomplish for himself. They are pancultural insofar as people around the world must come to terms with them in one form or another. Different practices in different societies affect the perceptions and resolutions of the tasks, but all must be faced.

Havighurst (1953) was one of the first to ascertain the tasks of life. He identified a series of developmental tasks for individuals to achieve in the life cycle. His principal aim was to provide a theoretical framework in opposition to the permissive theory of education that the individual develops best if left as free as possible. He emphasizes the importance and necessity of learning new roles as one progresses through the various stages of life. Each develop-mental task has its roots in biological, psychological, sociological, and cultural components of the necessities of human life. Development therefore is learning to live with yourself as you and your society change. This list of developmental tasks was worked out at the Institute of Human Development at the University of Chicago and is biopsychosocial. Other lists of develop-mental tasks are often either biological, psychological, or social. Havighurst's list combines some aspects of each. It is included here for reference when you are assessing maturity levels of patients (see Appendix A). The tasks are divided into six periods. Each period brings with it the new tasks and roles for that phase of life. The tasks and roles for infancy and early childhood (ages birth–6) are as follows:[5]

1. *Learning to walk*
2. *Learning to take solid foods*
3. *Learning to talk*
4. *Learning to control the elimination of body wastes*

---

[5] Robert J. Havighurst: *Human Development and Education*. New York: Longmans Green and Co., 1953, pp. 19–16, by permission, New York: David McKay Company, Inc.

5. *Learning sex differences and sexual modesty*
6. *Achieving physiological stability*
7. *Forming simple concepts of social and physical reality*
8. *Learning to relate oneself emotionally to parents, siblings, and other people*
9. *Learning to distinguish between right and wrong and developing a conscience*

Erik H. Erikson of the Institute of Human Development at Harvard describes a hierarchy of developmental stages of man that builds upon Freud's psycho-sexual theories. He describes eight ages of man that represent a continuum from the beginning to the end of life and discusses a stage-specific crisis for each phase (Erikson, 1963, Chapter 7). Each stage of life has a phasing out and a phasing in where psychic energy is used. Man has to face these crises wherever he is. Each phase has an aim and a crisis to overcome before movement on to the next phase. Healthy resolution of each crisis is essential for positive mental health and for the successful resolution of the succeeding phase.

Basic trust is developed where the infant knows that someone is there to meet his needs. The crisis is *mistrust*. Infants who have neglectful mothers or mother substitutes may not be able to resolve this phase. This stage of learning to trust others coincides with the oral phase of development described by Freud.

Autonomy is the next phase and is characterized by the achievement of defiance and independence. The crises are *shame* and *doubt*. It coincides with the period of life in which the child is in the "no, no" stage. Children in this phase will say "no" to almost everything asked of them.

Initiative is characterized by the development of love and hate for the parent of the opposite sex. The crisis is *guilt*. This phase coincides with the Oedipal and Electra phases of development as described by Freud.

Middle childhood

The next stage marks the midpoint of Erikson's eight ages of man; it is called *industry*. This phase corresponds with the latency period[6] described by Freud. Here the child is eager to learn and searches for reasons why things are as they are. The crisis is *fantasy*.

---

[6] Latency is the period between the phallic phase and the turbulence of puberty and adolescence.

FANTASY

Fantasy is one way of handling tension and anxiety. The infant probably has difficulty differentiating between wish and reality.

Later on, children may hit parents and berate them. Some parents need help to perceive that a child must relieve tension. There are dangers of over-permissiveness where a child is permitted to get into trouble and feels that the parent does not care for him. A confused superego may result. Some parents cannot tolerate expression of tension. The child may then retreat into fantasy. To him, to think his bad thoughts about his parents is often as bad to him as actually carrying out his thoughts. This is called *magical thinking* and is normal in certain amounts.

We tend to keep fantasies of the good parent. In fairy tales, the fairy godmother is the fantasy of the good mother. It is during infancy that one learns to wait. The ego wishes to integrate with the id. It is thought that hallucinated images of the mother permit momentary delay and temporary satisfaction. The infant may indulge in thumb sucking, which satisfies him temporarily. Where reality is denied for fantasy, schizophrenia may result. Handling anxiety by motor activity is thought by some clinicians to result in behavior disorders. It is through experience that one learns that real things have taste, odors, and are hot or cold. These real things are more vivid than those of the imagination. Our culture demands some sharp distinctions between the real and the unreal, but there are cultures where magic, symbols, and fantasies play a larger part in life. When symbolic action is a belief, magic exists. The play of the preschool child who reacts to his environment as though people and situations were present when, in actuality, they are not, gives impressions of hallucinatory activity. The imaginary playmate to whom the child speaks and does things for also has this quality. However, when asked, the child readily distinguishes his activity as play and as imaginary. The developmental tasks for the age group 6–12 are as follows: [7]

1. *Learning physical skills necessary for ordinary games*
2. *Building wholesome attitudes toward oneself as a growing organism*
3. *Learning to get along with age-mates*
4. *Learning an appropriate masculine or feminine social role*
5. *Developing fundamental skills in reading, writing, and calculating*
6. *Developing concepts necessary for everyday living*
7. *Developing conscience, morality, and a scale of values*
8. *Achieving personal independence*
9. *Developing attitudes toward social groups and institutions*

[7] Havighurst, *op. cit.*, pp. 28–40.

Excessive aggression in this phase may act as a defense against passivity or dependence (Engel, 1962).

Success in task attainment of the preceding developmental stages is considered necessary or desirable if the individual is successfully to meet later ones. There is variation between individuals in ways of attainment of specific developmental tasks. Different societies present unique patterns of developmental task attainment.

SCHOOL PHOBIA

School phobia usually involves children in the elementary grades, although it can and does sometime appear just before adolescence. It is not truancy and must be clearly differentiated from it. Children with school phobia are usually of average or above average intelligence; they respect authority and are from an achievement-oriented home environment. Truants usually come from home environments where there is little emphasis on achievement, where behavior is oriented against authority, and where there is general indifference to the school.

School phobia is most commonly seen upon entrance to school and usually revolves around separation from mother. The mother and child are excessively dependent upon each other, and the mother may unconsciously bind the child to remaining at home although she tells him he must go to school. The school phobic child verbally declares his avoidance of school and does all he can to remain in the security of the home. He will verbalize fear of school or somaticize with complaints of headache, nausea, fainting, or stomach pain.

In the treatment of school phobic children, the whole family is involved. Usually parents have not aided or permitted the child to achieve autonomy comparable to that of his peers. After assessment of the particular family situation, and development of rapport with the child himself, nurses may be able to help the family or to make a referral. The child may be able to relate directly why he is afraid.

Bulbulyan's (1966) work with school phobic children was part of her role in community mental health nursing. In communities where school nurses are employed, the school nurse may be this helpful figure. Treatment consists of returning the child to school as soon as possible. Accompanying the child to school or having him stay one day with the principal eases him back into the situation. Changing schools is not the answer. Going to the home at the time the child has to leave the house may give the emotional support to the mother and child that is required for the separation. Giving emotional support to the mother who must accept the separation will help her to adapt. Helping her to rebudget her time around other things when the child is absent may give equanimity to the family situation.

Adolescence

Trust thyself; every heart vibrates to that iron string.
   Ralph Waldo Emerson

In adolescence, the crisis of *identity* manifests itself. The young person searches for a unity for himself, a place in the social order. He also seeks to make two major decisions in life—what will his occupation be and whom will he love? The crisis is *nonidentity* or *identity diffusion* (Erikson, 1963). Nursing and other professional students such as those in medicine may have partly solved their identity crises by deciding upon their professions early in life. Others may not be so fortunate. Whom to love and what to be now have to be decided upon rather early in life. The requirements of specialization in a technological society demand that the adolescent decide in high school what he will do in college in order to take the necessary courses so that he will be able to compete with others in college entrance.

Adolescence, one of the most painful periods of life, is heralded by the relatively short puberty period. The legend of Romeo and Juliet epitomizes the intense feelings of the adolescent about self, family, culture, lover, and spouse. In this period, stereotyped behavior may serve as a defense against identity diffusion. There is doubt of self and of the future, there are strong emotions of shame about changes in one's body, guilt is prevalent, and feelings of inferiority are great. The formation of friendship groups or cliques aids in the establishment of identity. A negative identity may result in being a temporary thief or a member of a gang destructive in other ways.

There is a strong need to form an identity which is free of parental influence. New coping mechanisms are called for in the turmoil of relinquishing the latency period for heterosexuality.

Mass society makes its contribution to the identity crisis where most urbanized American schools are very large and daily contacts are with large numbers of people on a superficial basis. Young people are now handling aggressive impulses by the use of drugs, which help to counteract feelings of anger and frustration with parents and school.

The developmental tasks of the age group (12—18) are as follows:[8]

---

[8] Havighurst, *op. cit.*, pp. 111—47.

1. *Achieving new and more mature relations with age mates of both sexes*
2. *Achieving a masculine or feminine social role*
3. *Accepting one's physique and using the body effectively*
4. *Achieving emotional independence of parents and other adults*
5. *Achieving assurance of economic independence*
6. *Selecting and preparing for an occupation*
7. *Preparing for marriage and family life*
8. *Developing intellectual skills and concepts necessary for civic competence*
9. *Desiring and achieving socially responsible behavior*
10. *Acquiring a set of values and an ethical system as a guide to behavior*

Adolescence is a vulnerable phase for mental disorder. First admissions to mental hospitals in this age group and the resident population have increased within the past decade. Between 1963 and 1973 there will be a 15 percent increase among the 10- to 14-year-olds in proportion to the population of the United States. During the same period, a 16 percent increase in the mental hospital admissions will occur. Among the 15- to 24-year-olds, a 36 percent increase in the population as a whole has been projected; the mental hospital admission rate has been projected as 70 percent. (*Mental Health of Children*, Public Health Service Publication, No. 1396.)

During adolescence the general motto seems to be "live long and die young." The central problem of adolescence is definition of the self, for this is the period of life in which one learns who he is and identifies how he feels. It is the time that he differentiates himself from his family and detaches himself from his family. By becoming an individual in his own right, he is able to experience intense interpersonal relationships with others. He is often consumed with the intensity of his feelings toward others. It is the process through which the self is defined through experience and through clarification of experience. Maturity seldom arrives to those with minimal life experiences. Friedenberg (1959) pointed out that the basic unit of a continuing community is a stable self to respect. It is through this phase of life that the stable self emerges.

All of life's experiences are meaningful in the development of the individual. Resolution of one crisis prepares one for the next phase, a process that continues until death.

Early adulthood

Intimacy is the next stage and occurs in early adulthood (Erikson, 1963). It portrays the need for closeness and sharing and defines the stage of heterosexuality. The crisis is *isolation*. In the culture of the United States, intimacy is often never achieved. As adolescence is being phased out, intimacy is being phased in. Psychic energy is used both in phasing out and phasing in. In all these stages of man, overlapping may occur. There is no black-and-white line of demarcation. In adolescence, attachment to other boys and girls is likely to be one which fosters relationships that help define identity. In young adulthood, as a contrast, attachments involve real sharing. Our culture perhaps places little emphasis upon this stage, yet, earlier phases receive much attention. Thus, many young people never adequately solve the problem of development of intimacy. They may attain all other aspects but fail in intimacy and therefore be painfully isolated from others. This may account in part for the alienation felt in our society and for the popularity of encounter groups where individuals take off their clothes in efforts to be close to others. If the crisis of this stage, *isolation*, is not conquered, subsequent stages of life involve painful loneliness.

As a nurse you will have occasion for much physical contact with patients. What are *your* feelings about the intimacies associated with nursing? People confide in you, they bring their life's sorrows to your attention. In nursing, you perceive the inside of people, the intrapsychic functions. You also assist others with their body functions. In ordinary life you probably do not see the various parts of the body as you do in nursing. It will have an impact on you. Identify your own feelings about some of these experiences and discuss them with a friend. In nursing, you cannot avoid intimate contacts.

The young adult who is sure of his own identity can share satisfying intimate relations with others. The loneliness of subsequent stages of life may be due to the fact that the isolation crisis was never resolved.

The developmental tasks of this phase of life (ages 18—35) include: [9]

> *1. Selecting a mate*
> *2. Learning to live with a marriage partner*
> *3. Starting a family*
> *4. Rearing children*
> *5. Managing a home*

---

[9] Havighurst, *op. cit.*, pp. 259—66.

6. *Getting started in an occupation*
7. *Taking on civic responsibility*
8. *Finding a congenial social group*

University life for many young people is on a mass basis. Students may arrive on campus with hopeful expectations that they will be able to choose a variety of desired courses only to find a highly structured course requirement which gives little leeway to them as individuals. A student may also find himself in class with 1,200 other students who are in the same boat. Students living on the university campus in dormitories face the mass life at meal time, at the library, and in their living quarters. In the search for meaning, the university environment itself contributes to psychological numbness (Keniston, 1966). Students may be so unknown to faculty and administration that just being called by name is significant. During my student days, arrival on campus was designated "Berkeley Shock," and very little time was spent there except for classes and concerts. "Sitting in" at that time meant something entirely different from what it means now. To overcome the *ennui* of required courses in the constricted curriculum, "sitting in" meant attending other more interesting classes out of my major taught by prominent and internationally known professors on campus.

Rebellion against some of these aspects of university life is widespread in this country, following the example of the civil rights movement in the southern United States. Mass protests against rent, police power, and the rights of institutions in planning for the use of its property documented the Sixties.

As America becomes more and more urbanized, ways for young people to meet and select mates become increasingly difficult. Lonely hearts clubs and computer dating are indicators. It must be stated here that selection of a mate is not limited to early adulthood in any sense. The high divorce rate and the earlier death of men results in many people throughout the life arc selecting a mate. Nurses themselves are in this category and should be particularly aware of developing all aspects of themselves so that they are interested in and can discuss something more than their profession. The curriculum of most nursing schools and other preprofessional and professional students leaves little time for pursuit of other interests. The amount of required reading alone is enormous and the push for grades for eligibility for graduate school adds stresses. Keniston (1957) calls this compulsive professionalism. For the young man, there is the additional stress of spending time in the armed forces.

A balance of work, study, and play is necessary for positive mental health and should be achieved even if one has to take less than a full semester's load in college.

Taking up a new interest after high school and college or joining a club provides fun and an opportunity for meeting others.

In this phase of development, marriage brings a new set of adjustments and, as nurses, people confide in you. Cathartic listening can often aid the person with marital problems who, having a sympathetic ear, can then do his own problem-solving quite effectively. For more severe problems, referral to a marriage counselor may be required. Nurses also aid in family planning. The nurse may assist the family herself or help them to get the aid that they need. In turn, the nurse needs someone to whom to turn to discuss problems encountered in professional practice. The constant work with the crises and problems of individuals and families elicits needs in all professionals for checking perceptions with colleagues and/or consultants. Nursing students turn to their instructors and to their peers for this help.

In the rearing of children there are many facets which involve nursing. Helping mothers and children to be healthy is a traditional part of nursing all over the world. Helping parents to perceive the importance to children of love may set a firm foundation for the healthy emotional growth of the child. The needs of parents, especially young mothers, to have time to themselves for rest and relaxation cannot be overemphasized. The suburban housewife unable to find a babysitter may suffer stresses similar to those of the ghetto mother who lives in a crowded area and is constantly bombarded by stimulation from others.

Learning to manage a home, making a budget, and organization of the home to meet the needs of the various family members has to be learned. Cooking and managing a food budget are important items of homemaking. The knowledge that nurses have of normal nutrition can be used to assist families to develop normally.

The nurse may also be able to help the busy mother with many children find time to be alone with each child frequently. Some mothers are able to take yearly trips with each child. Others can use time for errands and outings to take a child along so he has some time all to himself to be with his mother. The husband and wife also need time alone together. The importance of space assignment to children is also vital—a room or some part of a chest of drawers—even a box where a little boy can keep his bugs or rocks where no one else has entry fulfills a basic need. Attention to this space for personal property aids the child to develop a sense of who he is and what he wants to be.

In some cultures, it is expected that women contribute to the economy of the country as well as to its progeny. In the Soviet Union, for example, women are given pregnancy leave and return to work within the year after the birth of a child. A well-developed and carefully run system of nursery schools enables mothers to do this. In our own country, nursery schools and child care centers are likely to be for the poor or the very rich or run on a cooperative basis by parents. Few provide weekend and overnight care, which means that the working mother has additional hardships to deal with if she works.

Suitable babysitters are both hard to find and expensive. The nuclear family has no old aunt, cousin, or grandparents to turn to for help. Some help is provided to families with handicapped children in certain communities. In Palo Alto, California, Respite House offers 24-hour care for retarded children from overnight stays to 2 weeks. This respite from the continuous task of caring for retarded children is also needed on a widespread basis. The working husband and wife who return to suburbia after a long day's work and often an even more stressful period of commuting may have few reserves for civic responsibility.

Some young people in this decade who have grown up in the affluence of a home environment where parents work to provide more material things for themselves and for their families are becoming disenchanted with the whole idea and establishing a life more meaningful to themselves in communes.

Middle age

Generativity is the stage in which one begins to look at what he has done and assesses it as worthwhile or as deficient (Erikson, 1963). If one feels his life is good and rewarding, he surmounts the crisis of *stagnation* or *self-absorption.* Generativity occurs in middle age and is related to productivity and creativity. It is during this period that individuals review what they have accomplished and what has yet to be done. It is a time where a life review occurs, and the individual realizes that, with the approach of the half-century mark, there is not much of life left to achieve all the hopes and desires of youth. One of the primary concerns of generativity is the guidance of the succeeding generations. The drive of generativity thus seems to be related to passing on one's influences to children, as in a family; to the next generation, as in teaching; to society, as in the Marxian sense, or to all succeeding generations, as Botticelli, Michelangelo, and da Vinci.

The *empty nest* phase occurs when the youngest child is in high school and the parents face their remaining years alone (Spence, 1969). It is the time when children leave the home for their own lives and parents face each other as a couple again. Mothers and fathers who have devoted themselves to their children to the exclusion of other interests may have a particularly difficult time in this phase.

The developmental tasks for this period of life (ages 35—60) are: [10]

---

[10] Havighurst, *op. cit.*, pp. 269—74.

1. *Achieving adult civic and social responsibility*
2. *Establishing and maintaining an economic standard of living*
3. *Assisting teen-age children to become responsible and happy adults*
4. *Developing adult leisure-time activities*
5. *Relating oneself to one's spouse as a person*
6. *Accepting and adjusting to the physiological changes of middle age*
7. *Adjusting to aging parents*

The empty nest phase of life and generativity seem to be part of the same period and relate to similar problems and growth points. However, the empty nest phase can only relate to individuals with children, whereas generativity relates to all individuals.

The middle years bring with them all the growth from the earlier phases of the life cycle; unresolved conflicts are also brought into this phase.

Middle age brings many physiological changes within the body. Vision changes and eyeglasses have to be worn. Hearing changes are evidenced and metabolism slows down. Jokes are made about gray hair, wigs and toupees are considered, and dyes are used in experimentation. In an attempt to keep up with the intensity and pace of earlier years, people of this age group often die on the tennis courts or during the furious early morning bicycle ride. Pursuit of earlier intense interests with moderation and with less competitive spirit should, however, be encouraged here.

CLIMACTERIUM

In women, the climacteric appears usually in the mid or late forties. Ovulation ceases and menstrual cycles may be irregular for 1 or 2 years; periods of heavy bleeding alternating with amenorrhea may occur. The hot flashes, associated with chilly sensations, perspiration, insomnia, muscle cramps, and manifestations of anxiety appear. Cyclic therapy with progestin regulates the cycle as the decline in ovarian function progresses to the stage of amenorrhea (Goodman and Gilman, p. 1548). Estrogen replacement therapy is used by most physicians. Others prefer to use small doses of phenobarbital and reassurance.

In men, although there is no consensus about the occurrence of the climacterium, the andropause has been fully described by Szalita (1966), who says that it is an inevitable phenomenon for every man who reaches advanced age. The gonads gradually decline in function, and there are disturbances in the endocrine balance, various emotional reactions, and a decline in sexual activity. The andropause is thought to occur later in men than menopause in women.

For men and women, there is a decline in physical capacity; depressive moods are prevalent, both depression and alcoholism are common to this age group.

Sexual activity may be increased with new partners or it may decrease. For some people the anxiety of proving themselves may lead to other impulsive behavior, e.g., exhibitionism. For further discussion of problems of this phase of life, refer to Chapter 7.

PREPARATION FOR GROWING OLDER

Each phase of the life cycle has a period of phasing in and phasing out. The attitudes of middle-aged persons toward growing older were studied by Neugarten (1959). In their sample, fear of aging meant fear of dependency involving loss of income and loss of health. Their data were analyzed for positive, negative, and neutral attitudes toward aging. Twelve percent of women and men in their study considered their health to be worse than others of the same age. These individuals also held negative attitudes toward the future. An interesting finding of the study was that the *fear of death was never alluded to,* nor was social isolation. Middle-aged people usually have to face death and the reminder of their own age and death through meeting the developmental task of adjusting to aging parents. Although Medicare now assists with their care, older people also need the care and concern of their children. Role reversal therefore occurs and offers opportunities for interpersonal growth and for regression as well. In this role reversal, the parent becomes dependent on the child, and the child relinquishes his longing for return to childhood (Sheps, 1959). The parent ceases to be seen as the all-powerful person and is, instead, perceived as a human being. Before the advent of Medicare, the financial strain of helping children through college and of assisting aging parents simultaneously was often a much more difficult problem.

The empty nest phase probably affects women more than it does men, but it involves both. Consideration of life without the children requires adaptation to new identities. Divorce is common at this point when readjustment to old roles often does not work out.

Older age

EGO INTEGRITY

Older age, the last phase of the life cycle, culminates all phases. *Ego integrity* is the last stage of man, the one in which he accepts his life as the one and only life, defends the dignity and meaning of his life style, and develops a new perspective of his parents (Erikson, 1963). The crisis is *disgust* or *despair*. Fear of death, despair, depression, and suicide are all related to disgust. Ego integrity implies a state of mind in which the person is involved in "follower-ship" in addition to the acceptance of leadership. Preparation for this phase of life begins with childhood; successful achievement of previous crises readies one for this last period.

It is often possible for a person to overcome earlier handicaps in his development and rather late in life achieve feelings of identity, intimacy, and integrity. Individuals with children and grandchildren may be better able to understand and work out their earlier conflicts as they interact with the two generations. Helping others to work out conflicts may also give insights into one's own. It is no longer thought that persons in their older years cannot undergo behavioral changes. Recent behavior is probably more amenable to change than behavior that has occurred many years previously. It is now held that new crises may call for new types of ego defenses in the older age group. The adage that persons in the older group will meet their problems with the same defenses that served them in their earlier years no longer holds. A new field of geriatric psychiatry has therefore emerged. The nursing care of people in the older age group calls on all the known psychiatric skills.

THE LIFE REVIEW

The point at which one arrives at the acceptance of his life is reflected dramatically in the later years. The reflection on the high and the low points of life—achievements as well as disappointments—occurs in this phase. The life review helps the older person perceive how his life has been spent and to see his own parents and himself as part of the flow of humanity. What one has done and cannot do and a review of these activities aids in the resolution of this phase. Depression is a form of disgust. It is not always manifestly expressed. An overconcern with body symptoms or psychological invalidism may indicate an underlying depression. A constant preoccupation with the state of affairs of being old and lonely indicates depression in the older person. Remarks such as, "I am just in the way," and "Why does someone like you want to visit the likes of me?" are common.

In aging there is a renewed ability to free associate (Bernfeld, 1951) and a reliving of earlier experiences while putting one's life in perspective. Butler (1968) and others refer to this process as the life review, which is part of the preparation for death. One older person at the age of 70 confided in me that she dreamed of her classmates in the second grade and woke up wondering where they all were. It is not uncommon for older people to give their life review from birth until the present within a few minutes whether it is at the bedside at the time of crisis or at other times when there is someone to listen.

The life review is a phenomenon of old age that, in the past, was thought to be due to the loss of recent memory and clearly one of the cardinal signs of senility. It is now clearly established to be a universal mental process of aging. The life review is not relegated solely to the years of later maturity but can come at times of stress and threat, such as impending death, during the earlier years. A salient point made by Butler (1968) is that retirement, along with removing the defenses of work, may provide the necessary time for the life review. Relationships with others are remembered and dreamed about. Yearnings to see former classmates and acquaintances and to know what they have done with their lives, whether they are alive or dead, become a preoccupation. Conflicts with others, especially with family members, are recalled and some-times a new and more mature perspective is attained through this introspective process.

Various ways are used to achieve the life review. "Pictures in one's mind" is one way; putting together a family album is another. Writing one's memoirs or relating the events of life to one who lends an interested ear may achieve the life review. Making a scrapbook of one's self is another approach. A study of one's genealogy may be accomplished as a legacy for living family members. Perceiving the progression of life from one phase to the next can result in a different feeling about one's identity, intimacy, autonomy, and all the other phases through which one has developed. Sharing life's experi-ences with another interested human being leaves one with the feeling of not being all alone and also of having an effect on that person. The relating of conscious past experiences helps one to see his life as it is and to accept it for its worth. It is important for the younger generation to remember this process and lend a patient ear to the reminiscing person. It lessens the alienation that an older person feels when there is no one else around who understands what times were like during the parts of his life when he was more ego-involved.

Taking photographs of older people aids them to perceive their changed self-image in comparison with younger years. A videotape made of a home visit by the writer to an older person living in a downtown hotel records the facets of his life review, beginning with his birth in a sod house.[11]

The developmental tasks of later maturity (ages 60–   ) follow:[12]

---

[11] The play "Krapp's Last Tape" by Samuel Beckett is a good example of the life review (*Krapp's Last Tape and Other Dramatic Pieces*. New York: Grove Press, 1960).
The epilogue by Arnold Toynbee in *Man's Concern with Death* provides a life review (London: Hodder and Stoughton, 1968).
[12] Havighurst, *op. cit.*, pp. 277–81.

1. *Adjusting to decreasing physical strength and health*
2. *Adjusting to retirement and reduced income*
3. *Adjusting to death of spouse*
4. *Establishing an explicit affiliation with one's age group*
5. *Meeting social and civic obligation*
6. *Establishing satisfactory physical living arrangements*

Older people now are mostly work oriented. They have lived through the Depression, where just having a job was sometimes a life saver. They have seen two World Wars, the Spanish American War, the Korean Conflict, and the war in Viet Nam. If they are from other countries, they are likely to have come to America in order to make better lives for themselves. Often a person's sense of identity is associated with his job and an organizational structure. Once a person loses his position by retirement, he no longer has a place in a meaningful organizational structure and therefore must make adaptations and adjustments to a new role.

RETIREMENT

Retirement age in this country is 65 for men and 62–65 for women. Preparation for retirement should begin early in life, and those who in their earlier years develop their inner resources will be better equipped for this period.

The older population in this country is becoming more isolated as their knowledge and skills become obsolete. Their world and their values have become increasingly irrelevant in a highly technological society with rapidly changing customs. If we are to counteract the dehumanizing aspects of contemporary society, one pathway is through care and concern for the aging members.

People now live longer and therefore have an increasingly higher number of retirement years. Twenty more years of life are expected now than at the turn of the century. Many Americans are unprepared for retirement and have numerous difficulties during this period of life. We need to know more about retirement and its effect upon persons and upon the society in which they live.

Persons who have the ability to obtain a good education, who have developed diverse interests, and who are in a high socioeconomic status group are more likely to adapt successfully to retirement.

The attitude that each person has toward the later years of life influences the quality of life of those years. The importance of time in our technological society points the way toward the need for planning the time of the retirement years. Carp (1968) emphasizes the need for more study of these emerging phases of the life cycle. Allocation of leisure time and taking on new careers are in order for the most effective use of the retirement time budget.

A variety of activities is necessary in any given community for effective use of leisure, due to the fact that different leisure activities can have the same significance for certain people (Havighurst, 1957). In this study, social class was determined to be an important factor in how people spent their leisure. Among the findings of the four social classes studied, for example, reading was favored equally by the two middle classes and the upper-lower. Since suitable leisure activity helps maintain life style and level of integration, it especially needs attention in the middle and later years. Kreps (1968) raises the question of the dilemma of increased leisure time in the older years when income is also reduced.

A target group of individuals who need special assistance in retirement planning are women who are social overachievers: "... they seem to have reached for statuses beyond their capabilities and, as a result, they tend to view themselves as failures (indicated by feelings of low self-esteem)."[13]

Preretirement education and counseling need to be done on a widespread basis. Nurses in occupational health practice have ready access to individuals at this time of life. The first longitudinal study of the effect of preretirement education was made at the University of Michigan's Division of Gerontology. Preretirement education reduced dissatisfaction with retirement and worry about health. It encouraged participants to engage in all kinds of activities but especially social activity with friends and family (U.S. Senate, 1969).

The retirement time budget should include renewal of social contacts with old friends, maintaining relationships with friends and family, and reaching out for new acquaintances. Plans for visits to the "old country" or to scenes of childhood and those of intervening years help to give perspective on life and a renewed sense of self. Perception of self in relation to these earlier contacts with friends, family, and place of birth aids in making the life review and surmounting the crisis of ego-integrity.

There is some evidence that the alternate generations get along better together than the contiguous ones; therefore, ways must be found for the older and the younger generations to get together. Much mutual education can be accomplished by this interaction (Evans, 1969). Friendly visiting programs are also helpful. The Foster Grandparents plan puts the two generations into contact with each other and, in addition, gives older people an opportunity to do community service. Foster grandparents may work in hospital pediatric units, helping with the sick children. Others work in

---

[13] Spence, Donald L.: "Patterns of Retirement in San Francisco," in Carp, Frances M., ed.: *The Retirement Process*. Washington, D.C.: Superintendent of Documents, 1968, p. 73.

juvenile centers giving love and help to children in trouble, or without parents themselves.

There are additional programs now being developed to provide continued usefulness. Large companies and other institutions such as universities use retired individuals for consultation, lecturing, and so forth. Retired vice presidents and presidents clubs exist in some areas. In the Soviet Union retirement age is 60 for men and 55 for women. Although they have an earlier retirement than we do, emphasis is put upon the retired person contributing to the economy of the country by helping in the nursery schools, museums, and other places. Returning to their old job for a few weeks each year is encouraged. This keeps the retiree in touch with his occupation, relieves others for vacations, and provides additional income. In our society, however, we have an unemployment rate which poses a different problem for us. In Denmark and Sweden, careful provisions are made for older people in terms of free health care, living arrangements in their home communities, and availability of health care in the place where they live.

For the nurse, preventive work is the focus. Find out what retirement means to each individual. There are cultural differences. In the American South, some professional workers still attempt to get retired older people to learn a hobby, join a club, or get involved in civic work. In practice, it is part of the culture to do nothing when one retires. The older person stays at home and others are expected to come to him, to seek him out for comments on life and for his connection with the past. A pattern learned early in life, that an older person sits in his porch swing and lets others visit him and seek him out for advice, is difficult to change overnight. In urban areas the activity rooms of churches in some instances have become "front porch swings." They provide places where older people living in crowded cities in their own homes, apartment houses, and residential hotels can get together to visit, talk, have a hot lunch, and create something with their hands if they wish. If retirement means time and money for travel, it should be obvious that most people either run out of money or get tired of traveling and eventually want a place to stay.

Helping the person who is retiring to talk about retirement, how his day will go when he no longer works, will help. In a time-oriented society, most people place high priority on this item. It is ironic that the retirement gift is often an elaborate and expensive watch! Wives who traditionally have done all the housework and who have had their days free to do as they please may find it particularly difficult to have a retired husband around the house all day with nothing to do. Many constructive tasks can be done around the house. Redoing the cabinet space, refinishing furniture, and gardening are all useful and creative. Rearrangement of living space provides room for each person to do his thing and asserts his territorial rights. Sharing household tasks and cooking may help solve this problem of some older couples; this practice is best begun in earlier years. Since women are more apt to fit into the household tasks upon retirement, they do not have the difficulty that men do in making adaptations. As more women enter the labor force, retirement begins to pose a different problem for them. Now, we are beginning to see a new phenomenon, the mother in her eighties who sees her children retire.

HOUSING

The cities are becoming more and more uncomfortable for retired people who may be repeatedly robbed of their purses and wallets, whose mail boxes are burglarized on the day that they receive their checks, and who may be knocked down and severely beaten if they do not have enough money to satisfy a thief. Even the elegant and expensive apartments with doormen and television observation of entering visitors are subject to terror. A person might be safe inside his tower, but the outside streets sometimes make it impossible for him to take a walk in his own neighborhood, shop, or go to church. Taxi service is expensive and not always as fast as the bus or subway.

Much housing for the elderly is being financed by private means and is therefore designed for profit. Older people who are well off financially have a greater choice of housing. The majority, however, do not have this choice, and therefore have to make other arrangements such as downtown hotels or public housing. A study by Wilner et al. (1968) of all the retirement housing in California concluded that this type of housing presents a solution for older persons who are alone and without families. The same study noted that the kind of retirement housing chosen was likely to reflect previous life arrangements. For example, those who owned their own homes were most likely to buy homes in their retirement years; those who had previously rented were likely to continue to rent. Mobile homes are popular in California, and although their communities may not be designated only for older persons, they may be described as "adults only" (for example, "Youngstown Adult Mobile Home Community—for the young in heart"). Diverse activities are planned within the mobile communities, and residents are encouraged to develop and pursue hobbies. A swimming pool is a "must" in California and golf, folk dancing, sewing, art work, and writing are encouraged.

Decreased income as well as other factors in the years of later maturity may require a move from a large to a smaller house for those who are able to afford their own home. For others it may mean moving from a rented apartment to a downtown rented hotel room either with meals included or without meals in which the older person must then depend on local restaurants for all of his meals. For people who live in cities, inclement weather poses additional hardships. The need for warm clothing and the navigation of icy streets can lead to serious problems for the older person. A change in life style may mean moving to smaller quarters and therefore giving up old furniture to which one has become attached. One older person living in a high rent area of the city attempted to keep all of her furniture in a small, expensive apartment and was desperately working long hours to maintain her former life style. Her money was so tight she could not afford even Part B of Medicare. This is an example of an inability to adjust to decreased income and a change in life style due to loss of spouse.

Older people from the southern states and from other countries need to live in an area where they have contact with language and other aspects of their earlier life. The older Italian or Chinese, for example, will surely wish to be in an area where he can speak his native tongue and where he feels a cultural affinity for those around him. Some older individuals are mobile enough to make the daily return by bus or on foot to Chinatown or the Italian area for sidewalk talks with peers about the price of food, what store closed and which one opened, as well as other changes in the old neighborhood. Newspapers and other reading material in their maternal languages are readily available, and nodding and speaking acquaintances are maintained. Other older people, in relocated neighborhoods and less mobile, may withdraw.

RELOCATION AND SEPARATION ANXIETY
Urban redevelopment and renewal have hit the central areas of cities and the retirement hotels where many old people have found places for themselves close to bus stations, other public transportation, inexpensive restaurants, physicians, and movie theaters with reduced rates for the older person. Emotional ties made with landlords, visiting nurses, the local church, and storeowners may help maintain independence at a time when physical vigor is declining. Once the older person is relocated, he may not be able to re-establish these kinds of relationships, and his desolation and separation anxiety therefore may be further increased. Forced by urban redevelopment to move to new areas even more convenient to them poses a threat to the self-system.

For single older persons who comprise one half of all relocated older individuals, and who have been somewhat neglected by relocation programs, catastrophic results are likely to ensue (Niebanck, 1966). A study by Smith (1966) of the relocation of elderly persons living in an area planned for redevelopment reports the wide spectrum of problems faced by older people who live in the central areas of cities.

The break with old neighborhood ties and acquaintances and the routine of the day can result in separation anxiety. Older people from ghettos containing many different ethnic groups may feel the loss of contact with their particular group in their daily associations with the others in the next door apartment, at the neighborhood drugstore, or grocery. Inability to secure foods that are common to a particular cultural group further adds to the separation. It may be manifest in an inability to participate in the life of the new location and a further withdrawal from those around him. Mistrust of new neighbors and a constant verbalization of a longing for old friends may be evidence of separation anxiety. Inability to participate in senior centers in new neighborhoods where one does not find members of one's own ethnic group may also be evidenced.

Middle class America creates some of its own problems—suburbia leaves the poor and the elderly in the cities. Retirement communities therefore become defensive reactions to noninvolvement in society. They have been built in large numbers over the country, often far away from medical care, public transportation, and hospitals. Health care facilities are needed more and more by the older age group, many of whom may have a number of chronic diseases.

Nurses have a responsibility to acquaint themselves with the various types of housing available for older people and to help them decide to move and find new places if their present living quarters are not suitable.

LOSS OF SPOUSE

The sickness or death of a relative, or of a *significant other*, may precipitate a crisis. Anderson's study (1964) of 600 well persons over 60 years of age and 600 older people in the same age group with a diagnosis of mental disorder showed that the death of a relative was the *most stressful event*. Older persons are therefore in need of aid relating to problems associated with grief, mourning, and bereavement. Grief work may take longer to accomplish than in the earlier years. The following is an example of what occurred with one older person upon the death of his wife.

> Mr. Altman, a somewhat melancholic man who has been retired from law practice for several years, lost his wife of 35 years. Although she had been ill for several months, her death came to him as quite a blow. Since he was the second husband, there was a question as to whether he would be able to remain in the house since the children of the dead wife were to inherit part of the estate.
>
> In his grief for his lost spouse, he felt that his pain was the worst that anybody ever had. He was also highly critical of the church where his wife had been a regular member. He felt that no one cared for him; no one came to see him, and he just did not know what to do. Nursing

interventions that helped Mr. Altman centered around the problem of loneliness. Going to visit with him, telephoning, listening, and encouraging him to speak of former times when his wife was alive built up a pool of *shared images* (see Chapter 7, p. 243) so that he could speak freely of times in which he had been happier.

Mobilizing the minister of his deceased wife's church to visit and telephone more often aided in emotional support which he also was receiving from his physician of many years. Although there were many contacts made by these caring people to Mr. Altman, it was his *feeling of loneliness* and of being abandoned that had to be worked through. All were in touch with each other by telephone and encouraged each other. He was encouraged to get someone to help him with the housework and cooking and subsequently found someone on his street to do this for him and thereby maintained his independence. With the passage of a year, his loneliness became less intense and he resumed his former pattern of life with daily walks, contacts with veterans of the Spanish American War, playing his guitar, and singing.

Many older people, in times of emotional need and great emotional stress, may not know that they need help or understand just what a psychiatrist can do to help. They have grown up in an era when there were few psychiatrists and where psychiatrists were used only for those who had to be admitted to the "asylum." They may have the idea that no one really needs a psychiatrist for the problems of life. Community mental health services now developing over the country make psychiatric care more accessible to older people whose needs may have formerly been unknown except to public health nurses and general practitioners.

Older people who have long depended upon a spouse to attend to certain business aspects of life such as filling out forms, cashing checks, and keeping books may be rather overwhelmed with the prospect of assuming this responsibility upon the death of the mate. Papers for Medicare, for example, are quite complicated for old eyes to read and fill out properly. Mt. Sinai Hospital, at Baltimore, Maryland, has a Service Center to help older people with the multi-agency problem, not just the medical care that they need. I have advised many older people to get their medical care at a clinic or a medical center where they only have to "open one door" and pay one fare for the trip. If an older person has many ailments, it is more convenient to visit physicians who have group practices with all offices of the specialists in one building.

Although older couples often speak of what each of them will do "if he (she) dies first" and have their funeral arrangements made and burial clothes in order, the full impact of losing a spouse only occurs upon return to the empty house.

POVERTY

Since Social Security only went into effect in 1935 in this country, we are only now learning about the financial problems of older people. One older individual who lived in a public housing project in a black ghetto stated, "It takes one generation to learn on; in this case, it happens to be my generation." She was ashamed of the place where she lived and reluctant to bring new friends to visit. At the same time she was very active in her community in two senior centers where she was much loved. She was also on the community relations bureau of the police department, where she worked hard to improve relations and thereby conditions in her area. Purse-snatchings were a regular hazard and taxi drivers were reluctant to enter the area.

For older persons living alone in 1967, the median annual income was $1310; for couples it was an income of $3370. The population aged 65 and over (noninstitutional) increased to 17,900,000 in 1966. Although the proportion of poor in this country for those under 65 is declining, the proportion for the aged poor remains the same (about 30 percent). In 1970, there were over 19 million people aged 65 and over in the United States. Their number is expected to exceed 21 million by 1975 and total 25 million by 1985. By 1990 about one person in eight will be of retirement age whereas in 1960 only one person in eleven was this old (Bogue, 1969, p. 893). In 1966 people over 65 made up 9.3 percent of the total noninstitutional population but 18.1 percent of the poor. Another large group of those over 65 are on the borderline between poverty and low income (U.S. Senate, 1969). Subsequent increases in Social Security have helped some keep up with the higher cost of living.

In this affluent society we have many poor older people. In a money-oriented society, older persons are economically useless and thereby without the status of a younger person. Through Medicare professionals are now more aware of older people, who, previous to its adoption, went without proper care and therefore were often invisible in the urban medical community. We are learning more about their needs and problems. More help is available from the federal government. For example, the Older Americans Act of 1965 (Public Law 89–73) was established "To provide assistance in the development of new or improved programs to help older persons through grants to the States for community planning and services and for training, through research, development or training project grants, and to establish within the Department of Health, Education and Welfare an operating agency to be designated as the Administration on Aging." The Older Americans Act Amendments of 1968 provided for service roles in retirement. The Office of Economic Opportunity provides aid to the older age group through various self-help projects.

The conclusions and recommendations of the U.S. Senate's Special Committee on Aging (1969) warned against the acceptance of low income among older persons as an inevitable component of life. The prevalence and persistence of poverty among older Americans raised the question of need for increases in Social Security and re-evaluation and reform of the Old Age Assistance payments. An Institute on Retirement Income was recommended. The Committee also asked for Medicare revisions and reforms in Medicaid to meet the need for health services and urged action to promote preventive medicine. The Bureau of Labor Statistics budget and use of consumer price indexes as a yardstick to determine adjustment in retirement benefits was advised. Attention to consumer protection for older persons and the usefulness of food stamps was advised. It was recommended that the use of meal service and nutrition projects as an avenue to other needs be evaluated. A comprehensive national program of community service by older Americans at federal, state, and local levels was advised to be considered by Congress and enacted into law as soon as possible. Other recommendations centered around (1) the integration of needs for older persons in the Model Cities program, (2) the federal government taking the lead in providing pre-retirement counseling as a model for use elsewhere, and (3) experimentation by the federal government in work programs to counteract arbitrary retirement. If effected, all these recommendations would decrease the alienation felt by older persons in our society and help provide them with a better life.

One of your principal tasks as a nursing student is to learn the needs and problems of each older person under your care and help him meet them. As you make an effort to get to know the older individuals around you, they become visible to you whereas before learning about them, you probably passed them up without scrutiny.

Proper nutrition becomes a problem for the older person who is poor, especially if he lives alone. It is not uncommon for older people to subsist on two meals a day or even one, eating dry foods as breakfast snacks in hotel rooms where cooking facilities are not permitted.[14] Rising food costs leave little leeway for food planning at lower costs, and changes in taste, denture problems, and eating alone are not conducive to the best nutritional states. Because of the cost of eating out, older people living in hotels that close their dining rooms on holidays and weekends often go without meals during these periods.

Senior centers may offer a hot midday meal to members. For some, this may be the main meal that day. Some cities have programs for the delivery of hot meals on a regular basis to those individuals who are homebound.

---

[14] A pamphlet "Food Guide for Older Folks" (Home and Garden Bulletin No. 17, U.S. Department of Agriculture, 1968) is an excellent guide to good nutrition. (Available for 10 cents from Superintendent of Documents, U.S. Government Printing Office, Washington, D.C. 2042.)

Classes in nutrition and meal preparation are often part of senior center programs.

The cost of medication may be a big item in the budget of an older person. Telephone shopping may prove valuable in the purchase of drugs and should be encouraged. Generic prescribing also helps in this cost since many drugs cost less when prescribed under their generic name instead of by brand name (Task Force on Prescription Drugs, 1968, p. 80).

Many older individuals without aid and sustenance are often ashamed to ask for assistance and should be encouraged to use resources that are set up for them. Wiltse (1963) found that the "hard to reach" client of later maturity for public assistance was the man on old age assistance. The fierce independence of the entrepreneurial system may keep needy persons on starvation diets, without electricity and without running water or gas, right in the middle of our cities. Trusting others may be the first hurdle to getting aid. After gaining trust, pride may be the intervening force unless persuasive arguments portray their right to aid.

INDEPENDENCE–DEPENDENCE

Older people now are maintaining independent existences longer than ever before. We are now in an era where parents may even see some of their own children retire.

Medicare gives a new independence to the elderly poor. Older people who previously were unable to receive medical care except through "charity" now can receive this by their Medicare cards. These enable them to receive cut rates at some downtown cafeterias and pay lower bus fares during designated hours in major cities. The card itself is shown proudly by some older people in the same way that a younger person might display his club card. Formerly, poor older patients in county hospitals were not likely to complain about any procedure, whereas now they feel more free to speak up since their care is financed differently.

Falling symbolizes loss of independence and the beginning of infirmity. Falls, however slight, are discussed and reviewed many times by the victim. Bringing to mind loss of sense of self, the possibility of a broken bone, hospitalization, and pictures of the incapacitated and bedridden older person, they are therefore a great threat to the ego and the sense of security. Outings such as visits to physicians and senior centers may be canceled due to fear of falling with its consequences.

Nurses, who have a definite role with the older person in helping him to prepare for dependence and helplessness, should be aware of available community resources. Listening to older peoples' fears and concerns about medical care, physicians, hospitals, convalescent centers, nursing homes, and other living arrangements helps them to sort out the real from the unreal and to accept help when it is needed. Talking about infirmity and what to do if it comes is important, along with discussing some of the positive aspects of various living arrangements. If possible, the older person should be in contact with his own culture; with orthodox Jews, for example, the availability of appropriate food and religious services gives a connection with self and the past.

Loss of independence can be a crisis and should be thoroughly assessed by the nurse. Adaptation from independence to dependence and vice versa varies with levels of wellness, motivation, and life style. In Clark's study (1967) of older San Franciscans, two basic goals were found in aging persons—survival and self-esteem. The study emphasized the linking together of self-esteem with the cultural and personal value of independence-autonomy and self-reliance for the present generation of older Americans.

Maintaining independence is therefore necessary for self-esteem. If institutionalization is required for survival, the challenge then becomes one also for society to help older institutionalized persons to maintain their independence in the way most meaningful to them and the preservation of their self-esteem.

The studies of Lieberman (1968) show that older persons require a year or more of preparation before entering a nursing home if they are to survive the first six months of adaptation. The preventive work of the nurse is therefore clearly drawn.

SOCIAL ISOLATION

Institutionalization brings with it a loss of status and social roles; independence is given up, and the older person feels abandoned by family and other loved ones. The reality of the nuclear family's limitations in being able to care for its aging relatives is manifest, and the older persons' feelings of being "in the way" and "unwanted" are reinforced. Visits, flowers, letters, and other contacts and symbols help, but they do not overcome the reality of social isolation by institutionalization.

Institutionalization   Institutionalization refers to the provision of custodial facilities for those individuals who can no longer care for themselves. Only small proportions of older persons live in institutions—3.7 percent in the United States (Shanas, 1968, p. 297). The sad element of this process is that it is often irreversible: institutions for the aged are seldom rehabilitative, and once the older person begins custodial care, he rarely returns to an independent state. The older individual in his own home who forgets to take his medication, whose special diet is not followed, who forgets to turn off the gas, and who seems unable to handle his money may be thought by nurses and other helping persons to be better off in an institution. There are two schools of thought on this point: some urge institutionalization, and others recommend it only as a last resort. What do we gain by having a well-fed older person in a communal dying house who loses his will to live? From a humanitarian point of view, even in the most cluttered and unsanitary hovel a person can maintain the identity and self-concept which are lost in an institution.

Older people who begin to lose their memory and ability to care for themselves are aware of the drawbacks of institutionalization and sometimes delay getting needed medical care in fear of being "put away in a home." Once the older person leaves his home for a hospital, he feels he has less and less to say about his own destiny. Some older persons, aware of this process, may finally agree to enter a hospital but will then sign themselves out after 2 or 3 days. Others, persuaded by family members to leave their houses and live in custodial institutions, simply leave them and return to their former homes. The question of institutionalization is a family crisis and various children hesitate to be the one to insist on it. Sometimes inheritance of property is a big issue and a deterrent to action due to fear of being disinherited.

Institutionalization, although providing for the physiological needs of the aging, in many instances leaves much to be desired in the psychosocial realm. The institutionalized older person may be cut off from his past and cared for by people who have little understanding of what life was like for him. With the advent of Medicare in 1966, convalescent homes became a common mode of living for the elderly who otherwise could not care for themselves. The use of the concepts of ventilation of feelings and verbal expression cannot be overemphasized as a part of nursing care in these settings. The switch from state hospital care to community care hopefully gives the older person who needs some help a chance to stay within his own community and thus maintain contacts with relatives and significant other persons.

Lieberman's study (1968) shows the deleterious effect of extensive change from residence in the community to an institution and transfer from one institution to another. He shows that the crucial time for the person who needs institutional care is the waiting period before he is admitted. At least one other study indicates the hazards of relocation (Aldrich, 1963). Nurses have an important job to do in this area—to help better prepare aging individuals for accepting assistance. Older people in this country speak of the "poor house" and remember what happened to family and acquaintances before them; such images are not easily removed from their memory. If nurses have visited the different kinds of homes for the aged, they are in a better position to explain what life is like in a rest home, boarding home, nursing home, convalescent hospital, or other type of living arrangement.

With institutionalization comes social impoverishment. There is likely to be little interpersonal behavior among peers when aged people are in institutions. Apathy therefore easily occurs, and regression is in full swing. With the lack of a future perspective, depression is imminent for some. An imposed construction of activities resulting in withdrawal from other activity leads any adult to preoccupation with himself. The institution may reinforce regression or immature behavior to aid in the passive adaptation to the process. The aged woman with her hair tied with a child's ribbon is one example; use of first names by nurses who are 50 or 60 years younger is another.

Older people in institutions are like displaced persons without hope of ever finding another place to live. The most critical period of adaptation and adjustment is in the first few months of institutionalization. The death rate following admission to an institution has been found by Lieberman (1961) to be two and one half times higher than in the waiting period.

Orientation Efforts by nurses to maintain orientation[15] can aid in healthy adaptation. The use of clearly visible calendars and clocks in rooms and lounges helps residents to maintain contact with time. Daily hometown newspapers help them to keep in touch with the events of their community.

Provision of recreational facilities aids the institutionalized person to better deal with his time. Television helps those who enjoy it. Music can aid the older person in catharsis where earlier and happier times are evoked by hearing a familiar tune. All can now have their own radio or television complete with earphones for individualized listening. At other times watching universally liked programs such as the news in a communal lounge encourages socialization and is an area where current affairs can be discussed with others. If childhood table games are available, some older people will spend hours at these pursuits. Many institutions, newly built, such as convalescent hospitals are unknown to older people. Knowing their location, who owns and operates them helps the older resident to maintain orientation as to where he is.

Acknowledgment of birthdays aids in maintaining identity. Nurses should find out about the life of each person and acknowledge to him some of his earlier achievements; encourage him to air his feelings about who he is and where he is. Bridging the gap between him and other residents through introductions and telling each a bit about the other may help the new resident to find a new friend. Grouping people together in the dining room who have similar interests and who know others in common is also important. Keeping one's clothes and some belongings and arranging these as desired within one's own room aids in the maintenance of some autonomy, which is essential to mental health. Use of the telephone as a means of contact with the outside world, both for incoming and outgoing calls is of central importance in the retention of sense of self. The institutionalized older person with decreasing emotional response needs to be encouraged to telephone others. Suggesting

---

[15] Orientation refers to awareness in three spheres—time, place, and person.

that he do so may be the impetus that he needs. Helping to get stationery and stamps and writing letters for those who are unable to do so themselves may result in receiving much desired mail.

Increased preoccupation with body responses can be diminished by listening to patients, investigating and assessing complaints, but also discussing something else. If the older person can make decisions about himself and his needs, the institution should encourage him to do so. If he has hope for return to an independent life, he will probably be more motivated toward autonomy than the individual who has no hope for independence. You may have to listen to the recital of malfunctions of each organ of the body before being able to move on to other subjects.

Some homes for the aging regularly have open houses and other programs which interested persons can attend, thereby seeing for themselves what it is like to live there. Older people can be helped to make a plan for themselves if infirmity comes. Human beings can adapt to great stresses in a more effective way if they have some time and help to prepare for them. Use of the reportorial approach here is useful in that the nurse can freely speak of what another person has done in preparation for the time when he can no longer manage things on his own. Older national figures who are going through illness, hospitalization, and infirmity can form the basis for preparation for accepting help. These are well known through the mass media. If the nurse is familiar with the peer group of the older person, talking about what plans others have made or not made for their helplessness aids the individual to come to terms with his own plans.

The Medicare programs under Title XVIII and the programs for help to older people in institutions for mental disorders under Title XIX should reinforce the efforts for local care in the older person's home community. Title XVIII discourages the use of state hospitals for long-term care; it facilitates the use of general hospitals, extended care facilities, and services provided by home health agencies for the care of the mentally disordered older person. A limit is made upon the number of days that an older person can spend in a psychiatric hospital during his lifetime; however, no limit is made on the number of illnesses that one may be treated for in a general hospital. Each hospital must have a hospital utilization committee which reviews admissions; length of stay is noted as well as the care provided for each individual who remains over a long period of time. The legislation is aimed toward reducing the custodial elements of mental hospital care by requiring treatment plans and programs for each patient and the use of alternative facilities for hospitalization. It is directed toward securing a variety of sources of care within the home community and a reduction of mental hospital long-term care. For a state to qualify for Medical Assistance under Title XIX, certain standards must be met.

Many older people were formerly sent to state mental hospitals simply because the state paid for their care and the counties had not developed any alternatives to state hospital care. A Geriatric Screening Program (Rypins *et al.*, 1968) was established in 1963 in my own county to provide alternatives to state hospitalization. Where an average of almost 500 older people were formerly committed to state mental hospitals annually, only one or two now have to be hospitalized by the state each year. A staff dedicated to helping older people find solutions to their problems saw the patients in their own home settings and not in the office. This practice was patterned after the Amsterdam Plan originated by Professor A. Querido.[16]

It is significant that the Geriatric Screening Project, without being involved in the direct care, mobilized community services to come to the aid of the disturbed older people; 44 percent were able to be maintained in their own homes.

CONSTRICTION

Because of the mental and sensory changes caused by aging in the individual, his circle of movement is likely to become constricted in some manner. Thought, movement, and activities are necessarily changed by the process of aging. Individuals who have been resourceful in their earlier years are likely to be more able to draw upon these resources in older age than those who lack them. Those who are financially better off and those with good education are also more apt to be able to avoid mental constriction. Patterns of involvement in early life may continue to the older phase—for example, membership in clubs or organizations. These continuing memberships may widen the horizons of older people and aid them in the establishment of an explicit affiliation with their age group.

Illness and infirmity are two conditions which cause constriction. The aging process itself produces changes in the sensory, motor, and mental activities of the individual. Arthritis, which is very common in older people, limits activity. One older woman, Mrs. Sanderson, depressed because of her physical decline, prayed every day that "the good Lord take me." Many older persons may have as many as four chronic diseases. The adaptations that older people must make because of illness may add to a diminishing circle of activities.

Pets and plants   In the lives of older people, pets and plants may assume great importance; they often become totems to older people. The nonhuman

---

[16] The reader is referred to F. M. C. Evans: *The Role of the Nurse in Community Mental Health.* New York: The Macmillan Co., 1968, for a description of the part that nurses have in this kind of work. As community mental health centers are developed in this country, mental health nurses will have a more prominent role in community care of the aging.

environment may become more important to the older person than ever before. The caged bird can be identified and sympathized with due to the fact that it also is a prisoner and unable to fly freely about the earth. Parrots can also be taught words to greet others who enter the home. Cats and dogs, although more expensive to care for, like to be caressed and cuddled, and they show steady affection.

Animals may become substitutes for affection for deceased spouses especially if the animal was also a pet of the deceased. They demand care and make the person feel needed and greet him on his return home. They also listen and give the older person the feeling of being understood. Plants are also alive and thrive under a careful green thumb. They grow, reproduce and die. Mrs. Angell spoke of removing leaves from the mother plant, planting the small leaves while the mother plant then died. She spoke of the mother plant doing work and not being needed any more, as if she were symbolically speaking of her own situation.

Cumming and Henry (1961) conclude that "disengagement is an inevitable process in which many of the relationships between a person and other members of society are severed and those remaining altered in quality." [17] Levine (1969) studied the relationship between the abandonment of life's central roles and disengagement. In this study disengagement was defined as decreased interaction between the aging individual and others in his social system. Levine showed that older persons have severed many of their relationships with other people; their low morale was found to be connected with living alone, widowhood, and retirement.

On the other hand, Clark's study (1967) did not find that acceptance of decreased social involvement in old age and willful disengagement from the social system was adaptive. Instead, it concluded that social engagement is more clearly related to psychological well-being and that without social contacts older persons become anxious and pessimistic.

EXPLANATION

When misfortune occurs and the older person cannot find an acceptable explanation for what has happened to him, he is in the crisis of explanation. The inability to explain the misfortune rather than the misfortune itself creates the crisis. This can happen to people who have not given any serious conscious thought to aging; they do not think of themselves as old.

The crisis of explanation was described by Kastenbaum (1964) as occurring when a person finds himself old and different from earlier years but cannot find any reason for it. It is the inability to explain the misfortune of old age.

---

[17] Elaine Cumming and W. E. Henry: *Growing Old—The Process of Disengagement.* New York: Basic Books, 1961, p. 211.

In this crisis the individual is faced with the very difficult task of explaining to himself and others that he is "not what he used to be," or is not, like the motto of one man's club in London "the older the bolder." Instead, the older person is more like the proverb "A man is as old as he feels and a woman is as old as she looks."

The following is an example of an individual experiencing the crisis of explanation and its resolution.

> Mrs. Rose, with fiery red hair, wears loud colors and brightly colored plastic earrings that dangle. Her skin is carefully made up, and when she goes out she always wears long gloves up to her elbow. She is found on weekends dancing until the wee hours at a local ballroom where she goes regularly with her daughter, who is introduced as her sister. She refers to her teenage granddaughters as "Mary's girls." Once religious, she has now removed expressive symbols of religion from her home. The nursing student gained rapport and trust, encouraged her to express her thoughts and feelings, and guided her visits to topics of family life—both present and past—her peers, and her health. It was felt that Mrs. R. had not accepted her age of 81 and that the work of the student for the year was to help her to accept her role as mother and grandmother to her family. On one visit, a family spat ensued in which the daughter was present, upset and drinking. The student remained with Mrs. R. throughout the episode, listening and showing concern for Mrs. R. and her daughter. The event seemed to be a turning point for Mrs. R. in her adaptation to aging. Clinical inference is that the supportive role of the student (accepting her as she was, listening, and showing concern) aided Mrs. R. in the resolution of her crisis of explanation. Subsequently, Mrs. R. began to sew for her granddaughters, referred to herself as a grandmother, and renewed her interest in religion. She also began to dress more like a grandmother, wearing pastels!

DESOLATION

The crisis of desolation, which may begin in middle age, continues until one's death. Desolation has been described by Townsend (1963) as being the underlying reason for loneliness in old age. He defined it in terms of deprivations by death, illness, or migration of the company of someone who is loved, e.g., a spouse or a child. Other dimensions may be added such as the requirement of the older person himself to change his ecological unit. For example, having to move from a condemned hotel or from an area that is being redeveloped or giving up a home for institutional living as in a nursing home. Desolation is expressed by many as: "I'm the only one left, all the others are dead." Or (as of a spouse) "I never thought she would die before me." One older person, Mr. M., who now lives in an area of the city formerly heavily populated by the Irish, said: "They are all dead now. Their children have moved away, and I have lost contact with them. There is no one to help me. There is no Irish mayor, and there is no one on the Board of Supervisors who is Irish. I don't know who to ask for help."

Relocation of older people from their familiar areas of the city can result in desolation since they can no longer visit old friends and familiar places.

Parents and siblings die, and desolation may be intensified if the individual himself has no progeny.

LONELINESS

> . . . man can fulfill himself only if he remains in touch with the funda-
> mental facts of his existence, if he can experience the exaltation of love
> and solidarity, as well as the tragic fact of his aloneness and of the frag-
> mentary character of existence.[18]

Loneliness has been described as a "state of mind in which hope that there may be interpersonal relationships in one's future life is out of the realm of expectation or imagination" (Fromm-Reichman, 1959). To be lonely is to be without the feeling that someone cares. Loneliness can occur at any time throughout the life cycle, but it is intensified in adolescence, early adulthood, and old age. It can be felt by émigrés and has been referred to as "cultural shock" by anthropologists. Loneliness felt upon the death of a loved one or by the dying person himself can be very intense. In the era of the organization man (Whyte, 1956) it can be felt when one loses his place through retirement.

One older person, Mrs. Parks, expressed her loneliness thus: "You come and visit me any time. You know when I start talking, I am just like a record, I can't stop. You know, the telephone doesn't ring very often." She had just spent forty-five minutes explaining in detail her sister's stroke, subsequent hospitalization and condition at this time, all staccato-like without stopping for a pause.

Loneliness is felt by everyone at some stage of life. Nurses can help older people lessen this feeling by being interested in them, caring about them, and sharing the thoughts of their generation with them. Some young people in our society have never really talked with an older person. Although the mass media now acts to keep older people in touch with the times, contact with others in the younger age group may be tenuous or nonexistent. Visiting with older people, showing care and concern for them, can aid in overcoming loneliness (Evans, 1969). Since people in the older age group are populations

---

[18] Erich Fromm: "Alienation Under Capitalism," in Eric and Mary Josephson: *Man Alone: Alienation in Modern Society*. New York: Dell Publishing Co., 1962., p. 71.

at risk in terms of being vulnerable to mental disorder, attention to their psychosocial needs and care is primary prevention. The interpersonal relationship is a means by which loneliness can be conquered.

Senior centers are places in which older persons can meet, plan interesting activities, and maintain usefulness and worth. Group work with older persons further encourages interpersonal well-being. Senior centers provide a place where one is known, expected, and missed when absent. When one is lonely, helping someone else may help relieve the pangs of loneliness. The Foster Grandparents idea is in this direction as are the organized helping groups within senior centers where homebound persons telephone others who live alone, at a designated time every day, just to see how they are and if they need anything. Those who are more well may organize monthly meetings and programs for the homebound themselves in which the Red Cross offers transportation to and from the centers.

Monthly birthday parties are given in the centers, and all who have a birthday in that month have a group party and cake. Each is therefore recognized and remembered. During holidays, when loneliness may become almost unbearable, members of senior centers may cook their dinner together or reserve a large banquet hall in downtown restaurants for this occasion.[19]

DEATH

Older people are most likely to be the age group where death is thought of rather frequently and openly and freely discussed. To die and not to die alone is a central issue of mankind and especially for the person of later maturity who lives alone and ponders about dying and the possibility of his death not being discovered for a long time. The beginning of grief and mourning for one's own death occurs in later maturity. Reading the obituaries becomes a daily habit, and interest in the details of funerals is manifest. One older widow, Mrs. Lucia, went to the funeral parlor and to all the funerals in her parish for several years, even though many of the deceased were strangers to her.

Funerals are important ceremonies in our culture and serve as social events as well as farewells to the deceased. Comments are made on the "natural look"

---

[19] An excellent monograph—Florence B. Vickery: *How to Work with Older People*, Division of Recreation, Department of Natural Resources, State of California, Publication 59–3, 1960—is a guide for professional and volunteer leaders of social activity programs for older people. The author did some of the pioneer work during her 20 years with older people at the San Francisco Senior Center (1947–1967). Another source of persons concerned with research and work on different aspects of aging from diverse disciplines is *International Directory of Gerontology*, U.S. Department of Health, Education, and Welfare, prepared by the Gerontological Society, Inc., for the National Institute of Child Health and Human Development, March 1968.

of the dead; cards are read and floral arrangements counted to determine which family and friends "remembered." The coffin is scrutinized for quality and cost, and comments are made on whether the children thought enough of the deceased to "put him away nice." Younger men are called upon to be pallbearers because the older ones are often too infirm to do the required lifting. Mourners view other mourners and wonder who will be next. Funerals bring to mind the need for preparation for one's own demise, and subsequent visits to the graveyard spur those remaining to write their own epitaphs.

To know that someone will mourn for them and to have an effect on younger people meet the need for *creative expansion* (Buhler, 1962).[20] Memorials may be established before death in the form of buildings and foundations, if the person is wealthy. For others, knowledge that one can live on in his progeny and in the memories of others may suffice. Most older people have mementoes of their past that they like to share with others. Helping them to decide to whom to leave their things is an important part of preparation for death.

Nurses can assist the elderly individual to arrange for a funeral suitable to his income and help him to talk about his own death. Every funeral director has an inexpensive funeral service if one demands it and refuses the four-car cortege and other expensive items. The return to the use of the plain pine coffin is refreshing. Some nurses may find the subject acutely uncomfortable and avoid it by keeping busy with other things. [This was a central finding of a study by Glaser (1966) of nurses in hospital settings.] Noting expressive symbols of religion in the immediate environment of the older person may help to raise the subject of whether the older person believes in an afterlife. In previous years it was commonly thought that the elderly immersed themselves in religion in preparation for death. While some may certainly do this, many, on the other hand, may feel that they have gone to church enough and can now pray at home. Many attend several churches or go to the churches of their friends. Clark's study (1967) of aging people in San Francisco supports this.

At the end of life, in this age group, the most that one can do is to help in the preparation for death, to provide as much comfort as possible, to stand by, and to be present when death comes.

COMMUNICATION WITH OLDER PERSONS
In communicating with older persons, conversations should deal with (1)

---

[20] Buhler described the tendency toward creative expansion first occurring in the child at about 8 months. The child begins to realize his own potentialities and will choose a toy that he can do the most with—e.g., a rattle that he can swing best. Although Buhler describes old age as a contracting tendency, I think creative expansion continues as long as there is life.

something of the past, (2) something of the present, and (3) something of the future. Discussion of the past emphasizes times that the older person was perhaps more ego-oriented and involved.[21] Discussion of the present relates to how things are now, and discussion of the future relates to hope.

Older persons may not hear all you have to say, so speak slowly, use short sentences, enunciate clearly, and pause for response. Face-to-face communication will help those who have hearing problems. If they are in bed, position them to face you. All aspects of therapeutic communication apply in your relationships with older people (see Chapter 5).

There are various aids and devices available to help compensate for failing sight and hearing. For example, a flashing light on the telephone for the hard-of-hearing draws his attention to the instrument. Special earphones for television sets amplify sound for the viewer who watches with others. Amplifiers for telephone conversations help, as do lip-reading classes given by various adult education programs. Hearing aids and eyeglasses assist many older people to maintain social contacts.

Telephone visits are often welcome and very much enjoyed if they are timed appropriately. A bedtime hour of 8 P.M. or even earlier is quite common for older persons. Letters and cards for special holidays and other events are symbols of love to older people who may receive very little mail.

Discussion of all the little things that happen in life aids in health maintenance. Having a confidante helps relieve loneliness.

The use of touch is essential; shaking hands as you come and go aids communication. Effective communication is also achieved through control of the complexity, timing, and amount of communication. A topic that requires serious consideration should be mentioned at the beginning of a contact so that all facets of it can be reviewed. If an older person brings something to you which you cannot handle, you will help him get assistance elsewhere. For the older individual, anticipating a visit, the visit itself, and thinking about the visit help overcome loneliness.

Blocks to communication with the older individual include your own feelings. Persons in the therapeutic role are sometimes irritated that they must shout to be heard. There may be difficulty in acceptance of limited goals and the fact that very small things mean so much and count a lot in therapeutic care. There may be a feeling of futility that change is not possible. Stereotypes may block us in that we expect an older person to behave in a certain manner. Our feelings about parent-child or grandparent-grandchild

---

[21] In later years, the ego has less energy to involve in activities outside the self; there is a decreased investment in living in that gratifications tend to be more vicarious than direct (Rosen and Neugarten, 1960).

get in the way. This is called countertransference.[22] It may be difficult to accept the social, physical, psychological, and economic dependency that one sees in aging. Attitudes of professionals toward older people have often been developed by contact with those in nursing homes where symptoms have been labeled as being due to senility with the feeling that nothing further can be done.

A new cadre of professionals is needed—and fortunately is being developed—which will provide for better care of our aging population.

Summary

This chapter emphasizes the developmental tasks and stage-specific crises for all the phases of the life cycle from infancy through old age. Crisis is presented in terms of expected and unexpected crises. As nursing concerns itself more and more with the care of individuals from womb to tomb, knowledge of life's crises is required for better nursing care. Some of the crisis points in each developmental phase are thereby included here to aid the nursing student to recognize these crises so that help can be provided to patients and families in the attainment of developmental tasks, life's crises, and in early crisis resolution.

References

Aldrich, C. K., and Mendkoff, E.: "Relocation of the Aged and Disabled: A Mortality Study," *Journal American Geriatrics Society*, **11** : 3, March 1963.

American Psychiatric Association: *A Psychiatric Glossary*. Washington, D.C.: American Psychiatric Association, 1969.

Anderson, Barbara Gallatin: "Death as a Subject of Cross-Cultural Inquiry," Paper presented at the First International Congress of Social Psychiatry, London, 1964.

Beckett, Samuel: *Krapp's Last Tape and Other Dramatic Pieces*. New York: Grove Press, 1960.

Bernfield, Siegfield: Notes taken from Case Presentation, 1951.

---

[22] Countertransference refers to the conscious or unconscious reaction of the nurse toward the patient, as if he were a significant other in the nurse's earlier life. It is a temporary identification with the patient.

Bogue, Donald J.: *Principles of Demography*. New York: John Wiley & Sons, 1969.

Bowlby, John: "A Two-Year-Old Goes to the Hospital," *The Psychoanalytic Study of the Child*, **7**:82—94, New York: International Universities Press, 1952.

———— *Attachment*. New York: Basic Books, Inc., 1969.

Buhler, Charlotte: *Values in Psychotherapy*. New York: The Free Press of Glencoe, 1962.

Bulbulyan, Agavni: Notes taken from paper presented at the American Nurses' Association Convention, June 13—17, 1966, San Francisco.

Butler, Robert N.: "The Life Review: An Interpretation of Reminiscence in the Aged." in Neugarten, Bernice L., *Middle Age and Aging*. Chicago: University of Chicago Press, 1968, pp. 486—496.

Carp, Frances M., ed: *The Retirement Process*. Washington, D.C.: Superintendent of Documents, 1968, pp. 1—26.

Clark, Margaret, and Anderson, Barbara Gallatin: *Culture and Aging*. Springfield, Ill.: Charles C Thomas, 1967.

Cumming, Elaine, and Henry, W. E.: *Growing Old—The Process of Disengagement*. New York: Basic Books, 1961.

———— "New Thoughts on the Theory of Disengagement," in Kastenbaum, Robert; *New Thoughts on Old Age*. New York: Springer Publishing Co., 1964.

Eissler, K. R.: *The Psychiatrist and the Dying Patient*. New York: The International Universities Press, 1955.

Emerson, Ralph Waldo: "Self Reliance" in Londeman, Edward C.: *Basic Selections from Emerson*, New York: A Mentor Book, 1954.

Engel, George L.: *Psychological Development in Health and Disease*. Philadelphia: W. B. Saunders Co., 1962, p. 134.

Erikson, Erik H.: *Childhood and Society*. New York: W. W. Norton and Co., Inc. 1963.

Evans, F. M. C.: "Visiting Older People—A Learning Experience," *Nursing Outlook*, **17**:3:20—23, 1969.

———— *The Role of the Nurse in Community Mental Health*. New York: The Macmillan Company, 1968.

Friedenberg, Edgar Z.: *The Vanishing Adolescent*. New York: Dell Publishing Co., Inc., 1959.

Freud, Sigmund: *The Ego and the Id*. standard edition. London: The Hogarth Press. Vol. 19, 1961.

Fromm, Erich: "Alienation Under Capitalism," in Josephson, Eric and Mary: *Man Alone: Alienation in Modern Society*. New York: Dell Publishing Co., Inc., 1962.

Fromm-Reichman, Frieda: "Loneliness," *Psychiatry*, **22**:1—16, 1959.

Glaser, Barney: *Awareness of Dying.* Chicago: Aldine Publishing Co., 1966.

Goodman, Louis S. and Gilman, Alfred: *The Pharmacological Basis of Therapeutics*, 3rd ed. New York: The Macmillan Co., 1965, p. 1548.

Gorman, Warren: *Body Image and the Image of the Brain.* St. Louis: Warren H. Green, 1969, p. 104.

Havighurst, Robert J.: *Human Development and Education.* New York: Longmans, Green and Co., 1953.

————— "The Leisure Activities of the Middle-Aged," *American Journal of Sociology*, **63**:152–62, 1957.

Kastenbaum, Robert: *New Thoughts on Old Age.* New York: Springer, 1964, p. 318.

Keniston, Kenneth: "Drug Use and Student Values," in Hollander, Charles, ed: *Background Papers on Student Drug Involvement*, United States National Student Association, 2115 S. Street, N.W., Washington, D.C., 1967.

Kramer, Morton, Taube, Carl, and Starr, Sheldon: "Patterns of Use of Psychiatric Facilities by the Aged: Current Status, Trends & Implications," Paper presented at the American Psychiatric Association, Regional Conference on Aging in Modern Society, San Francisco, California, 1967.

Kreps, Juanita M.: "The Allocation of Leisure to Retirement," in Carp, Frances M., ed.: *The Retirement Process.* Washington, D.C.: Superintendent of Documents, 1968, pp. 137–45.

Levine, Rhoda: "Disengagement in the Elderly—Its Causes and Effects," *Nursing Outlook*, **17**:10:28–30, October, 1969.

Lieberman, Morton A.: "Psychological Effects of Institutionalization," *Journal of Gerontology*, **23**:343–53, July, 1968.

————— "Psychological Correlates of Impending Death: Some Preliminary Observations," in Neugarten, Bernice L.: *Middle Age and Aging.* Chicago: The University of Chicago Press, 1968.

————— "Relationship of Mortality Rates to Entrance to a Home for the Aged," *Geriatrics*, **16**:515–19, 1961.

Menninger, Karl: *The Vital Balance.* New York: The Viking Press, 1963.

Neugarten, Bernice L., and Garron, D.: "The Attitude of Middle-Aged Persons Toward Growing Older," *Geriatrics*, **14**:21–24, 1959.

Niebanck, Paul L.: "Knowledge Gained in Studies of Relocation," in *Patterns of Living and Housing of Middle-Aged and Older People.* Washington, D.C.: Superintendent of Documents, 1966.

Potter, Ralph: Notes taken from lectures on "Growth and Development from the Psychoanalytic Point of View," Napa State Hospital, Imola, Calif., 1962.

Ribble, Margaretha Antoinette: *The Rights of Infants*, 2nd ed. New York: Columbia University Press, 1965.

Rosen, Jacquelin L., and Neugarten, Bernice L.: "Ego Functions in Middle

and Later Years: A Thematic Apperception Study of Normal Adults,"
Journal of Gerontology, **15**:1:62–67, January, 1960.

Rypins, Russel F., and Clark, Mary Lou: "A Screening Project for the Geriatric
Mentally Ill," *California Medicine*, **109**:273–78, October, 1968.

Shanas, Ethel: "Family Help Patterns and Social Class in Three Countries,"
in Neugarten, Bernice: *Middle Age and Aging*. Chicago: The University of
Chicago Press, 1968.

Sheps, Jack: "New Developments in Family Diagnosis in Emotional Disorders of Old Age," *Geriatrics*, **14**:443–49, 1959.

Smith, Wallace F.: *Preparing the Elderly for Relocation*. University of Pennsylvania, Institute for Environmental Studies, 1966.

Spence, Donald L.: "Patterns of Retirement in San Francisco," in Carp,
Frances M., ed.: *The Retirement Process*. Washington, D.C.: Superintendent
of Documents, 1968.

——— Notes taken from lecture "Psychiatric Problems of Aging," Mendocino, Calif., 1969.

Spitz, Rene: "Hospitalism. An Inquiry into the Genesis of Psychiatric Conditions in Early Childhood," in *The Psychoanalytic Study of the Child*,
Vol. I. New York: International Universities Press, 1945.

Szalita, Alberta B.: "Psychodynamics of Disorders of the Involutional Age,"
in Arieta, Silvano, ed.: *American Handbook of Psychiatry*, Vol. III. New York:
Basic Books, Inc., 1966, pp. 69–74.

Task Force of Prescription Drugs: *The Drug Users*. U.S. Department of Health,
Education, and Welfare, Washington, D.C., 1968.

Townsend, Peter: *The Family Life of Old People*. Baltimore: Penguin Books,
1963.

Toynbee, Arnold: *Man's Concern with Death*. London: Hodder and Stoughton,
1968.

Tunstall, Jeremy: *Old and Alone*. London: Routledge and Kegan Paul, 1966.

U.S. Department of Health, Education, and Welfare: *The Mental Health of
Children*. Washington, D.C.: Superintendent of Documents, 1965.

U.S. Department of Health, Education, and Welfare: *International Directory
of Gerontology*. Washington, D.C.: Superintendent of Documents, 1969.

U.S. Senate: *Developments in Aging, 1968. A Report of the Special Committee on Aging*. Washington, D.C.: Superintendent of Documents, 1969.

Vickery, Florence: *How to Work with Older People*. Sacramento, Calif.:
Division of Recreation, Department of Natural Resources, State of California Publication 59-3, 1960.

Whyte, William H.: *The Organization Man*. New York: Simon and Schuster,
Inc., 1956.

Wilner, Daniel M., Walkley, Rosabelle, and Sherman, Susan: "Psychological Factors in Housing for the Aged," in U.S. Department of Health,

Education, and Welfare, *Mental Health Program Reports No. 2*. Public Health Service Publication No. 1743, U.S. Government Printing Office, Washington, D.C., 1968.

Wiltse, Kermit: *Group Methods in the Public Welfare Program*. Palo Alto, Calif.: Pacific Books, 1963.

Suggested readings

Barad, M., Altschuler, K. Z., and Goldfarb, A. I.: "A Survey of Dreams in Aged Persons," *Archives of General Psychiatry*, **4**:419–24, 1961.

Bettelheim, Bruno: *The Children of the Dream*. New York: The Macmillan Co., 1969.

Blenker, Margaret, Jahn, Julius, and Wasser, Edna: *Serving the Aging*. New York: Community Service Society of New York, Institute of Welfare Research, 1964.

Bolman, William M.: "Systems Theory, Psychiatry and School Phobia," *American Journal of Psychiatry*, **127**:25–32, 1970.

Branstetter, Ellamae: "The Young Child's Response to Hospitalization: Separation Anxiety or Lack of Mothering Care," *American Journal of Public Health*, **59**:1:92–98, January, 1969.

Brockington, Fraser, and Lempert, Suzanne: *The Social Needs of the Over-80's*, Manchester, England: Manchester University Press, 1966.

Bulla, Clyde Robert: *Flower Pot Gardens*. New York: Thomas Y. Crowell Co., 1967.

Butler, Robert N.: "The Healthy Aged Versus Cherished Stereotypes," *Geriatric Institutions*, January-February, 1963.

Deykin, Eva, Jacobson, Shirley, Klerman, Gerald, and Solomon, Naida: "The Empty Nest: Psychosocial Aspects of Conflicts Between Depressed Women and their Grown Children," *American Journal of Psychiatry*, **122**:1422–26, 1966.

Dunn, Halbert L.: "Significance of Levels of Illness in Aging," *Geriatrics*, **13**:51–57, January, 1958.

———— *High Level Wellness*. Arlington, Va.: R. W. Beatty Co., 1961.

Erikson, Erik H.: *Young Man Luther*. New York: W. W. Norton, 1962.

———— *Identity, Youth and Crisis*. New York: W. W. Norton, 1968.

Evans, Richard I.: *Dialogue with Erik Erikson*. New York: Harper & Row, Publishers, 1967.

Fried, Barbara: *The Middle-Age Crisis*. New York: Harper & Row, 1967.

Friedenberg, Edgar Z.: *The Vanishing Adolescent.* New York: Dell Publishing Co., 1959.

———— *Coming of Age in America.* New York: Vintage Books, 1967.

Fromm, Erich: *The Art of Loving.* New York: Bantam Books, 1956.

Gesell, Arnold: *The First Five Years of Life: A Guide to the Study of the Preschool Child.* New York: Harper & Row, 1940.

Goldfarb, Alvin I.: "Problems of Psychotherapy of the Aged," in *Proceedings of the Third World Congress of Psychiatry.* Toronto: University of Toronto Press, 1963, pp. 232–37.

Gunter, Laurie M.: "A New Look at the Older Patient in the Community Through the Eyes of Nursing Students," *Nursing Forum,* **8**:1:50–63, 1969.

Hallstrom, Betty J.: "Contact Comfort: Its Application to Immunization Injections," *Nursing Research,* **17**:2:130–34, March-April, 1968.

Keniston, Kenneth: *The Uncommitted: Alienated Youth in American Society,* New York: Harcourt, Brace & World, 1965.

———— *The Young Radicals.* New York: Harcourt, Brace & World, 1968.

Lidz, Theodore: *The Family and Human Adaptation. Three Lectures.* New York: International Universities Press, 1963.

———— *The Person.* New York: Basic Books, Inc., 1968.

Loether, Herman J.: *Problems of Aging.* Belmont, California: Dickenson Publishing Co., Inc., 1967.

Neugarten, Bernice, *et al.: Personality in Middle and Late Life.* New York: Atherton Press, 1964.

Pappenheim, Else and Sweeney, Mary: "Separation Anxiety in Mother and Child," *The Psychoanalytic Study of the Child,* **7**:95–114. New York: International Universities Press, 1952.

Pulkkinen, Susan D.: "A Focus on Feelings," *Nursing Outlook,* **17**:12:7–71, December, 1969.

Rochlin, Gregory: *Griefs and Discontents: The Forces of Change.* Boston: Little, Brown & Co., 1965.

Rose, Arnold M., and Peterson, Warren A.: *Older People and Their Social World.* Philadelphia: F. A. Davis Co., 1965.

Rudd, T. N.: *Human Relations in Old Age.* London: Faber and Faber, 1967.

Shanas, Ethel: *Family Relationships of Older People.* New York: Health Information Foundation, 1961.

Snook, Leslie: *Gardening for the Elderly and Handicapped.* London: Pan Books Ltd., 1968.

Spitz, Renee: *The First Year of Life: A Psychoanalytic Study of Normal and Deviant Development of Object Relations.* New York: International Universities Press, 1965.

U.S. Senate: "Health Aspects of the Economics of Aging," Washington, D.C.: Government Printing Office, 1969.

U.S. Senate: "Economics of Aging: Toward a Full Share in Abundance," Washington, D.C.: Government Printing Office, 1969.

Vischer, A. L.: *On Growing Old*. Boston: Houghton Mifflin Co., 1967. University of Florida Press, 1959.

Vogel, Ezra F. and Bell, Norman W.: "The Emotionally Disturbed Child as the Family Scapegoat," in Bell, Norman W., and Vogel, Ezra F., eds: *A Modern Introduction to the Family*. New York: The Free Press, 1968, pp. 412–27.

Wheelis, Allen: *The Quest for Identity*: New York: W. W. Norton, 1958.

3 The family

Although other professionals have been concerned for many years with family work, it is only within the past decade that psychiatrists and psychiatric nurses have been involved in working with families. In order to be able to identify interaction within the family group, it is helpful to learn about healthy families. The best way to do this is by getting involved with families without deviant members and studying them closely over an extended period of time. In family-centered nursing, it is essential to have a clear understanding of the constituents of health; the healthy family is the model that the family with mental disorder is attempting to achieve. Nursing students who learn family dynamics in addition to the intrapsychic viewpoint of individuals will be more effective practitioners.

The number of families in the United States has been increasing steadily since World War II. In March, 1967, 181.1 million people or 92 percent of the country's resident population were members of families. The average family size at this time was 3.70 persons (Metropolitan Life, 1969).

A family is defined as a group of two or more persons living together and related by blood, marriage, or adoption. There are at least six dimensions of a family: (1) It is composed of individuals, each of whom has needs and expectations. (2) It is a group and must be viewed also in this dimension— the action of one individual has an effect on the entire family. (3) It is a primary group and as such is (usually) small, with considerable emotional involvement and shared goals. (4) It is the basic unit of society and thus must be studied in the context of the total social system. (5) It is a medium for transmission of values of the social system of which it is a part. (6) It has a geographical and occupational status, as is evidenced by the differences in urban and rural settings (Kluckhohn, 1954; Parsons, 1952). On the whole, heads of families in the United States are relatively young; over 25 percent are under 35 years of age. About another 25 percent are in the age group 35–44, and approximately one seventh of the heads of families are at least 65 years old. The proportion of families headed by women increases with age, thereby reflecting the higher mortality rate among men (Metropolitan Life, 1969).

Life style

Life style refers to the ways in which families cope with conflicts, needs, and crises. Depending on how they resolve it, some families emerge from a crisis stronger; others become weaker. When the family as a group is threatened with disruption, there are several processes which restore the equilibrium. Spiegel (1957) delineates the following techniques of resolution of conflicts and restoration of the balance of the family group.

Role complementarity

The fundamental idea in the study of the family system refers to description of the behavior of a person in his relations with others. Every role ties in with the role of another. In the nuclear family, there are fewer roles than in the extended family.[1] The basic roles of the nuclear family are mother, father, lover, child, spouse, brother, and sister. Role concepts may vary markedly within different cultural groups. For example, in the Italian culture, it is expected that the new husband provides for his bride, who in turn cares for the home, provides nurture for the husband, and bears the children. Shortly after World War II, many G.I.'s brought home Italian wives. Conflicts occurred when the American husband expected his new bride to work during the first years of marriage to help make payments on a new home, car, and other objects. Added to the handicap of her cultural expectation of what a wife should be were linguistic and educational problems, and cultural shock.

Complementarity is necessary for role integration. For any one person who holds a particular role in a group, there is a role partner. An example of the role of performer and the role of the listener follows: A grandmother invited her family to her piano concert. They gathered around her living room, she played some unpublished Schubert and just before the end of the piece, everybody began talking. In a loud voice, she exclaimed, "Quiet! *I'm* still the main person!" and restored the complementarity. All behavior in interpersonal

---

[1] The nuclear family refers to the smaller family of contemporary society in which there are at most two generations with conjugal parent-child and sibling relationships. Extended family refers to the two-generation nuclear family plus either a third generation or relatives such as uncles and cousins.

relations has this idea of complementarity built into it. If complementarity is not maintained, disruption occurs within the family. Since no family remains the same for very long, it is likely that complementarity changes.

Speigel (1957) has described five sources of strain: (1) *Cognitive*. Individuals cannot carry out roles unless they know what is expected of them. Parents have to learn how to interpret cues from the child and to learn what to expect as children develop; likewise, the child also learns expectations as he matures. Knowledge of life's crises and what each phase has in store greatly helps the individual within his family. Courses in marriage and family life, for example, assist in a smoother transition from familial limbo to the married state. Family conferences at periodic intervals also help individual members.

(2) *Conflict in goals*. Roles enable one to work toward goals, and if different goals are being pursued, conflict occurs and complementarity is lost. Agreement on mutual goals restores the equilibrium. Biological deficiencies and limitations also affect pursuit of goals, as do genetically determined and other handicapping conditions such as poverty, fatigue, and malnutrition.

(3) *Differences in culture*. How one is to behave as a husband or wife or parent may be different depending on the cultural background of each. Some parents plan ahead so much that a bank account is opened for an infant before it is born. We have been said to spend so much energy on planning for the future that we cannot enjoy the present. In the melting pot of the United States cultural conflict is widespread. The American bride who expects to do the grocery shopping is surprised to find that her Persian husband insists that it is his job.

(4) *Instrumental*. This strain is very marked in our money-oriented society if such necessities as money and transportation are lacking. Food, clothing, shelter, furniture, and money are necessary in our consumer society for individuals to carry out roles.

(5) *Allocative*. Some roles are *ascribed*, e.g., age and sex (Parsons, 1964). No one can get out of an age or sex role without conflict. An older person cannot act young or a child act old without violating certain sanctions. Although surgery now permits some individuals to change their sex and transvestitism is rather common, the conflicts remain. Other roles have to be *achieved*, and some can be assumed by *adoption*. The older brother who adopts the role of protector toward a younger brother is an example. If he can protect the younger brother and be the hero in action, he has both achieved and adopted the two roles.[2] Another kind of role is *assumed*, as in play.

---

[2] See *The Autobiography of Malcolm X*. New York: Grove Press (p. 24) for a vivid example of these roles.

Assumed roles have a vital part in family equilibrium because through play, cues can be responded to and tested out in moving toward change.

Spiegel (1957) describes techniques of equilibrium maintenance in families as falling within two categories: *role induction* and *role modification.* In the resolution of conflict by role induction, one or the other family members agrees with, submits to, or goes along with the role. One takes the complementary role without a change occurring, and equilibrium is restored. Role induction is based upon manipulative techniques. On the other hand, role modification involves a change in both parties to the conflict. Complementarity is achieved once more, but it is mutually agreed upon. Role modification is based upon insight.

The following six steps are grouped together as a process; the sixth is an intermediary between role induction and role modification.

1. **Coercing**   One person forces the other to accept roles by threats or punishment. It may be neutralized by defiance.
2. **Coaxing**   Asking, promising, pleading, and begging. This involves the manipulation of rewards and may be neutralized by refusal.
3. **Evaluating**   Praising, blaming, shaming, approving, and disapproving. Some elements of this may be influenced by a perfectionistic childhood of parents. "Stop behaving like you were born in a barn" and "In your former life, you must have been a pig" are typical comments. The specific neutralizing technique is denial.
4. **Masking**   Correct information is withheld or some other incorrect information is substituted. It includes behavior such as pretending and evading; unmasking is the neutralizing element. (Spiegel [1957, p. 558] notes the belief that masking is as significant to the function of the social system as repression is to the function of the personality.)
5. **Postponing**   Time permits changes to take place that solve the conflict. During this time, intrapsychic processes reduce tension that bring about a change in attitude. "I'll think about it" is an example and the old adage "When in doubt, do nothing." Provoking is the specific neutralizing technique and incites the conflict to emerge.
6. **Role Reversal**   This can lead to induction or modification. One person puts himself in the position of the other.

Because role induction is primarily defensive, the same conflict can occur repeatedly. It is like a method that treats the symptom instead of the disease.

Role modification, which leads toward insight, begins with (7) joking; (8) referral to a third party; (9) exploring (this is the testing phase and describes the work of the helping person who is involved in assisting the family to find solutions to conflicts); (10) compromising, the phase in which parties to the conflict perceive the need for a change of goals; and (11) consolidating, learning how to make the compromises work. Roles are modified through redistribution of goals.

The foregoing frame of reference provides a method for systematic observation of processes within families that may otherwise go unobserved. Miller's (1963) study of family dynamics was based upon these processes. Her primary emphasis was upon *masking*, which seemed to be the technique most often used in the family studied. In her paper, a dramatic picture was drawn of the deleterious effects of masking upon the mental health of the family.

Mental health of families

Families serve to provide values, roles, tension management, emotional support, and communication. However, emotional neglect or emotional exploitation may occur. *A healthy family provides perception of needs of others, respect accorded to these needs, and satisfaction of them.*

Maternal deprivation

Today it is generally accepted by those working with families that one of the essential ingredients for mental health of the individual is "... that the infant and young child should experience a warm, intimate, and continuous relationship with his mother (or permanent mother-substitute) in which both find satisfaction and enjoyment."[3] A situation in which the child does not have this relationship is called maternal deprivation. Deprivation can be partial or rather complete; it can also occur in the presence of the mother.

Ainsworth (1962), in a review of findings and controversy over what constitutes maternal deprivation and its effects, summarized the findings as follows: the effects of deprivation are now thought to be more reversible than they were in 1951, but cases of long-standing deprivation have limited improvement. The conclusion remains that early deprivation is of such magnitude that all efforts should be made toward prevention. In Bettelheim's

---

[3] John Bowlby: *Maternal Care and Mental Health.* Geneva: World Health Organization; 1952, p. 11.

(1967) work with Joey, an autistic boy, it was discovered, after several years, that behind Joey's anger at his parents was not the bad things they did to him but the fact that they had not even cared enough to be "bad" (p. 259). At Joey's birth, his mother was so terrified at the new responsibility that all her emotions were bound up in controlling her anxiety. She did not want to see Joey because she felt he was more than she could manage. Although parental deprivation as with the case of Joey is possible, emphasis is placed upon the mother figure because she is most likely to be the one to care for his needs in our culture.

Two cases of extremely isolated children demonstrate the effect upon an individual of lack of social influence. Both cases were illegitimate and had been hidden away and given little attention from anyone for about 6 years. Both acted like infants and were without speech (Davis, 1948).

Basic needs of individual members

Many of the basic needs of individuals are met in families. Levels of need have been classified by Maslow (1954), who put basic needs into the following hierarchy: (1) physiological, (2) safety, (3) love and belonging, (4) self-esteem, and (5) self-actualization. Another function of the family is to provide for the mental health of its members. The need to be secure can be provided by the family unit. Every child needs to learn to love and to be loved, something he can be taught within his family.[4] He can also gain a sense of belonging and can achieve impulse control from his family. Impulse control may be one of the most difficult things to teach disadvantaged children. They find it very difficult to delay gratification because of their many experiences in which they never had anything unless they took it when they first saw it.

The growing child needs to be accepted for what he is at all phases of development and must receive personal recognition, both of which can be provided within the family. The need for expansion or achievement can be observed and commented upon, and facilities and materials can be provided for the child to develop his potentialities. Encouragement, approval, and other forms of emotional support can be given. Children need to belong to a group in which they share their experiences; the family can constitute such a group. Ego integration depends on awareness of one's own identity and self-assurance in knowing who one is. The family is the group that provides

[4] A provocative account of peer group influence within the kibbutz and without the constant attendance of family members has been given by Bettelheim (1969).

roles to carry out, tasks to perform, and reflection of the mirror-image self, all important in the identity maintenance which is the mainstay of mental health. It is thought by most mental health professionals that a secure childhood provides the individual with the necessary psychological armor for the remainder of his life.

Characteristics of positive mental health

In assessing positive mental health of the individual members of a family, Jahoda's list of indicators is useful (1958). She synthesized psychological theory into six major points. How these characteristics are developed in the individual in infancy and childhood affect his life behavior. The first indicator of positive mental health relates to *the attitudes of an individual toward himself.* An objective view of the self, an acceptance of self including the high points and the shortcomings, and a sense of identity are included under this heading. Erikson's (1963) eight stages of man included the crisis of identity versus role confusion (see Chapter 2). The behavior of the individual, his phenomenal self, gives clues to the assessment of this characteristic. The child who knows who he is and who is secure in his family constellation will manifest this characteristic of positive mental health.

The second indicator is the individual's style and degree of *growth, development, and self-actualizing* as expressions of mental health. The psychosocial developmental milestones of man described by Havighurst (1953) and Erikson (1963) are measuring sticks for this indicator. Non-attainment of developmental tasks may result in maladaptation. The attention, interest, love, and other ingredients of a healthy family aid the individual child toward an adequate self-concept which is a strong component of this characteristic. Conditions within the family can assist each individual member meet his need for expansion and reach his highest potential.

The third indicator of positive mental health is a central synthesizing function or *integration* incorporating some of the two preceding aspects. Integration emphasizes an equilibrium of intrapsychic forces, a philosophy of life, and an ability to resist stress and tolerate anxiety.

The subsequent indicators are all a part of reality orientation. *Autonomy* refers to the individual's independence from others. Singling out the person's degree of independence from social influences is most revealing of the state of his mental health; it is the ability to manage for one's self. The autonomous person is self-directed. Although in infancy and early childhood the individual is totally dependent on others for sustenance and life, he moves rapidly toward independence. Autonomy refers to the ability to make a choice between different factors within situations. Autonomy versus shame and doubt has also been described by Erikson (1963) as the second stage-specific crisis which man encounters.

Mental health is also expressed in the *adequacy of the individual's perception of reality.* Perception of his environment as it is without distortion and supporting what he perceives are included under this heading, along with empathy or social sensitivity. Jahoda (1958) states that "the major requirement of the healthy person in this area is that he treat the inner life of other people as a matter worthy of concern and attention." [5] Moving from the real world to the unreal world is an indicator of mental disorder. Perception of reality is strongly influenced by culture, which must be included in the assessment of each individual's mental health in relation to his family, to himself, and to the social system to which he is attached. Psychiatry reflects the tenor of the times; and the father who brought his son to the psychiatrist because the son had registered as a conscientious objector can be said to have distorted reality.

The sixth criterion of positive mental health is *environmental mastery.* Inherent in this indicator is the ability to love and adequacy in love, other interpersonal relations, work, and play. The ability to meet the situational requirements of life, to adapt, adjust, and problem-solve effectively are all aspects of this characteristic. Three dimensions of healthy problem-solving are (1) an individual goes through the process and all the stages, (2) maintains an appropriate feeling tone, and (3) directs an attack on the problem. In a technological, industrial society, this indicator may become more and more complex. For example, toward the end of life, what does environmental mastery mean to the individual who is in retirement? The basic need to do purposeful work remains, yet there are many years left without employment for hundreds of thousands of older people in their retirement years. Retirement enforces a reduction in striving and therefore a redistribution of energy from work to new purposes.

Some characteristics of families

The role of the family in the maintenance of mental health is crucial. In contemporary society, there is a downgrading of the authority of parents,

---

[5] Marie Jahoda: *Current Concepts of Positive Mental Health.* New York: Basic Books, 1958, p. 52.

currently referred to as the "generation gap." There is also a move toward an egalitarian family: more wives are working at public work than ever before and the traditional roles of men and women are merging. Men no longer return home after a day's work to evenings of leisure; they are expected to participate in recreation with children, help to care for them, and even do housework. Margaret Mead says that husbands are so tamed domestically that they are losing their sense of adventure.

There is a relative decrease in the authority of the father in the modern family. In our money-oriented society, where the symbol of power is the dollar, the father often turns over all his earnings to his wife to manage and will carry only a few dollars in his pocket. The suburban husband is simply not present most of the time to discipline the children. Even when he is present, there is now a deemphasis on discipline; both parents and children are "nice." Parental uncertainty is widespread, and there is hesitancy to set limits.

Although marriages without procreation may conflict with the conforming mode of the family in this country, some students of the ecological revolution and population explosion now advocate a shift from emphasis on procreation as a function of the family to the smaller or childless family. Influences and changes within the smaller family on a wide scale remain for the future. Knowledge of availability and social acceptance of birth control methods will undoubtedly influence the sizes of future families.

Since nursing students tend to come from middle-class families and have their own opinions about what constitutes family life, attitudes toward unconventional living arrangements may interfere with objectivity. The nonjudgmental attitude of the professional does not develop overnight but has to be acquired gradually before one can be of much assistance to patients and families.

During my experiences with nursing students and their child psychiatric patients, some have been profoundly moved coming into contact with children who are unwanted by their parents, who may be suffering from the battered child syndrome, or evidence other types of neglect and abuse. New knowledge arises from contact with both nonconforming families and those exhibiting deviant behavior. Knowledge of the ways of life of different groups within one's own social system as well as those of other cultural groups aids in identification of healthy components of families as well as deviant behavior. Discussion with others also helps to foster self-understanding.

The decrease in importance of the grandparents is new in this society; the nuclear family often has no place for older people. Box houses, labor-saving devices, the pace of modern living, and facilities outside the home providing social and recreational activities for different age groups instead of family activities contribute to lack of place for older family members. The time budget, so highly valued in our society, often does not include the older person. Vertical and horizontal mobility[6] tend to leave out the grandparents.

War has increased distances between people. In their travels, servicemen meet people wherever they are, some marry and locate in a distant area instead of nearer to their own homes. The career military man and his family move many times from country to country, often at great distances from grandparents. These factors all contribute to the absence of interaction during ceremonies, holidays, and other times important to all, especially for the young; in the failure to establish family identity; and cause the loss of a sense of connection with the past. For the older person, love, acceptance, belonging, and aid in meeting the crises of aging may not be so readily available as they can be for the young.

Interdependence, independence, and dependence

Although in the nuclear family older people may not live under the same roof as their children, patterns of mutual help and assistance remain as they exist in the extended family, where the generations live near each other. The family that does not have proximity to the older generations often forms peer group associations in which members of other families become substitutes and are even exchanged temporarily (as in the husband and wife swapping).

A national study of patterns of help to the elderly within families was found to relate to family size, structure, and living arrangements (Shanas, 1968). Shared living arrangements are often initiated by children. Older people are more likely to ask their daughters to help them than their sons (Shanas, 1962, p. 113); but where there are no daughters, help comes from the sons. Living arrangements of older individuals differ by social class—middle-class white-collar parents in the United States are likely to live independently of and at some distance from their children. The majority, however, live close enough to a child to get help if it is needed.

The kinds of mutual aid given relate to general assistance during illness and other emergencies. Older people help by giving gifts, assisting with grandchildren, doing home repairs, gardening, and yard work, and helping with the housework. In turn, the children help their parents by giving economic support, personal care, transportation, gifts, outings, and assistance with household chores (Shanas, 1968, p. 304).

---

[6] Vertical mobility refers to movement from one social class to another. Horizontal mobility is the movement from one place to another.

In an earlier national study, it was found that less than 3 percent of persons over 65 preferred to live in institutions (Shanas, 1962). It was also found that almost all older people feared and were hostile to a move to an institution because it signified (1) loss of independence, (2) a prelude to death, and (3) rejection by children. On the psychological effects of waiting for institutionalization, the central position of the family in the world of the older person is supported (Prock, 1969). A cluster of characteristics of the waiting list group was found to show that what had been termed "effects of institutionalization" actually occur before these people become residents of institutions. Helplessness, powerlessness, low interaction with others, depressed mood, low self-esteem, little hope for the future, disorganization of experience, low ego energy, tension, and anxiety were evidenced by the waiting list group. Comparison of persons on and off a waiting list showed that for the waiting list group "the intimacy and mutuality of family ties were decidedly weaker. . . ." (Prock, p. 1841). This suggests an intrafamily disequilibrium and complements the work of Lieberman (see Chapter 2, p. 37) that the critical period of need for the older person to be institutionalized is within the 6 months or more preceding the institutionalization itself. Not only does the older person himself need help with his feelings, but the family must be helped to combat feelings of guilt, anger, ambivalence, helplessness, and powerlessness.

The contemporary family is a dependent consuming unit, different from the independent economic unit which existed in the past. The emphasis now is not so much on making something one's self (e.g., a toy or a garment) but to make enough money to buy these articles. Families are no longer held together by the necessity of cooperation in the maintenance of a life style. More and more facilities are being developed that draw individuals away from family activities, thereby fragmenting togetherness. Since members of families are now mouths to feed instead of each contributing to the economic unit of the family, grandparents may also be viewed as consuming members. Children no longer have economic responsibilities in the family and thereby also assume the consumer role.

Family developmental tasks

No family stays the same for very long. Duvall (1967) and others have aptly described the developmental tasks of American families, which are basically: (1) *physical maintenance*; (2) *allocation of resources*; (3) *division of labor*; (4) *socialization of family members*; (5) *reproduction, recruitment, and release of family members*; (6) *maintenance of order*; (7) *placement of members in the larger society*; and (8) *maintenance of motivation and morale.* Duvall also describes families in terms of expanding or contracting and outlines specific tasks for all phases.

To help the family with mental disorder, one needs a parallel concept of the healthy family since that is what the family with mental problems must achieve. Psychological disruptions in families must be compared and contrasted with the functions, developmental tasks, and interactions of healthy families. Assessment, interaction, and communication therefore become the focus for the nurse.

Alienation

In the contemporary middle-class family, there is an emphasis upon being sensible, talking things through, and being tolerant. Rebellion toward such a family is not easily accomplished. Therefore, new forms of rebellion have appeared—e.g., campus demonstrations, freer sexual practices, the use of drugs and the hippie culture. What could irritate middle-class parents more than such behavior?

Our culture is marked by discord between the individual and the larger society—alienation, identity confusion, and the search for self through con-formity. Peace and civil rights marches, riots in the cities, survival days, and communes manifest the disharmony. One effect of this is that the individual now depends more on the family group for self-renewal, acceptance, sense of self, and belongingness. Alienation from the larger society requires more tenderness and closeness from the nuclear family. To keep in touch with the psychic pulse of each of its members is an added task for the modern family. Is it able to provide for these needs?

Togetherness is a familiar topic; we hear about it everywhere. But when the family gets together on a Sunday, it is very tense. Accustomed to individual activities, its members find doing things together difficult.

In urban areas, large numbers of families live in close proximity without knowing each other. The lack of support from others within the immediate community affects family relationships. New suburban housing estates may also contain similar elements of anonymity where kinfolk do not precede families in long residence to help bridge the gap between the nuclear family and the wider community. This situation requires that more psychological glue be given to each individual from the family itself. The disharmony between rural and urban life is exemplified below:

The Williams family recently moved from the bayous of Louisiana to a large urban area. They knew no one around their block, and their only acquaintances were the minister, the teachers, and the visiting nurse. When the mother hung her clothes out to dry, they were stolen. She feared letting the children go out of the house or to summer camp because of the possibility of trouble. One of the current acts of vandalism was breaking windshields with baseball bats, and she was determined that her children would not do that. The husband, who worked at construction out of the city, left home very early in the morning and returned late at night. He worked long hours and as many days per week as possible during the dry season, because he was out of work when the rains came. The house in which the family lived was condemned and better housing was unavailable at what they could afford to pay. The move from a rural area to an urban area was a difficult adjustment to make. Superficial adaptation had been made, but the whole family felt lonely and out of place.

Because the values, beliefs, and social relations of the city are vastly different from those of the country, the use of psychic energy is required in the adjustment and adaptation process.

When the equilibrium of the family interrelationships is upset, emotional isolation occurs. Tenderness is gone and the family seeks equilibrium in conformity; there is an unusual preoccupation with issues of control and discipline. Security, gratification, and family unity are not present. Attempts to solve intrafamilial conflicts revert to enforced family group activities, compulsive care of children, moving, or the use of alcohol or drugs. Roles may be so circumscribed that role complementarity is absent; for example, a parent may be more like a child than an adult. Adults who have not learned how to be parents perhaps have the most difficulty in learning to communicate with children, accepting their changes as they mature, separating from them at school age, and accepting rejection and building a new life for themselves at the empty nest phase.

Familial limbo [7]

While most people in the United States live with families, there are many who do not. When teenagers break the ties with their family of orientation there may be a period of many years before they are members of a family of pro-

[7] This term is borrowed from Cumming (1959).

creation. After forming a family of procreation, there are more years for many people in which they live alone either due to separation, divorce, or the death of a spouse. Little attention is given in the literature to the effect upon individuals involved in these particular situations of familial limbo. Often, substitute family members are secured, particularly if there are no living members of the original family. On the other hand, when family members live at a great distance from each other, substitutes are found in their home communities and mutual assistance patterns formed. Communes, popular in the nineteenth century, are again being organized; other rather loose living arrangements are frequent in the hippie culture. Stop now and think of the members of your own family. If you are away from home or without a family, who are the substitutes? Compare your findings with others in your situation.

Impact of disequilibrium

Healthy families complement rather than tear apart each other's thoughts and ideas. Criticism of others can be rationally made without loss of emotional control, and each family member is clear about his position within the group. The environment of the healthy family aids in the process of each individual member carrying out his required developmental tasks and those of the family as well. Members of healthy families are supportive to each other and have a respect for the needs and manifestations of the different generations. Variations in multiple cultural backgrounds of the American family make it an impossible task to describe criteria and standards for the mental health of any one family; each family has to be assessed against its own patterns.

At the time of illness of one of a family member, the equilibrium of family interaction is disrupted and new adjustments and adaptation are required. *Behavior expressed by any one member of a family is related to the state of the whole family.* Examples are given as follows:

> Mrs. Morgan married a writer 30 years her senior. In his seventies he had a stroke which incapacitated him. He was paralyzed and required total care, i.e., feeding and bathing. Speech therapy helped, but daily physical therapy brought few changes. Mrs. Morgan, in addition to her usual role of housewife and spouse, now took on the role of provider and manager of the sick room. These roles continued until her husband died 3 years later.

Other wives in similar situations may not be able to withstand the role reversal and will drop out of the situation. Periodic relief from all responsibilities of work and care and emotional support from friends and the health team enabled Mrs. Morgan to carry out her unanticipated role functions.

A Persian family composed of Mr. and Mrs. Khan, Mr. Khan's sister, and his mother, adapted to the helplessness and senility of the mother simply by assigning her full care to the unemployed sister. In this instance, nurses were occasionally brought in so that she could go away on trips for rest and relief from responsibilities.

The structure, organization, socioeconomic status, and cultural background of the Khan family aided it in equilibrium maintenance.

Mr. and Mrs. Jackson lived in the ghetto. There were five children: Catherine, 10; Edward, 8; Curtis, 6; Clarence, 3.5; and Julian, 2. Curtis had shown aggressive behavior in school, disrupted the class, and had also kicked his pregnant mother in the abdomen several times. Subsequently, he was admitted to the children's service of the local state hospital. In his absence, he was cited by the children and the mother as the cause of all the family quarrels; no efforts were being made either to visit him or to take him back into the family unit. This family was dealing with its emotional problems by scape-goating[8] and temporarily maintained itself by excluding the "acting out" member.

Scapegoating may be conscious or unconscious. It may be found within the group or outside the group. Whole families may displace their hostility onto one of their members, as did the Jackson family onto Curtis, or they may find something or someone outside the family to serve the same purpose. Confusion, irritability, and other aspects of insecurity may result in scape-goating. Parts of a family may team up and use other members as scapegoats. Scapegoating is common among adolescents. Other groups undergoing stress and conflict may find a scapegoat to hide behind instead of resolving the conflict.

If the Jackson family could have been seen as a family before the aggressive behavior of one member was directed toward the pregnant mother, perhaps it could have been helped to resolve its many problems.

Problems of mental disorder may either be hidden from the visiting nurse or difficult to discern. Depression, for example, is not always obvious, and it is not uncommon for depression—even of the type leading to suicide— to go undetected by family members and the uninitiated nurse.

----

[8] Scapegoating refers to "a person or thing bearing the blame for others." *Webster's Seventh New Collegiate Dictionary*. Springfield, Mass.: G and C Merriam Co., 1965.

Family therapy

Family therapy is the treatment of the family simultaneously in the same psychotherapeutic session on a periodic and continued basis. The assumption underlying such therapy is that mental disorder in one member of the family may be an indication of dysfunction within the total group.

Ackerman (1958) says, ". . . the family becomes a source of sick emotional contagion."[9] Psychiatric patients, he adds, ". . . come from disordered families, and the first family member referred for psychiatric care may prove to be the most or the least sick member of the group."[10]

Several methods of treatment are used, with the trend being toward including the nuclear family members. Some family therapists, however, also include others. After several joint sessions, the children may be dropped while the parents continue. The principal focus is toward knowing the interactions among the various family members in the best way possible to aid them with their problems.

The Mental Research Institute at Palo Alto, California, is organized to do research and conjoint family therapy (Satir, 1964). Further discussion of family therapy may be found in Kalkman (1967, Chapter 21).

Treatment in the home involves combined elements of group therapy, activity therapy, and role playing (Francis, 1968). The use of this psychiatric nursing technique with the urban poor emphasizes concern with the family as a whole unit within the home. The therapist brings play materials that the family can use together which will help elucidate their conflicts. During the session the therapist acts as a catalyst to pinpoint conflicts, intervenes if necessary, and demonstrates other ways family members can relate to each other.

The nurse as a primary agent in home treatment, assisting with supervision of patients on pharmacotherapy, conducting individual and family therapy and supervising the general needs of patients and families is outlined by Weiner (1967). Orientation of the nurse to the giving role helps in reaching individuals and families where approaches by other professionals may fail.

Application of the concept of interdependence within families is presented by Hover (1968) in her work with a family with many problems. Her first impression was the need for hospitalization of one member. Subsequent visits involved an assessment of the total needs of the entire family, a diagnosis

---

[9] N. W. Ackerman: *Psychodynamics of Family Life.* New York: Basic Books, Inc., 1958, p. 101.
[10] Ackerman, *ibid.*, p. 104.

of the family problems, setting priorities, and providing help. Busch (1968) describes the use of the home visit with a child and mother in follow-up care after hospitalization and in collaboration with the child psychiatrist and the school nurse. Special techniques used in therapy were operant conditioning and role playing.

The effect upon a family of hospitalization of the mother with emphasis on how the father manages has been studied by Merrill (1969).

The systems approach in family therapy, in which the nurse works with the "here and now" interactions in every family interview, is applied by Anderson (1969). In this approach the behavior of the individual is perceived in its relationship to other members of the family and discussed in this context. The nurse-family relationship is emphasized in the report by Kovacs (1966) of her work with an acutely disturbed man whom she followed, together with his family, through hospitalization and aftercare.

Home visits

One of the challenges that confronts the nurse is how to collect meaningful data in identifying the needs of families. There is no substitute for the home visit; facades are often unveiled by the family when it is in its familiar setting. Nurses perhaps more than any other professionals are accepted in the homes of their patients, although such visitation is a comparatively new role for the psychiatric nurse. As community nursing becomes a reality, more and more nurses will be involved in this kind of work. Currently it is most likely that the nurse works in collaboration with others on the mental health team—a psychiatrist, a psychologist, a social worker, and the family physician. There may be still others, depending upon philosophy and availability. Therefore, data collected are usually combined with that taken by the other members of the clinical team. One of the unique facets of home visiting is that it is relatively unstructured; it is informal, direct observations can be made, and the professional is in the territory of the family.

The following information from a home visit speaks for itself.

> The father of my patient, Miss Miller, stated in a home visit that her illness would not have happened if he had not become ill. (He had a sudden convulsion before my patient's hospitalization and surgical removal of a brain tumor that left him deaf and paralyzed on one side.) Mr. Miller felt that if he had not been ill he could have visited her in the remote logging community of northern California and taken her to a doctor sooner. He now thinks that she needs individual attention

which she cannot get at home. "She needs someone there to make sure she stays interested and is doing something all the time. My oldest son is just now ready for marriage, so he should have his chance and not be forced to support his sister." Mr. Miller seems to be a stern disciplinarian. He did exercises regularly and regained partial use of his left side. When my patient is at home she does things so fast that it upsets him; consequently she tends to go to the cleaning shop which the mother operates and to remain there all day. He does not believe in drinking alcohol, so my patient and her mother have a beer at the cleaners before they come home. Mrs. Miller wants to have my patient at home, but there is conflict between the parents on this issue. The father feels that he has lost his place in the family, and the mother feels that she has to do everything. The younger son is filing for divorce, and the mother says, "He felt guilty about deserting his parents by marrying." The father says that he doesn't feel bad about his physical condition—he just thanks God that he is alive. My patient avoids her father. She doesn't talk with him and will not stay in the same room with him. The older son works and lives at home. The younger son is under psychiatric care.

The patient, now 36, had been hospitalized off and on for ten years. The numerous conflicts in the intrafamily relationships were unknown until the home visits were made. In this situation, family therapy was recommended.

The influence of the home on the individual can be perceived best by a home visit. For example:

Mrs. M., who is deaf and speaks little English, lives in a rooming house near the civic center. It is neat but needs painting, as do all of the buildings surrounding it. The lighting within is poor, and religious statues and paintings adorn the lobby where older ladies sit and chat on old chairs and a modern green leather couch. The place struck me as having a morguish type of atmosphere. The elevator is old and slow and makes loud noises. Mrs. M.'s room is on the third floor at the end of a narrow hall carpeted with a worn rug. The walls are faded red. A statue of Mary holding Jesus below the cross is on a stand outside Mrs. M.'s door. Every time she passes she touches her hand to her lips and then to the statue. The room itself is drab beige. Many of the rooms have sinks on the wall but Mrs. M.'s doesn't. The curtains are of faded gaudy purple and brown. The old nightstand supports a shrine of Our Lady, and several pictures of Jesus of the Sacred Heart are scattered on the cracked walls. The bed against one wall wears a bright pink flowered spread with homemade pillow dolls thrown on top. A card table with an old lace cloth and two wooden chairs take up the space in the middle of the minute room. A large dresser near the window displays more religious statues and a crucifix hangs above it. She displays her sewing machine over her full bookcase. As I looked around the room, I compared it with the plush surroundings of her son's office.[11]

Students who have visited a family will probably have less anxiety in subsequent family visiting than the highly skilled professional who has never made any home visits. The best time to visit a family to assess its interactions is during a meal, because this is probably the only time that the whole family is together (except for Sundays, which are usually not used for visiting). To study family interaction patterns, it is necessary that all members be present. The nurse acts as a participant observer. Notetaking is not done because it takes attention away from observation.

Some work can be done beforehand with regard to the ecological unit of the neighborhood and the larger community. Cities are divided into census tracts with data available about the demography of the tracts and the city itself.[12] A cursory survey of the immediate block in which the family lives may yield valuable data. It is important to build upon the census tract data which, for example, does not deal with mobility within neighborhoods subsequent to the census count; neither does it describe the quality of the life within a particular community which itself influences well-being. The human aspects of life in a neighborhood should be added to the census figures. Individuals and families may live in a congested area but still suffer from social isolation.

Community mental health services should be based upon the demographic characteristics of the population which is being served. These data aid in the identification of "populations at risk."

Before going out into the city alone, nurses should make certain preparations. As the American city becomes more and more uncomfortable as a place to live, individual safety is a factor. Nursing students may never have been alone in the interior of a big city or in a ghetto area; many come from nonmetropolitan areas. The first thing to do is to know where you are going, the transportation schedule, how to get there, and how to get back. A good city map with block numbers is a must. If you know where you are going you will not only feel purposeful, but you will convey self-assurance. Carry some dimes in a pocket for telephone calls, and do not forget to carry your professional calling cards. Spot the places within the areas you are visiting where there are telephones— the grocery store, gas station, drugstore, or bar. If you are to be in the neighborhood regularly get acquainted with others—firemen, for example, or local business people.

---

[11] By Jacquelyn Lippitt, nursing student, University of San Francisco.

[12] This book does not purposely omit problems of rural areas. Focus is upon the urban/suburban setting because that is where most people live now and where many more will live in the future.

There are many ways to structure home visits. One guide is comprised of the following parts:

I. A sequential summary of the elements of the visit.
II. Description of the ecological unit of the family. This includes:
   A. A short description of each member of the household (including pets), living arrangements (space to sleep, work, and play), developmental tasks, health and safety hazards, and cultural background.
   B. The family as a group (interactions, developmental tasks, and role behaviors); occupation of members; economic status; and adequacy of the family.[13]
   C. Interfamily and community relationships—how the family relates to other families and friends; activities shared; memberships in church, school, and other community groups; and dependence on community agencies.
   D. Communications—the use that the family makes of television, radio, newspapers, magazines, films, and books and their influence upon the family.
III. Strengths within the family. Also, is the family democratic, matriarchal, or patriarchal?
IV. Problems presented within the family.

Because specific recall fades rapidly, the written report should be made as soon as possible after the visit. Evaluation and use of relevant data and information about families are important parts of family diagnosis. Another aspect is the assessment of problems presented by the family which require assistance. No family can be expected to do much work on its interrelationships if resources such as food, shelter, and clothing are lacking. It is the work of the helping person to assist with needs on a priority basis conducive to the total health of the family. No program of mental health services is effective unless it is supported by multiple health and welfare resources.

The skills of the nurse who may carry out the goals for the family set by the mental health team require assessment. Students are often torn between meeting the demands of the curriculum and meeting the needs of particular families with whom they are involved. The abilities to set realistic goals, time interventions, carry out specific techniques, recognize one's limitations, know

---

[13] Criteria for an adequate family include (a) the personalities of the members afford giving of affection and emotional security to each other; (b) the family provides for the needs of its members; (c) each individual accepts his roles and also the roles of the others within the family; (d) the family has group goals and is working toward them; and (e) the members of the family are willing to accept the goals of the family as theirs and be willing to give up individual goals for the goal of the family group (Koos, 1959).

when the family needs others, be aware of one's own reactions, and withdraw when the needs are met are not learned all at once. Each nurse, each home visit, and each family is different. There are no formulas for action; each situation requires individual assessment, action, and evaluation.

Summary

This chapter deals with some aspects of families in the United States. Emphasis is made upon ways that nurses can systematically study families, and role complementarity within families is described in equilibrium maintenance. Mental health of families is presented in terms of the role of the family group in influencing itself as a group and also in its effect upon its individual members. Some characteristics of the contemporary family are described, including alienation and familial limbo. Developmental tasks are outlined. The concept of interdependence is discussed in terms of the impact of illness and the involvement of nurses in work with families.

References

Ackerman, Nathan W.: *Psychodynamics of Family Life*. New York: Basic Books, Inc., 1958.
———— "The Family as a Unit in Mental Health," *Proceedings of the Third World Congress of Psychiatry*. Toronto: University of Toronto Press, Vol. 3, pp. 109–112, 1963.
———— *Treating the Troubled Family*. New York: Basic Books, Inc., 1966.
Ainsworth, Mary D., Andry, R. G., Harlow, Robert G., Lebovici, S., Mead, Margaret, Prugh, Dane G., and Wootton, Barbara: *Deprivation of Maternal Care—A Reassessment of its Effects*. Geneva: World Health Organization, 1962.
Bettelheim, Bruno: *The Empty Fortress*. New York: The Free Press, 1967.
Bowlby, John: *Maternal Care and Mental Health*. Geneva: World Health Organization, 1952.
Busch, Karen D.: "The Use of the Home Visit by the Child Psychiatric Nurse," *American Nurses' Association Clinical Sessions*. New York: Appleton-Century-Crofts, 1968, pp. 352–57.
Caplan Gerald: *An Approach to Community Mental Health*. New York: Grune and Stratton, 1961.

Coser, Rose Laub, ed.: *The Family: Its Structure and Functions*. New York: St. Martin's Press, 1964.

Cumming, John H.: "The Family and Mental Disorder: An Incomplete Essay." in New York: Millbank Memorial Fund; *Causes of Mental Disorders: A Review of Epidemiological Knowledge*, 1959.

Davis, Kingsley: *Human Society*. New York: The Macmillan Co., 1948.

Dunn, Halbert: "High Level Wellness for Man and Society," *American Journal of Public Health*, **48**:6:786–89, June, 1959.

Duvall, Evelyn Millis: *Family Development*, 3rd ed. Philadelphia: J. B. Lippincott Co., 1967.

Erikson, Erik H.: *Childhood and Society*. New York: W. W. Norton, 1963.

Francis, Toni M: "Treatment in the Home as a Psychiatric Nursing Technique," in *American Nurses' Association Clinical Sessions*. New York: Appleton-Century-Crofts, 1968, pp. 286–95.

Haley, Alex: *The Autobiography of Malcolm X*. New York: Grove Press, 1964.

Havighurst, Robert J.: *Human Development and Education*. London: Longmans, Green and Co., 1953.

Hover, Dorothea Eitel: "The Theory of the Interdependence of Family Members and Its Application in an Emotionally Disturbed Family," in *American Nurses' Association Clinical Sessions*. New York: Appleton-Century-Crofts, 1968, pp. 46–52.

Jahoda, Marie: *Current Concepts of Positive Mental Health*. New York: Basic Books, Inc., 1958.

Kalkman, Marion: *Psychiatric Nursing*. New York: McGraw-Hill Book Co., 1967.

Kluckhohn, C. and Spiegel, John P.: "Integration and Conflict in Family Behavior," Report No. 27, *Group for the Advancement of Psychiatry*, August, 1954.

Koos, Earl Lomon: *The Sociology of the Patient*. New York: McGraw-Hill Book Co., 1959, p. 67.

Kovacs, L. W.: "A Therapeutic Relationship with a Patient and Family," *Perspectives in Psychiatric Care*, **4**:2:11–21, 1966.

Levine, Rachel: "Treatment in the Home; An Experiment with Low Income Multi-Problem Families," in Riessman, Frank, Cohen, Jerome, and Pearl, Arthur, eds.: *Mental Health of the Poor*. New York: The Free Press, 1964.

Maslow, A. H.: *Motivation and Personality*. New York: Harper and Bros., 1954, pp. 80–106.

Merrill, Georgia: "How Fathers Manage when Wives Are Hospitalized for Schizophrenia," *Social Psychiatry*, **4**:1:26–32, 1969.

Miller, Sally: "A Study in Family Dynamics," *Perspectives in Psychiatric Care*, **1**:3:9ff. March-April, 1963.

Parsons, Talcott: "The Transmission of Values," *Psychiatry*, **15**:1:15—25, February, 1952.

———— "Status and Authority," in Coser, Rose Laub, ed.: *The Family: Its Structure and Functions*, New York: St. Martin's Press, 1964, pp. 251—66.

Prock, Valencia N.: "Effects of Institutionalization: A Comparison of Community, Waiting List and Institutionalized Aged Persons," *American Journal of Public Health*, **59**:10:1837—44, October, 1969.

Ruesch, Jurgen: *Therapeutic Communication*. New York: W. W. Norton, 1961.

Satir, Virginia: *Conjoint Family Therapy*. California: Science and Behavior Books, 1964.

Shanas, Ethel: *The Health of Older People: A Social Survey*. Cambridge, Mass.: Harvard University Press, 1962.

———— "Family Help Patterns and Social Class in Three Countries," in Neugarten, Bernice L., ed.: *Middle Age and Aging*. Chicago: The University of Chicago Press, 1968, pp. 296—305.

———— Townsend, Peter, Wedderburn, D., Friis, H., Milhoj, and Stehomwer, J.: *Older People in Three Industrial Societies*. New York: Atherton Press, 1968.

Spiegel, John P.: "The Resolution of Role Conflict Within the Family," in Greenblatt, Milton; Levinson, Daniel J. and Williams, Richard H. eds.: *The Patient and the Mental Hospital*. Glencoe, Ill. The Free Press, 1957, pp. 545—64.

Stampp, Kenneth M.: *The Peculiar Institution*. New York: Vintage, 1956.

Statistical Bulletin. Metropolitan Life Insurance Co., Vol. 50, June 1969, pp. 7—9.

Townsend, Peter: *The Family Life of Old People*. Baltimore: Penguin Books, 1957.

Weiner, Leonard, Becker, Alvin and Friedman, Tobias T.: *Home Treatment. Spearhead of Community Psychiatry*. Pittsburgh: University of Pittsburgh Press, 1967.

Young, Michael and Willmott, Peter: *Family and Kinship in East London*. Baltimore: Penguin Books, 1957.

Suggested readings

Bell, Norman W., and Vogel, Ezra: *A Modern Introduction to the Family*. New York: The Free Press, 1968.

Bulbulyan, Ann Agavni: "The Psychiatric Nurse as Family Therapist," *Perspectives in Psychiatric Care*, **7**:2:58—68, 1969.

Clark, Kenneth B.: *Dark Ghetto*. New York: Harper and Row, 1965.

Cohen, Yehudi, ed.: *Man in Adaptation*. Chicago: Aldine, 1968.

De Young, Carol D.: "Nursing's Contribution in Family Crisis Treatment," *Nursing Outlook*, **16**:2:60—63, February, 1968.

Dumas, Rhetaugh: "This I Believe. . . . About Nursing and the Poor," *Nursing Outlook*, **17**:9:47—50, September, 1969.

Harrington, Michael: *The Other America*. Baltimore: Penguin Books, 1963.

Henry, Jules: "Family Structure and the Transmission of Neurotic Behavior," *American Journal of Orthopsychiatry*, **21**:800—18, 1951.

Lewis, Oscar: *Five Families*. New York: Basic Books, Inc., 1959.

———— *The Children of Sanchez*. New York: Alfred A. Knopf, Inc., 1961.

Liebow, Elliot: *Tally's Corner*. Boston: Little, Brown and Co., 1967.

Mezzrow, Mezz: *Really the Blues*. New York: The Dell Publishing Co., 1946.

Morley, Wilbur E., Messick, Janice M., and Aguilerra, Donna C.: "Crisis: Paradigms of Intervention," *Journal of Psychiatric Nursing*, pp. 531—44, November-December, 1967.

Nimkoff, M. F.: *Comparative Family Systems*. New York: Houghton Mifflin, 1965.

Nye, F. Ivan: *Emerging Conceptual Framework in Family Analysis*. New York: The Macmillan Co., 1966.

Office of Policy Planning and Research, U.S. Department of Labor: *The Negro Family. The Case for National Action*. Washington, D.C.: Superintendent of Documents, 1965.

Potter, Minerva C.: "The Nurse as Community Crisis Counselor," *Nursing Outlook*, **17**:9:39—42, September, 1969.

Smoyak, Shirley A.: "Threat: A Recurring Family Dynamic," *Perspectives in Psychiatric Care*, **7**:6:267—74, 1969.

Theobold, Robert: *Free Men and Free Markets*. Garden City, New York: Anchor Books, 1965.

Toole, Ben, and Boyts, Harold: "New Roles for Mental Health Personnel II. The Nurse Therapist," *Hospital and Community Psychiatry*, **18**:1:21—22, January, 1967.

Wiltse, Kermit, ed.: *Group Methods in the Public Welfare Program*. Palo Alto, Calif.: Pacific Books, 1963.

4   Social psychiatry

Although the orientation of this book is toward social psychiatry, this chapter includes specific concepts recently incorporated into the field of psychiatry and toward which new programs are being directed. It relates to some of the social factors associated with the living experiences of psychiatric patients in institutional settings and to the potential psychiatric patient in the wider society. Social psychiatry encompasses identification of the effects of social conditions upon the mental patient and his family; it also refers to the involvement of the patient, his family, and his community in the treatment plan.

Epidemiology of mental disorder [1]

Mental disorder is America's major health problem. The list of the ten leading causes of death includes suicide but omits mental disorder *per se*. Yet the incidence and numbers of suicides are considered to be one barometer of the mental health of a population. The epidemiological approach identifies populations at risk within communities and detects origin of diseases and the ways they spread. The distribution of mental disorder is studied in relation to "... time, space, or the distinguishing characteristics of individuals or social groupings affected." [2] Once the history of mental disorder within a population has been determined, preventive methods are established.

For the past decade, psychiatric professionals have been taking a broader view of mental disorder. Not only are they concerned with the intrapsychic dynamics of individuals, but they are focusing as well on the family and the community.

We need to know more about the dynamic interconnections of individual, family, and community. Where there is a family, mental disorder is thought to be regularly preceded by interpersonal conflicts within the family group.

---

[1] The study of the mass aspects of mental disorder.
[2] D. D. Reid: *Epidemiological Methods in the Study of Mental Disorders*. Geneva: World Health Organization, 1960, p. 8.

Therefore, the more that is known about family development, family dynamics, and the interrelationships of culture, the better we will be able to identify etiology of mental disorder. Nurses who practice in these settings can add data to the much-needed research in this area.

Classification of mental disorders

A classification is needed to study epidemiology. The first classification of mental disorder was made by Emil Kraepelin toward the end of the nineteenth century (Deutsch, 1937), although a division into two main groups of mania and melancholia had been made previously by Hippocrates. Kraepelin described two entirely new groups of patients with mental disorder—manic depressives and what were later termed schizophrenics by Bleuler (1911). Kraepelin's classification, introduced into the United States in 1896, provided the basis for the classification used today.

Any science requires a system of classification; therefore, the adoption of a classification of mental disorder was a move toward development of a science of psychiatry. It provides a method of studying the spread of mental disorder in a specified population. Some of the interconnections between the population—its biological, demographic, psychological, and socioeconomic aspects—and mental disorder lead to the study of etiology.

The data of classification are also useful in preventive and treatment services. Despite the late start of psychiatry in medicine, it adopted a standard nomenclature in 1917 and cooperated in the establishment of the *Standard Nomenclature of Disease*, published in the Thirties. Most psychiatric problems encountered in World War II did not fit the old nomenclature, so the Veterans Administration, the army, and the navy each devised its own system. After World War II, a new classification was made [3] by the American Psychiatric Association; this was recently revised in cooperation with the *International Classification of Diseases*, eighth revision.[4] An international committee worked together to reach consensus on the diagnostic groupings. The DSM II coincides for the most part with the international classification, although there are some differences. Some changes have been made for national use which do

[3] *Diagnostic and Statistical Manual of Mental Disorders*, American Psychiatric Association, 1952.
[4] *Diagnostic and Statistical Manual of Mental Disorders, II.* American Psychiatric Association, 1968.

not, however, interfere with the broad international divisions (see Appendix B). The section on mental retardation is very complete and includes a category "with psychosocial deprivation." The old category "sociopathic personality" has disappeared from the new manual; an addition is "psychosis with childbirth." The new categories for children allow the diagnostician greater flexibility. Adoption of the international classification aids in the accumulation of data which is basic to the study of the epidemiology of mental disorder on a world-wide basis.

The new classification requires an initial classification as to whether or not a syndrome[5] in a patient represents a psychosis but does not require a specification as to whether or not it is acute or chronic.[6]

All patients with mental disorder, except for mental retardation, are divided into two major groups:

1. a. Those in whom there is mental disorder resulting from or precipitated by a primary impairment of the brain tissue function.
   b. Those who have organic brain syndromes but are not psychotic.
2. Those in whom there is difficulty in adjustment and adaptation and in which any associated brain disturbance is secondary to psychiatric disorder.

The existence of an international classification is expected to result in increased understanding of the use of the diagnostic categories which, in turn, will provide a basis for standardization. The availability of this classification will also assist in the development and improvement of statistics, particularly in the developing countries. It will aid those who are working with the problems of human mental disorders to be sure that they are counting the same things.

For the past few years (1966–1970), a comparative study of patients with schizophrenia has been made with eight countries participating: Colombia, Denmark, the United Kingdom, India, Nigeria, Taiwan, the Soviet Union, and the United States. Results of this study are forthcoming.

With the convergence of sociology, anthropology, psychology, and psychiatry there has been a gradual widening of concepts of mental dysfunction. A classification which would include such dysfunction is advocated by some persons in the field.

---

[5] *Syndrome* refers to a group of signs and symptoms that occur together and characterize a particular abnormality. *Sign* refers to objective evidence of abnormal nature in the individual. *Symptom*, on the other hand, refers to subjective evidence of abnormality, i.e., evidence related by the patient.

[6] *Acute* refers to being reversible; *chronic* refers to being irreversible.

Ecology of mental disorder

Within the last decade emphasis in psychiatry has turned toward the study of man in relation to his environment. This approach is now added to the consideration of the intrapsychic self (Evans, 1968). Knowledge about the self or the patient and the effect man has upon man is fundamental to the understanding of patients with mental disorder. Although there are many aspects of ecology that can contribute to mental disorder (e.g., genetics and the *Treponema pallidum*), this book limits its emphasis to some of the sociocultural concepts.

MIGRATION AND RELOCATION[7]
These two aspects of finding a new home do not necessarily result in mental disorder, but they do add stress to the family unit. A disrupting event such as migration can bring about stress and emotional reactions which can result in a variety of mental problems. The father's change in jobs, loss of job, discrimination in the labor market, the family's change in life style, and loss of friends may result in adverse reactions. Immigrants face learning a new language and establishing an economic standard of living.

The relationship between migration and mental disorder varies with the characteristics of the migrants, the sending and receiving communities, and the situation of the migration (Kantor, 1969). In a study of hospital admission rates, it was found that rates of first admissions to mental hospitals in New York were higher for migrants than for nonmigrants (Malzberg and Lee, 1956). In a later paper, Lee (1963) found that widowhood was more likely to be followed by institutionalization in migrants than in nonmigrants. Opler (1959) cites sociocultural stress as one of the prominent explanations for higher rates of mental disorder in migrants. The study of Faris and Dunham (1960) showed that most of the foreign-born in Chicago had higher hospitalization rates for schizophrenia than the native-born. Malzberg (1969) recently analyzed the reports on high rates of first admissions to mental hospitals of the foreign-born. He found that when the factors of age, sex, and urban-rural

---

[7] *Migration* refers to a change of residence from one community to another, whereas moving is simply a change of residence within the same community. *Relocation* refers to forced moving, usually thought of in relation to urban renewal or some other event such as disaster.

distribution differentials were considered, the rates of first admissions to mental hospitals were almost equivalent for native- and foreign-born, although the foreign-born are reported uniformly as having higher rates. Migration is now changing character since 75 percent of migrants to metropolitan areas come from other big cities or their suburbs (Tilly, 1968).

In migration, the attitude toward the change is important in the adjustment of the family members. Disintegration of patterns of communication, cooperation, help, and support has occurred. New patterns must be developed if mental health is to be maintained. In families who are prepared to move and have a favorable attitude toward the move, adjustment and adaptation are perhaps better than for those who are not. Favorable attitudes of parents can influence the children. In the case of relocation, the primary prevention is clearly to assist families to be prepared to make the move. Migrants of low socioeconomic status are perhaps harder hit than those in the higher status group. Changes in status sometimes accompany migration and may be perceived as a threat to the ego, thereby adding to the stress.

Relocation has been found to result in a sense of loss with intense grief reactions (Fried, 1965). The varieties of problems affecting isolated older persons in relocation have been presented by Smith (1966), who pointed out that the greatest deficiency in community resources was the link between such people and the services themselves. Self-help groups such as the Salvation Army have long recognized the needs related to migration and relocation and are organized to provide some of the material aid required at these times; various other organizations also assist.

Relationships and forms of communication within a community take time to develop. In some instances after migration and relocation they may never be developed, and alienation and other problems will emerge. Nurses in community mental health can aid in prevention of mental problems by (1) case finding (knowing who these families are), (2) helping them to know their community and its resources, (3) helping them get needed help, (4) organizing regular community meetings in relation to the needs of a community, (5) referral, and (6) provision of emotional support. Forced migration or relocation as at the time of a disaster involves local, state, and federal aid and the assistance of many agencies. These agencies are generally not functioning well, if at all, in a country torn by war, and the suffering endured by those fleeing battle zones is severe.

POVERTY
The high incidence of mental disorder among the poor has been documented and studied by Hollingshead and Redlich (1958). In the Midtown Manhattan Study's Home Survey, a sample population of 1660 individuals, somewhat

more than 80 percent, were found to have some kind of psychiatric symptoms. The best mental health occurred in persons whose parents were in high socioeconomic status groups, and relatively poor mental health was found in persons whose parents were of low socioeconomic status (Srole, 1962, Chapter 12). More people in the low status groups were exposed to disintegrative influences (Leighton *et al.*, 1963). Poverty adversely affects the mental health of our nation's children (Joint Commission on Mental Health of Children, Inc., 1970).

The problem of delivery of mental health services to the American poor is now being attacked from several directions. The Office of Economic Opportunity is helping in many ways to assist these people to become self-supporting, and the developing community mental health centers make services available to all, poor and rich. The idea of decentralized neighborhood services involving people within the neighborhood in the diagnosis of needs and provision of its services can aid in removing threads of alienation from the wider society. Professionals are now calling on indigenous workers to assist in the identification of needs of lower status groups, and other groups as well, in the delivery of services. Other innovative arrangements are being made, including, for example, the use of the indigenous nurse as a crisis counselor.

OTHER CULTURAL CRISES

Striving and *interference* with striving are both related to mental disorder (Leighton, 1966). Not only the poor but also some of the foreign-born and their children have high rates of mental disorder. *Cultural conflict* between the parental culture and the American culture is important in the etiology of mental disorder; *social isolation* is another factor. The inner American city is likely to be populated with older persons who live alone, prostitutes of both sexes, schizophrenics, alcoholics, and drug addicts. All, in some sense, suffer social isolation and alienation from the wider society.

There is a heightened appreciation in psychiatry that mental disorder does not result from a single agent but is multidetermined. Although the precipitating event may truly be, for example, automation resulting in loss of job, money, and therefore loss of status and security, the stresses of war, or forced migration, such episodes do not occur in isolation from the usual ways of reacting, as well as the cultural background of the individual and of the family. There are many other cultural conditions that can lead to crises.

A disruption of the basic needs of the individual and of the primary functions of the family results in a crisis. The principal focus of nursing is related to helping individuals and families to meet such needs and functions or to find suitable substitutes for them.

Milieu therapy

It is widely accepted by the health team that the nurse is responsible for the milieu in psychiatric treatment. Milieu therapy is presented here in reference to the conscious use of the social setting or environment in the treatment of psychiatric patients. It is concerned with physical environment, atmosphere within the psychiatric setting, attitudes, interaction among staff and patients, interaction among patients, and social organization. It adds use of the social system[8] to individual therapy. In milieu therapy, the patient becomes an active participant instead of passively receiving treatment. His strengths are emphasized together with those areas in which he needs help; he is recognized as part of a community that has a culture of its own.

Appearance

The nurse's white uniform, symbol of the sick role to the patient—symbol of *non compos mentis*, hospitals, and helplessness—is disappearing in psychiatric nursing. Although children's services discarded uniforms many years ago, the practice did not readily spread to adult psychiatric services.

If we are to emphasize the well part of the patient who is mentally disordered, to look for his strengths, and to build upon them, we must consider all aspects of the environment surrounding the patient, including the uniform. After substitution of street clothes for nursing uniforms in one institution, the treatment environment was judged more therapeutic by patients and staff (Brown and Goldstein, 1968). Other professionals in psychiatry—i.e., psychiatrists, psychiatric social workers, and psychologists—do not wear the traditional hospital white.

Since staff members act as role models for patients, it is accepted as part of milieu therapy that their appearance influences the patient. An attractive, vitally alive staff carries much nonverbal impact.

---

[8] Two major approaches to the study of social systems are: (1) the study of functions, requirements for the functions of the system, communication, and role structure and (2) the study of interaction within the social system. The latter is more frequently used in the psychiatric field.

In the use of milieu therapy, the environment is modified to facilitate more satisfactory patterns of interaction; full use is made of the social environment and social interaction as part of treatment of the psychiatric patient. A milieu program that is well planned and organized includes provisions for patients and staff to make decisions on matters concerning themselves through the medium of community and small group meetings. Group therapy and patient-centered activities which are planned and carried out by patients are essential to a complete program. Work therapy or vocational rehabilitation is also an integral part of milieu therapy. It receives more attention in the Soviet Union than in the United States; the philosophy guiding Soviet citizens and patients is: "If you don't work, you don't eat."

Milieu therapy emerged from and is a part of the therapeutic community concept formulated by T. F. Main (1946), Joshua Bierer and Maxwell Jones (1948, 1953). The role of the nurse in the therapeutic community has been described by Holmes (1966). In a wider context, the principles of the therapeutic community began when Philippe Pinel, during the French Revolution, removed the chains from the mental patients at the Hotel Salpetrière. The period of reform was continued by William Tuke and others in England.

The era of moral treatment of the American mental patient comprised the years 1800–1850. A significant period of urbanization began in 1850, and at this time the size of mental hospitals increased. This heralded the period of custodial care in the 1880's which lasted until approximately 1945.

Joshua Bierer started the first therapeutic social club in England in 1938. It was organized in a hospital setting for acute and convalescent neurotic and psychotic patients. The principal function of the therapeutic social club centered around provision of rehabilitative social activities for mental patients.

Fountain House was the first therapeutic social club in the United States. It was started after World War II by a group of patients from Rockland State Hospital, and today, with a membership of 1000, it is the largest center in this country (Grob, 1968). Therapeutic social clubs offer former mental patients the opportunity to participate in a program of varied activities. Staff emphasize reality orientation and ego-strengthening by doing things together with the patients. Without the impetus of the therapeutic community concept, the idea of the therapeutic social club would probably have never been spread.

Slavson (1961) describes an experiment in using principles of a therapeutic community with delinquent boys and girls in 1935. The therapeutic community concept served as an impetus to humanize many large institutions in this country. The use of milieu therapy in family-centered nursing is portrayed at Cassell Hospital, England. Grounded in psychoanalysis and group dynamics, nurses worked with whole families within the institutional setting (Barnes, 1968). Further development of the therapeutic community concept emphasizes social learning and multiple leadership for patients and staff (Jones, 1968).

Group psychotherapy

Group psychotherapy was introduced in this country by Joseph Pratt in 1905 at a Boston dispensary. He worked in internal medicine with groups of patients with tuberculosis, diabetes, and hypertension, in a program designed to assist them with problems of morale (Bowman, 1958). Although group techniques were used by various physicians thereafter, the push in group psychotherapy came about during World War II, due in part to the great shortage of psychiatrists. The involvement of nurses in this kind of therapeutic work was made possible by the federal funds available for education of nurses through the National Mental Health Act of 1946 and establishment of the National Institute of Mental Health. An important contribution to group psychotherapy in nursing practice has been made by Armstrong and Rouslin (1963).

The boom in group work of all kinds is evident in all phases of life. For example:

T-groups or sensitivity groups
Synanon groups
Rap groups
Activity group therapy
Marathon groups
Encounter groups
Group work
Group psychotherapy
Intensive group psychotherapy

Some types of groups used in the treatment of psychiatric patients are given below. These may be comprised of families, couples, patients with the same diagnosis, relatives of patients, or a number of other combinations.

Didactic   This is a group in which content is introduced by a leader; the material might consist of a lecture about the relationship of emotion to bodily changes, or a movie which will subsequently be discussed. This was the type of group used effectively during World War II for patients with neuroses; it is now used for various types of patients—alcoholics, for example. It may be especially helpful to those patients who need an authority figure. Remotivation groups used in many public mental hospitals for long-stay patients fall under this heading; lectures on nature with nature walks are an example. The aim of the didactic group is to motivate the patient toward recovery.

Repressive-Inspirational   In this type of group coercion, persuasion, and other techniques are used to assist the patient in giving up a symptom or a way of life for other things. It is used, successfully in many cases, by Alcoholics Anonymous. Inspiration is used to aid the patient to repress his problems.

Nondirective   Encouragement of free expression on any topic related to the problems of the patient is the main focus of this group. Rogers (1969) has made the major contribution to nondirective techniques. The therapist, who listens and tries to empathize deeply with the group members, gives feedback about what he perceives from others and about his own feelings toward them. The group members gain trust and therefore can be more open and gain a more objective view of self.

Analytic   In this group, the classical concepts of psychoanalysis are used: catharsis, resistance, analysis of transference, interpretation, insight formation, and reality testing. It requires a highly skilled therapist.

Nonverbal   Emphasis in the nonverbal group is upon art materials, music, body movement, or other types of activity. Slavson (1943) originated activity group therapy from his work with children with behavior disorders. Play therapy is included under this heading (Baruch, 1964). In no instance does the activity itself receive emphasis; rather, it is the interaction with others, the therapist, and/or the group members that receives primary focus.

Testing   Opportunity to test out relationships with others is provided in this kind of group. It may take many forms. Psychodrama was developed by Moreno (1949) and is used with some patients who can benefit from it. Sociodrama and role playing are other ways of testing relationships. One technique of psychodrama is self-presentation, on a stage, in which the individual is asked to portray conflicting situations in his own life. Psychodrama focuses on the individual and sociodrama centers on the group.

Confrontation which involves a face-to-face meeting of the involved participants is included under this heading. Confrontation affords a minimum of distortion in interpersonal relationships.

Sociograms

For the person who is beginning the study of groups, a method of visualization of the quantity and quality of communication without the group structure can be helpful. An example of the communication within a psychotherapy group is shown in *Figure 1*. The observer in this instance only recorded the quantity of remarks. Qualities of communication could also be visualized through the use of various configurations or colors.

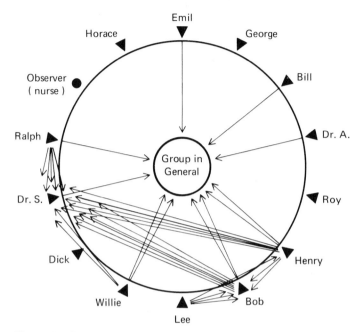

Figure 1   Communication within a psychotherapy group.

Role playing

Role playing is a technique useful in solving human relations problems. Relatively nonthreatening, it is fun and can be part of group work. The steps in role playing are as follows:

   "Warming" up the group
   Selecting the participants
   Preparation of the audience to observe
   Role playing
   Discussion and evaluation
   Replaying the revised roles
   Sharing the experiences and generalizing

  1. **The warm-up—for awareness and identification**   The warm-up serves several very important functions. It acquaints the participating

group with the problem at hand and arouses awareness of their need to learn ways of dealing with the problem. It involves the group emotionally in a specific situation and thereby helps each to identify with individuals coping with the tangle of human relations. In the warm-up, a group member describes a particular situation in which he has a problem of human relations.

2. **Selection of participants for the role playing** After a short discussion, the leader asks the group to describe the characters of the story briefly and to tell how they felt as trouble weighed upon them. Then he asks for volunteers to play these characters' parts in acting out an ending to the story.

3. **Preparation of the audience to observe the enactment** Before the role playing starts, the leader prepares the listening group to observe the enactment and to participate through observation.

4. **The enactment** The role-players then put on their enactment. The actual performance may be brief or quite extended; length is not necessarily important. The actors may end the story with a mere question-and-answer session; or they may see so many facets of the problem and have such mixed feelings about it that finding a solution is a matter of *working one out* in an emotional conflict of values and ideas.

5. **Discussion and evaluation** The next step is discussing and evaluating how well the actors portrayed the roles they assumed and how well the problem of human relations was solved.

6. **The re-enactment** Re-enactment is the next step in role playing. It is not always necessary, and some leaders omit it. So often in life one wishes for a second chance to solve a dilemma. In role playing, this second chance is forthcoming. Facing problems on a practical level you have all the chances that you need. You can arrive at a solution to a human difficulty through as much trial and error as is necessary.

7. **Sharing experience and generalizing** This is the last step and is self-explanatory.

T-groups[9]

Although T-groups are not therapeutic groups, discussion of them is included here because of their relevance to learning.

The T-group differs from the therapy group in that it is concerned with conscious or preconscious behavior rather than unconscious motivation.

---

[9] T-groups are *training* groups.

T-group participants are presumed to be well rather than ill (Bradford, 1964). In T-groups a participant learns human relations, communication, and leadership skills. He learns about behavior of himself and the other group members by being in the group under the guidance of a trainer. The T-group is not designed or practiced as therapy.

T-groups originated at the National Training Laboratory (NTL) at Bethel, Maine, in 1947; the focus was on using this method in human relations training. Subsequently, regional laboratories were established, and the initial summer laboratory of 1947 has expanded into a year-round program. Other countries have established laboratories, and participants come to NTL[10] from all continents.

Broad objectives of training are self-insight; better understanding of other persons and awareness of one's impact upon them; better understanding of group processes and increased skill in achievement of group effectiveness; increased recognition of the characteristics of larger social systems; and greater awareness of the dynamics of change. At NTL, other laboratories are held in areas such as community leadership training, school administration, and higher education. Some of the early work on the integration of the school system in St. Louis was done by a group of teachers in consultation with the late Hilda Taba, an NTL alumna.

The T-group is composed of 12 to 15 individuals who work together on an intensive schedule perhaps 6 hours a day for 2 weeks. To meet personal goals of improvement in sensitivity and skills, the following conditions should be met: (1) *presentation of self*—the individual shares his thoughts and feelings; (2) *feedback*—a continuously operating system which reflects relevancy of behavior; (3) *climate*—a group atmosphere of trust is necessary for persons to be able to reveal their thoughts and feelings; (4) *cognition*— knowledge from theory and research aids the individual to understand his own experience; and (5) *experimentation*—an opportunity to try new behavior is necessary for it to become part of a person. A chance to practice new approaches also aids in helping the individual accept being different. Unless these new learnings can be applied at home, they will probably not last very long.

The process of learning from this presentation-feedback-experimentation process has to be learned and is one of the most valuable aspects of the experience. Peculiar to the T-group is its process of inquiry, exploration, and experimentation relative to its own activities. As the trainer creates a vacuum by abandoning the usual leadership role, other members of the group enter into the act.

Nursing students can benefit from T-group experience or modifications of it. Some nursing schools offer T-groups to all students as part of the curriculum.

---

[10] NTL is now the NTL Institute for Applied Behavioral Sciences.

They are an aid in the identification of feelings and in the fostering of the conscious, therapeutic use of self. This kind of group also assists students to become aware of the universality of feelings. The following comments from students about what they got out of such groups speak for themselves:

> From the group, I learned to look for the patient's feelings rather than concerning myself with what the patient thought of me.

> Last Friday, I conducted a patient-centered conference so I had an excellent opportunity to find out the facets of a group. It isn't easy when there is opposition in a group. I used all I had learned to bring out the ideas of the opposition without antagonism within myself. It worked!

In such groups, feelings of confusion, worry about grades, fear, pressure, anger, inferiority, and identification with the problems that patients have can all be aired. Awareness and sharing of such feelings develop an ability to respond to peers and the needs of patients. Students demonstrate to each other ways of helping people surmount stress and of caring for their patients.

Implications for nursing

The move toward prevention and community care for patients and families is resulting in new roles for nurses (Evans, 1968). The merging of public health and social psychiatry is an exciting era in health care in the United States. Nursing students of today will have the opportunity as graduates to practice in a variety of settings outside the walls of hospitals and to provide continuity of care for patients and families.

Between 1955 and 1956, the first drop occurred in the state and county mental hospital population of this country. In 1955, the hospital population was 558,922. Tranquilizers were widely used for the first time during that year. The decrease in this population has been consistent since then. At the end of 1967, the resident population was 426,000 or 24 percent less than in 1955 (Public Health Service Publication No. 1921, 1969, p. 4). Patient-care episodes[11] for 1966 were 2,687,000; they were made by 2,392,761 individuals or 1.2 percent of the American population. Mental hospitals treated

---

[11] The sum of the numbers of residents at the beginning of the year or on the active rolls of the outpatient clinics plus admissions during the year is called patient-care episodes.

39 percent of the total (1,035,000 patient-care episodes). Thirty percent (806,000) of the total patient-care episodes were in state and county hospitals, 5 percent (125,000) were in Veterans Administration Hospitals, and 4 percent (104,000) were in private mental hospitals.

Other settings provided for treatment for the remaining 61 percent (1,652,000) of the episodes, which were distributed as follows: 17 percent (466,000) were in general hospitals with psychiatric services, and 44 percent (1,186,000) were in psychiatric outpatient clinics.

On the other hand, in 1955, mental hospitals treated 61 percent; general hospitals with psychiatric services, 16 percent; and outpatient clinics, 23 percent. These figures demonstrate the decrease in the number of patients treated in mental hospitals. Treatment in the general hospital psychiatric departments has not changed appreciably, but treatment in psychiatric outpatient clinics has greatly increased. The move toward treatment within the community is therefore obvious; the developing community mental health services are intended to continue this pattern.

With respect to age, patients in each age group of 25 years and over have contributed to the decrease in state and county mental hospital populations. Although the number of patients who are 65 or older in state and county mental hospitals is decreasing at an annual rate of 1.1 percent, this age group comprises approximately 30 percent of the population of these institutions. For those under 15 years and between 15 and 24 years, the annual rates have been increasing at 9.5 percent and 5.3 percent, respectively.

Patterns of use of psychiatric facilities show that outpatient clinics provide for those under 35 years of age; mental hospitals provide services for those 35 and over. For those over 65, there is a high patient-care episode rate in mental hospitals resulting from two factors: (1) those long-stay patients who have grown old in an institution and (2) the high admissions rate for patients with cerebral arteriosclerosis and senile brain disease.

The increase in nursing home beds since 1963 and a drop in the number of persons over 65 in state and county mental hospitals have great implications for nursing and planning at a community level. The number and proportion of older persons with mental disorders in nursing homes have increased and, under the benefits of Medicare and Medicaid they will continue to rise. The Social Security amendments of 1965 provide insurance for the care of the older person with a mental disorder. Section A of Title XVIII encourages the use of general hospitals, extended care, and home health services. This change in care and residence of older persons with mental disorders is planned to provide better care at a local level. For example, for nursing homes to be licensed, definite standards must be met and the provision of qualified nurses and nursing care plans, unknown in some large public mental hospitals, is mandatory.

The clinical specialist

The clinical specialist in psychiatric nursing is now moving into community mental health work and also into institutional positions. Preparation at the graduate level is required for this professional who, following such study, is well prepared to provide direct care to designated patients and families. In community mental health, the patient may be the total community which the nurse organizes into a neighborhood for the purposes of identifying its needs and meeting them.

An example of neighborhood organization in which a clinical specialist played a prominent part in setting up task forces to study its needs resulted in the formation of several ongoing groups of interested and concerned citizens. The work of the task forces centered around planning, emergency services, children, youth, and family; outpatients; the aging; race relations; and research and program evaluation. It is noteworthy that class officers of the schools in the catchment area were invited to a special meeting designed to inform them of the newly available mental health services and to enlist their aid in combating the problem of drug abuse.

Other changes are occurring rapidly in nursing. For example, the health nurse clinician is being developed at a master's level to help fill the gap between nurse and physician. Health nurse clinicians will assess health needs of people, carry out health examinations and be trained to work in a variety of health care settings. A family health practitioner program is being developed at the University of California at Berkeley, to assist in filling the gap between nursing services and the services of physicians. Other different kinds of programs related to better delivery of health care are also in progress.

The *feldscher* (assistant medical officer) was developed and used by the German Army during World War I and is now widely used in the Soviet Union. There, the career ladder includes nurse, feldscher, and physician. In practice, the feldscher is likely to be stationed in more remote areas of Russia, where physicians may not be so readily available. He assesses health status, does health examinations, and calls on the physician when needed.

Nursing practice will eventually be changed to permit nurses to do the things they are prepared to do. As a substitute for constant amendment of licensing laws, nurses, physicians, and hospitals now get together at a state level and issue "joint statements" clearly delineating the functions of nursing.

The direct nursing care provided by the clinical specialist in psychiatric nursing involves individual psychotherapy, group psychotherapy, family therapy, and sociotherapy (American Nurses Association, 1967). Legal issues involved for nurses who practice psychotherapy have been aptly described and the appeal for legislative reform made by Stachyra (1969).

A survey that investigated the duties of the registered nurses employed in 187 American psychiatric outpatient clinics showed that the majority are involved in individual and group psychotherapy and that more than two thirds make home visits (Reres, 1969). The same study also showed that the nurses in half of the cases were graduates of diploma schools who had no additional educational preparation. The need for nurses from all educational levels to practice within the local community mental health facilities will continue to increase.

Clinical specialists in day treatment centers act as catalysts in assisting new patients to become acculturated into the patient group. Using the social system of the day treatment center, the clinical specialist assists in establishing therapeutic patient-patient and staff-patient interaction. The staff interaction is also set up in such a way that all relationships within the center help patients learn about themselves and work toward improvement of their relationships with people. Role modeling by the clinical specialist is an important aspect of treatment; participating in intake conferences is also a contribution (Churchill, 1969). Many other diverse areas of practice for clinical specialists are now available.

If you, as a nursing student, are interested in the provision of more in-depth care to patients and families, these new tracks are open to you in your field of interest. Traditional bureaucratic social systems of hospitals, professions, and communities are gradually being invaded by a cadre of well-prepared professionals who can provide new types of care to patients and families. As community mental health centers are developed, a wide variety of services within the local community will provide new areas and settings for practice. One such example is the Crash Pad program in the high schools of San Francisco which is designed to help students with problems of drug abuse. An interdisciplinary staff provides this service.

The idea of community involvement in the provision of care is not new but has somehow been lost with urbanization. The focus on self-determination by the poor in the United States gives an added impetus to the work of professionals in the provision of quality health services.

Summary

In this chapter an attempt has been made to present some aspects of social psychiatry. The necessity for a classification of mental disorder which extends to all countries is shown in the study of epidemiology. The revised classification of mental disorder which corresponds to the eighth revision of the *International Classification of Diseases* is given in Appendix B. Some aspects of the ecology of mental disorder are discussed, with emphasis upon migration, relocation, and poverty. Milieu therapy is presented in terms of the therapeutic community and the use of group psychotherapy. Implications for nursing are discussed.

References

American Nurses Association: *Statement on Psychiatric Nursing Practice.* New York: American Nurses Association, Division on Psychiatric-Mental Health Nursing, 1967.

American Psychiatric Association: *Diagnostic and Statistical Manual of Mental Disorder, II.* Washington, D.C.: American Psychiatric Association, 1968.

Armstrong, Shirley, and Rouslin, Sheila: *Group Psychotherapy in Nursing Practice.* New York: The Macmillan Co., 1963.

Barnes, Elizabeth, ed.: *Psychosocial Nursing.* London: Tavistock Publications, Ltd., 1968.

Baruch, Dorothy: *One Little Boy.* New York: Dell, 1964.

Bettelheim, Bruno, and Sylvester, Emmy: "Milieu Therapy: Indications and Illustrations," *Psychoanalytic Review*, 36:1:54–68, January, 1949.

Bierer, Joshua: "Social Experiments in Social and Clinical Psychiatry in Great Britain," published by the Committee on the Celebration of the 60th Birthday of Professor S. Naka, Japan, 1960.

Bleuler, Eugen: *Dementia-Praecox.* Leipzig and Vienna: F. Deuticke, 1911.

Bowman, Karl M.: "Group Psychotherapy—Historical Perspectives," in *Proceedings of the Second Annual Western Regional Meeting*, American Group Psychotherapy Association, 1958, p. 42.

Bradford, Leland, Gibb, Jack R., and Benne, Kenneth D.: *T-Group Theory and Laboratory Method.* New York: John Wiley and Sons, Inc., 1964.

Brown, Julia S., and Goldstein, Lester S.: "Nurse-Patient Interaction Before and After the Substitution of Street Clothes for Uniforms," *International Journal of Social Psychiatry*, 14:1:32–43, 1967–68.

Churchill, Julia E.: "The General Clinical Division," Department of Nursing, New Haven, Conn., Connecticut Mental Health Center, 1969.

Deutsch, Albert: *The Mentally Ill in America.* Garden City, N.Y.: Doubleday, Doran and Co., Inc., 1937.

Erikson, Erik H.: *Childhood and Society*, 2nd ed. New York: W. W. Norton and Co., Inc., 1963.

Evans, Frances Monet Carter: *The Role of the Nurse in Community Mental Health*. New York: The Macmillan Co., 1968.

Faris, R. E. L., and Dunham, H. W.: *Mental Disorders in Urban Areas*. New York: Hafner Publishing Co., 1960.

Fried, M.: "Transitional Functions of Working-Class Communities: Implications for Forced Relocation." in Kantor, Mildred B., ed.: *Mobility and Mental Health*. Springfield, Ill.: Charles C Thomas, 1965.

Grob, Samuel: "Psychiatric Social Clubs Come of Age!"*Proceedings of the Institute of Social Clubs for Former Psychiatric Patients*. Hartford, Conn.; The Connecticut Association for Mental Health, 1968.

Hollingshead, August, and Redlich, Frederick C.: *Social Class and Mental Illness*. New York: John Wiley and Sons, 1958.

Holmes, Marguerite J., and Werner, Jean A.: *Psychiatric Nursing in a Therapeutic Community*. New York: The Macmillan Co., 1966.

The Joint Commission on Mental Health of Children, Inc.: *Crisis in Child Mental Health: Challenge for the 70's*. New York: Harper & Row, 1970.

Jones, Maxwell: *Beyond the Therapeutic Community*. New Haven: Yale University Press, 1968.

———— and Tanner, J. M.: "Clinical Characteristics, Treatment and Rehabilitation of Repatriated Prisoners of War with Neurosis," *Journal of Neurology, Neurosurgery and Psychiatry*, **11**:53–60, 1948.

————, Baker, A., Freeman, Thomas, Merry, Julius, Pomryn, B.A., Sandler, Joseph, and Tuxford, Joy: *The Therapeutic Community*. New York: Basic Books, 1953.

Kantor, Mildred B.: "Internal Migration and Mental Illness," in Plog, Stanley C., and Edgerton, Robert B. eds: *Changing Perspectives in Mental Illness*. New York: Holt, Rinehart and Winston, Inc., 1969, pp. 364–93.

———— *Mobility and Mental Health*. Springfield, Ill.: Charles C Thomas, 1965.

Kennedy, Mark C.: "Is there an Ecology of Mental Illness?" *International Journal of Social Psychiatry*, **10**:2:119–33, Spring, 1964.

Kramer, Morton: *Applications of Mental Health Statistics*. Geneva: World Health Organization, 1969.

Lee, Everett: "Socio-Economic and Migration Differentials in Mental Disease," *Millbank Memorial Fund Quarterly*, **41**:249, 1963.

Leighton, Alexander H.: "Psychiatric Disorder and Social Environment," in Bergen, Bernard J., ed.: *Issues and Problems in Social Psychiatry*. Springfield, Ill.: Charles C Thomas, 1966, pp. 155–97.

Leighton, Dorothea C., Harding, John S., Machlin, David B., Macmillan,

Allister M., and Leighton, Alexander H.: *The Character of Danger: The Stirling County Study, III.* New York: Basic Books, 1963.

Main, T. F.: "The Hospital as a Therapeutic Institution," *Bulletin of the Menninger Clinic,* **10**:3:66–70, May, 1946.

Malzberg, Benjamin, and Lee, E. S.: *Migration and Mental Disease.* New York: Social Science Research Council, 1956.

——— "Are Immigrants Psychologically Disturbed?" in Plog, Stanley C., and Edgerton, Robert B.: *Changing Perspectives in Mental Illness.* New York: Holt, Rinehart and Winston, Inc., 1969.

Moreno, J. L.: "Psychodrama," in Arieti, Silvano, ed.: *American Handbook of Psychiatry,* Vol. II. New York: Basic Books, Inc., 1959, pp. 1375–95.

Opler, Marvin K., ed.: *Culture and Mental Health.* New York: The Macmillan Co., 1959.

Public Health Service Publication No. 1921; "Patients in State and County Mental Hospitals," Washington, D.C.: Government Printing Office, 1969.

Reid, D. D.: *Epidemiological Methods in the Study of Mental Disorders.* Geneva: World Health Organization, 1960.

Reres, Mary E.: "A Survey of the Nurse's Role in Psychiatric Out Patient Clinics in America," *Community Mental Health Journal,* **5**:5:382–85, October, 1969.

Rogers, Carl: *Client-Centered Therapy.* Boston: Houghton Mifflin Co., 1951.

——— "The Group Comes of Age," *Psychology Today,* **3**:3–27, December, 1969.

Ruesch, Jurgen: "Creation of a Multidisciplinary Team," in Bergen, Bernard J., ed.: *Issues and Problems in Social Psychiatry.* Springfield, Ill.: Charles C Thomas, 1966.

Shepherd, Clovis R.: *Small Groups.* San Francisco: Chandler Publishing Co., 1964.

Slavson, S. R.: *An Introduction to Group Therapy.* New York: The Commonwealth Fund, 1943.

——— ed.: *The Fields of Group Psychotherapy.* New York: International Universities Press, Inc., 1956.

——— "Are there 'Group Dynamics' in Therapy Groups?" *International Journal of Group Psychotherapy,* **7**:2:131–54, April, 1957.

——— *Re-educating the Delinquent Through Group and Community Participation.* New York: Harper and Row, 1955.

Smith, Wallace F.: *Preparing the Elderly for Relocation.* Philadelphia, Pa.: Institute for Environmental Studies, University of Pennsylvania, 1966.

Sprott, W. J. H.: *Human Groups.* Baltimore: Penguin Books, 1958.

Srole, Leo, Langner, Thomas S., Michael, Stanley T., Opler, Marvin K., and

Rennie, Thomas A. C.: *Mental Health in the Metropolis*. New York: McGraw-Hill Book Co., Inc., 1962.

Stachyra, Marcia: "Nurses, Psychotherapy and the Law," *Perspectives in Psychiatric Care*, **7**:5:200–13, 1969.

Szurek, S. A.: "Emotional Factors in the Use of Authority," *Public Health Is People*. New York: The Commonwealth Fund, 1950, pp. 206–24.

Tilly, Charles: "The Forms of Urbanization," in Parsons, Talcott, ed.: *American Sociology: Perspectives, Problems, Methods*. New York: Basic Books, Inc., 1968, pp. 75–92.

World Health Organization: *Manual of the International Statistical Classification of Diseases, Injuries, and Causes of Death*. Geneva: World Health Organization, 1967.

Suggested readings

Bales, Robert F.: *Interaction Process Analysis*. Cambridge, Mass.: Addison-Wesley Press, Inc., 1950.

Bartlett, F. Lewis: "Institutional Peonage," *Atlantic*, **214**:1:July, 1964.

——— "Present-Day Requirements for State Hospitals Joining the Community," *New England Journal of Medicine*, **276**:90–94, January 12, 1967.

Bettelheim, Bruno: *Love Is Not Enough*. Glencoe, Ill.: Free Press, 1950.

Beukenkamp, C. F. J.: *Fortunate Strangers*. New York: The Grove Press, 1958.

Bion, W. R.: *Experiences in Groups*. New York: Basic Books, 1959.

Brown, Myrtle Irene: "Social Theory in Geriatric Nursing Research," *Nursing Research*, **17**:3:213–17, May-June, 1968.

Caplan, Gerald: "The Mental Hygiene Role in Maternal and Child Care," *Nursing Outlook*, **2**:1:14–19, January, 1954.

Caudill, William: *The Psychiatric Hospital as a Small Society*. Cambridge, Mass.: Harvard University Press, 1958.

Coleman, Jules V., and Dumas, Rhetaugh: "Contributions of a Nurse in an Adult Psychiatric Clinic: An Exploratory Project," *Mental Hygiene*, pp. 448–49, July, 1962.

Coles, Robert: *Children of Crisis*. Boston: Little, Brown and Co., 1964.

Corwin, R. G.: "Professional Employee: A Study in Conflict in Nursing Roles," *American Journal of Sociology*, **66**:604–15, May, 1961.

Deutsch, Albert: *The Shame of the States*. New York: Harcourt, Brace and Co., 1948.

Dubos, Rene: "Human Ecology," *WHO Chronicle*, **23**:11:499–504, November, 1969.

Fleming, C. M.: "Participation as a Therapeutic Element," *International Journal of Social Psychiatry*, **4**:3:214–19, Winter, 1958.

Foulkes, S. H., and Anthony, E. J.: *Group Psychotherapy: The Psychoanalytic Approach*. Baltimore: Penguin Books, 1959.

Freud, Sigmund: "Group Psychology and the Analysis of the Ego," (1921) standard ed. Vol. 18. London: Hogarth Press, 1955.

———— *Civilization and Its Discontents*. London: Hogarth Press, 1953 (first published 1930).

Goffman, Erving: *Asylums*. Garden City, N.Y.: Doubleday and Company, Inc., 1961.

Hanlon, John J.: "An Ecologic View of Public Health," *American Journal of Public Health*, **59**:1:4–11, January, 1969.

Hinckley, Robert G., and Hermann, Lydia: *Group Treatment in Psychotherapy*. Minneapolis: University of Minnesota Press, 1951.

Homans, George C.: *Social Behavior: Its Elementary Forms*. New York: Harcourt, Brace & World, 1961.

Kiening, Sister Mary Martha: "Use of Community Mental Health Facilities by Baccalaureate Programs," *Perspectives in Psychiatric Care*, **8**:2:79–83, 1970.

Klerman, Gerald L.: "Mental Health and the Urban Crisis," *American Journal of Orthopsychiatry*, **39**:5:818–26, October, 1969.

LeBon, Gustave: *The Crowd*. London: Ernest Benn Limited, 1896.

Luft, Joseph: *Group Processes*. Palo Alto, Calif.: The National Press, 1963.

Malzberg, Benjamin: "Internal Migration and Mental Disease Among the White Population of New York State, 1960–61," *International Journal of Social Psychiatry*, **13**:3:184–91, Summer, 1967.

Olmsted, Michael: *The Small Group*. New York: Random House, 1961.

Opler, Marvin K.: *Culture and Social Psychiatry*. New York: Atherton Press, 1967.

Parsons, Talcott: *The Social System*. New York: The Free Press, 1951.

Peck, Harris B.: "The Small Group: Core of the Community Mental Health Center," *Community Mental Health Journal*, **4**:3:191–200, June, 1968.

Querido, Arie: "The Shaping of Community Mental Health Care," *International Journal of Social Psychiatry*, **7**:5:300–11, May, 1969.

Reeder, Sharon Ringholz, and Deck, Edith: "Nurses' Participation in a Group Psychotherapeutic Approach to Antepartal Management," *Nursing Forum*, **2**:4:62–80, 1963.

Reuck, A. V. S., and Porter, Ruth: *Transcultural Psychiatry*. Boston: Little, Brown and Co., 1965.

Schutz, William C.: *Joy*. New York: Grove Press, Inc., 1967.

Schwartz, Morris S., and Schwartz, Charlotte G.: *Social Approaches to Mental Patient Care*. New York: Columbia University Press, 1964.

Stokes, Gertrude, Williams, Florence Stolz, Davidites, Rose Marie, Bulbulyan, Ann, and Ullman, Montague: *The Roles of Psychiatric Nurses in Community Health Practice: A Giant Step*. Brooklyn, N.Y.: Faculty Press, Inc., 1969.

Thompson, Naida D., Lakin, Martin, and Johnson, Betty Sue: "Sensitivity Training and Nursing Education: A Process Study," *Nursing Research*, **14**:2:132–38, 1965.

5 Therapeutic communication

It is estimated that people commonly use about 800 words and that these words may have more than 15,000 meanings. Words developed for use in science have more precise meanings than those used in everyday life. The scientific jargon of medicine and nursing is for the convenience of the professions in communicating among themselves, not for the edification of the patient. Communication with patients requires the use of the ordinary words of daily life, with their multiple meanings. Therefore, effective communication requires work from the professional level—an ability to analyze behavior both of the patient and of self—and an interest in the patient under your care. It also requires that all the senses of the nursing student be intact.

Students entering nursing make a transition between the student role and the professional role. Emphasis upon development and refinement of communication skills early in the nursing career aids in professional identification.

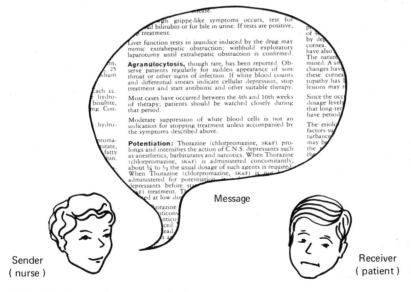

Figure 2 Face-to-face communication.

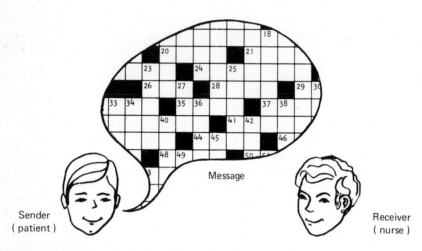

Figure 3 Reciprocal behavior of the receiver is necessary for communication.

Nursing itself is concerned not only with the sick person and his family but with the promotion and maintenance of health; it is more than ministration to the physiological needs of the dependent, helpless, horizontal patient. In order to consider the needs of the whole person, it is important to be comfortable in one-to-one relationships with patients where the emphasis is upon communication.

In face-to-face communication, there is a sender, a message, and a receiver (see *Figure 2*). Both the nurse and the patient assume the roles of sender and receiver at different times. Listening is the principal task of the receiver. The sender (speaker) should know what he wants to say and be able to say what he means. There are several aspects to each message: what the sender wants to say, what he really says, what the receiver hears, and what the receiver thought was said, all referred to as metacommunication (Ruesch and Bateson, 1951). Since the mind works faster than the mouth, the thought processes have a jump on words. The reciprocal behavior of the receiver is necessary for communication and allows for verification of the effectiveness of communication.

Some methods of teaching and learning in nursing may omit consideration of psychological needs of the patient and overemphasize physiological needs. If you have a clean, well-fed patient who is unhappy, what have you gained? Emphasis upon the development and analysis of communication skills may help you to better perceive the holistic needs of your patients and their families. Keeping busy with the "tangibles" of nursing may be a defense against involvement with the needs of patients that may be adversely affecting their lives. As a nursing student, you should get involved with patients and learn how to cope with your feelings about patients and events that occur while they are under your care.

Although nurse-patient relationships have elements of other types of interpersonal relationships, they differ in their conscious application for a specific purpose related to promotion and maintenance of health, and prevention of disease. Communication skills may be practiced on persons other than patients in order to effect higher levels of professional competence. Students report that their communication skills with friends also improve after concentration on this aspect of nursing.

Kinds of communication

It is through behavior, both verbal and nonverbal, that people communicate. Verbal behavior refers to spoken words; nonverbal behavior may consist of written words, signs, symbols, and other behavior—i.e., affect, perceptions, dreams, moods, fantasy, thoughts, and body language (intonations, facial expressions, and gestures). Behavior includes overt actions of individuals and the more intangible psychological processes of the mind such as learning, perception, and dreams.

Cultural components of communication

Emphasis upon what the nurse brings to the interaction with her patients is of great importance in communication. What is the mirror-image self? The cultural background of the nurse asserts itself silently. Imposing one's own likes and dislikes on the patient, for example, because this is important to the nurse, may violate the mores of the patient. Avoid the trap of deciding what patients need on the basis of your own experience.

Ethnocentrism

Nurses who are able to relate to all kinds of people are better practitioners than those who may have prejudices or idiosyncrasies related to working with certain age and cultural groups. In nursing, one should be familiar with one's own country, its subcultures, and its foreign cultures. The social screen between the nurse and the patient who is from a different class or culture can be overcome, although some discomfort may be incurred in the process. Choosing patients who are different from yourself for your assignments and studying everything you can about them, including your own reactions, is one approach. Travel within your own country and others is another way to become more objective about your own culture.

Time

Time represents one of the most significant cultural components of communication in this country. Think of the fantastic timing, down to the millisecond, of the astronauts in their lunar orbits. We tend to schedule every minute of our waking hours, striving for efficiency of effort and achievement (DeGrazia, 1962). Roth (1963) emphasizes the stress incurred by the hospitalized individual who tries to make up a timetable of his own progress or regression. Share your hospitalized patient's schedule with him as a courtesy to him and his time budget.

Waiting

In our culture, waiting communicates a great deal. It is unfriendly to keep people waiting. No one seems to like to wait very long for anything. Punctuality is important in our culture, and lateness should be avoided at all times in your contacts with your patients. To keep patients waiting increases their frustration and decreases their sense of worth. Notification of delay is essential to the maintenance of trust in your nurse-patient relationships.

In hospitals, times of events that we usually control ourselves are often not known to the patient—e.g., delivery of mail and mealtimes. It is not uncommon to visit a convalescent home and find that patients confined to their rooms have no clocks or calendars. I once visited an elderly friend in the local county hospital where all the patients were in one large room, with 25 beds on each side. Over the doorway to the ward entrance hung a large clock. My friend, whose old eyes could not see the clock, asked the time of day from the orderly, who replied, "What do you wanna know for? You're not going anywhere!" Ways of determining the time of day and night, the date, and the year are necessary for the well-being of patients. Those who are hospitalized spend a lot of their waking hours discussing time. In a mental hospital, dates of entry and exit are compared and contrasted; many queries are made to others with regard to departure dates.

Territoriality

Territoriality is important to most of us, particularly if we have not been raised in a collective or in some other type of communal living arrangement. We have our own houses, rooms, and cars—comforts are often given up when we enter hospitals as patients. The impact of one's territory being constantly invaded by strangers in a hospital unit has an effect on patients which should be recognized by the nurse.

Several different types of space are relevant to nursing practice. Thermal space is the area immediately surrounding a person. Our thermal detectors in the skin, olfaction, and visual images all inform us when we are within the patient's thermal space. One human being feels the warmth of another when they are in close proximity. When there is a fast turnover of patient population in a hospital unit, nurses often refer to "keeping the beds warm." In fact, we make sure that all traces of preceding patients are removed from a hospital room that a new patient will occupy.

Hall (1966) identified four principal categories of space distances: intimate, personal, social, and public, symbolizing each with a bubble. Nursing involves all these distances, with particular emphasis upon the first three. Visual, kinesthetic, tactile, and thermal aspects of the patient are affected by his environment, and feelings of well-being or irritation can be evoked depending upon how the nurse enters into his space distances. If the patient can have some control over his territory, he will be better able to maintain his identity. Territorial rights of those in mental hospitals have long been ignored, and the lack of such rights has contributed to the dehumanizing of the mental patient. New legislation in California[1] requires institutions to provide for individual locker space, for example, in recognition of the importance of this concept in therapeutic care. The patient without control over his own territory may become irritable and defensive.

Rest from this constant invasion is a necessity for some people. If the patient in a ward constantly pulls his curtains around him, find out why. He may not be withdrawing at all; he may be asserting his territorial rights! The need for retreat to one's intimate space bubble should not only be provided for within the nursing care plan but scrupulously honored by the nurse.

Perception

Perception, which relates to what is taken in through the senses, also refers to the process that occurs between sensing and thinking. It uses the immediate sensory experiences and experiences from the past; one sense is modified by the other. Nursing is concerned with the elimination of misperception; if we want to help our patients, we have to perceive each one as a human being. Nursing is also concerned with understanding sensory defects and deprivation and their effects upon patients. Preceding events influence us and must be considered in ourselves as well as the patient. The individual's biological needs are factors in perception. It is well known that experience influences perception. Some other factors influencing perception are intactness of the sense organs, direct suggestion, intelligence, surroundings, anxiety level, culture, and the influence of others. Perception usually involves symbolic and emotional processes. During an exciting event, for example, we do not usually think of details. Perception and interaction are reciprocal; therefore the patient also perceives the nurse in his own way. Preceding knowledge may have created a perceptual set. *Perceptual set* refers to the expectations we have of a sensory experience similar to a previous experience, even though the two may involve different circumstances or people. For example, in the process of grief and mourning, the bereaved widower, accustomed to hearing his recently deceased wife's footsteps on the garden walk, hears the nursing student's approach and asks, "Betty, is that you?" Be aware that previous experiences affect perception, and keep your senses ready for new and different perceptions; be open to new experiences with different patients and under varied circumstances.

---

[1] The Lanterman-Petris-Short Act, effective July 1, 1969.

Therapeutic interaction:
the helping relationship in nursing

Therapeutic interaction is conceptualized here as being beneficial or helpful to patients and their families. Nursing interventions that are aimed toward helping the individual, family, and community maintain health status and move toward positive mental health and those that help the patient regain health are all included in therapeutic tasks and interventions.

The desire to help others seems very strong and powerful in a civilized society, especially with teen-agers, who yearn to attach themselves to "causes" and whose fantasy life may be rich. To be willing to help others is a beginning; to know how to help others is an art and a science. The science lies in the knowledge of human behavior, the art in the ways of helping man solve his problems.

The motivation to be a nurse emerges from the maternal instinct. Others in the helping professions may also have this motivation.

A question that students sometimes pose is that of involvement. "Should I get involved with my patients?" "How much should I get involved with my patients?" Unless there is involvement in the nurse-patient relationship, nothing of consequence can happen. Help with involvement, however, requires supervision by or consultation with an experienced person. In some instances, seeing a person through whatever he is undergoing requires years. The ways in which most nurses work *at this time* requires termination either at the end of the curriculum for students or at the discharge of the patient to his home or another agency.

It is important to understand that although not all contacts with patients are therapy, each has the potential of being therapeutic, of promoting inter-personal growth, changing behavior, or benefiting the patient in some other way.

Interviewing

Although nurse-patient relationships are as old as the profession of nursing itself, interviewing in nursing is relatively new. Even 20 years ago most interviewing in nursing was thought to be done by those in public health nursing. In this era of transitory relationships in life as well as in nursing, interviewing has a new emphasis.

Interviewing is conversation with a purpose. It is primarily the verbal communication within the interaction between the nurse and the patient, family, or other members of the health team which is directed toward the maintenance, promotion, or restoration of health (Bermosk, 1964). In this book, interviewing in nursing and therapeutic communication are considered inseparable.

Therapeutic communication differs from other communication in purpose. As a professional, your responsibility is to help others. In therapeutic use of self, the secret of caring for your patient is *to care* about him; the techniques used in therapeutic communication draw from methods of communication that we use every day. Some special methods may be used, as, for example, the technique of free association used in psychoanalysis in which the patient relates his life history. Therapeutic communication is not limited to the couch of the psychoanalyst; it can occur at home, at the bedside, in the outpatient clinic, on the street, or at work. If you are yourself with your patient you encourage him to do the same. As a nurse, you incorporate the idea of therapeutic communication into your role concept. Listening and ego-strengthening behaviors exhibited by the nurse are two major components of nursing practice.

Interviewing includes the interaction (behaviors and other communication—i.e., symbols, cultural components) between the nurse and the patient and is an integral part of every contact the nurse has with the patient and his family. Three main purposes of interviewing are (1) to gain information, (2) to give information, and (3) to motivate.

To gain more information about the patient, nurses may interview a newly admitted patient for a history which is then placed on the patient's record for use by all professionals, or used to help in establishing the nursing care plan. Information required from patients entering crisis clinics may be secured by the nurse member who may then give assistance or make an appropriate referral.

. Many examples of nurse-patient interaction—help with diet, preparation for surgery, lectures on mental hygiene to teachers and mothers—show the purpose of giving information. Orientation of patients to the hospital or to new services offered is giving information, as is health counseling.

Interviewing for the purpose of motivation involves some aspects of both giving and gaining information. Encouraging one's patient to schedule a yearly health examination or to have hope of recovery is part of the nurse's work. Motivating the regressed schizophrenic patient toward recovery is also included under this heading, along with one-to-one nurse-patient relationship therapy.

The impetus for better interviewing technique has come from psychoanalysis. Emphasis is upon relating to the patient and understanding his phenomenal self and that of the nurse rather than cataloguing behavior.

In the process of interviewing, basic aspects of the teaching-learning experience relate to the thoughts, feelings, and perceptions of both the patient and the nursing student. Through relating to patients in a goal-seeking way, the nursing student undergoes a human experience that is more successfully achieved in this manner than through formal lectures given by the instructor. The formal content is not omitted but is better retained and used in a more creative manner when it is learned in relation to a perceived problem. There is an attempt through social interaction with patients to try to achieve a quality of reciprocal influence that improves the learning of student and patient. Since learning also involves changes in people's thoughts, feelings, and perceptions, analysis of nurse-patient interactions is one of the most effective ways to become conscious of the feelings involved in learning and discover ways to help others.

Interacting with a patient enables the nursing student, with guidance, to reflect upon his actions, perceptions, thoughts, and feelings and thereby increase one's own reactions to an event. The most effective content to begin with is the feelings that the student is aware of experiencing. Relationships with patients and families offer the nursing student the opportunity to feel the process of finding meaning in the experience and to learn new ways of looking at one's own place in the profession and in the universe. Literature, music, and drama also add to this learning process.

A culture within the classroom which is experimental and which focuses upon the feelings of both patient and student aids in the achievement of personal security and growth in the emerging professional.

Recordings of interactions with patients and families are made by all professionals. Verbatim reconstructions are the greatest aids in learning the nuances of the helping relationship. Some students may choose to use a tape recorder if the permission of the patient is secured and such a practice is within the policies of the agency. However, finding time to listen to tapes and having them transcribed present problems. Reports of interactions can be written immediately after contact; key words are quickly jotted down in a pocket notebook after the nurse-patient contact is closed and are later translated into a full report. These kinds of data, which should include verbal and nonverbal behavior, provide the basis for analysis of nurse-patient interaction. The recording gives the instructor, who guides the student in the nurse-patient relationship, a comprehensive view of the interaction and can be used in individual conferences with the student with regard to the analysis of communication and the rationale for nursing action. It can also be very helpful to the student who keeps a copy and reads it over before conference or reads it in a group for critique.

Nonverbal behavior, such as gestures, inflection of the voice, and movement, should be included in the write-up of interactions with patients. If a long period of time has elapsed from the event of the nurse-patient contact and the conference with the instructor, much is lost because recall has faded. The best work is done by students through the following timing and sequence: (1) patient contact, (2) recording, (3) thinking it over, (4) evaluating, (5) discussing with instructor, (6) achieving new understandings, and (7) renewing patient contact.

Phases of the helping relationship

Every relationship has a beginning, a middle, and an end. Patient contacts also have an establishing phase, a middle phase, and a terminating phase. These phases are not clearly demarcated from each other; as you and your patient go through each phase, you will find some aspects of the other two phases contained in it. The strategy and tactics of the contact with your patient depend upon his needs. There are no formulas, no programming, no predetermined roads to follow; what happens in that contact is effected by you.

ESTABLISHING PHASE
Purposes and goals of interviewing in the helping professions are different from those of other types of interviews in that you can only have a general objective before your contact; it has to be acted on as it happens. This calls for a great deal of flexibility and alertness—what Theodor Reik (1956) called *listening with the third ear*. It is not so much hearing the actual words of your patient as *what he is trying to tell you.*

The purpose of the first contact is to get acquainted. It is important to state clearly who you are, why you are there, and how long you will stay. During this first contact you also begin to prepare your patient for termination. It is here that you set the limits of the relationship by noting the time span that you will be with the patient. Is it just for one morning? Is it three times a week for 2 weeks? Is it for the full length of his hospital stay? Is it for the full academic year, or for as long as help is needed? At this time you and your patient agree on when you will see each other. It is important not only to define the time limit of the relationship right from its beginning, but to discuss termination openly during the relationship. (Do not use the word *termination* itself with your patient; it has a different meaning for him!) During this phase of the relationship, the establishing phase, you set the tone of subsequent contacts. To be effective in your communication skills, you control the time, complexity, and amount of communication.

In nursing, contacts with patients may be prolonged or they may be very transitory. If we value continuity of nurse-patient relationships, it is the responsibility of the nurse to ascertain something about the duration of the relationship with each patient and family under her care wherever this is possible.

In most instances in nursing, the patient does not choose his nurse.[2] This may help clarify a finding of Duff and Hollingshead (1968) that patients did not get as much satisfaction from the nursing care they received as the nursing personnel did from the care they gave. The fact that the patient in most instances does not choose his nurse makes it particularly important during the first contact for the nurse to state who the nurse is, why present, what the nurse and the patient will do together, and so on. Nothing should be taken for granted—patients are often unaware of the expressive symbols of the profession and require exact information as to what is expected of them and what the nurse intends to do. If someone else has preceded you in the care of your patient, it is important for you to define your relationship with him.

Stating your purpose of contact and how you happened to come to the patient also gives him and his family a chance to clarify their position. If you have been preassigned, asking your patient to tell you why he thinks you are there may be helpful. One community patient thought the nurse had come to help her with the housework; another thought the nursing student would be his "girl friend" who would go to Chinatown with him every Friday for lunch. One patient thought the assignment of the student meant that she was becoming more helpless and going downhill. If there are other patients in the hospital units who do not have students assigned to them, it is important for them to be informed of the purpose of the student-patient assignments so that they do not feel left out or think that their illness is a stigma which makes them inaccessible to the students.

Confidentiality   Patients need to know that their confidences will be honored. This does not mean that you withhold information from your instructor or that you are committed to secrecy. Telling your patient that a general record is made of nurse-patient contacts and assuring him that recordings are for purposes of teaching and learning and are read only by your instructor is usually enough. Give the general purpose of recording, withholding details. All professionals do this. The use of professional calling cards with your name, address, and telephone number is important in a non-institutional setting.

---

[2] Patients may employ private duty nurses, and if a patient does not like his nurse, he can dismiss her and ask for another until he gets one who is compatible.

PROFESSIONAL ATTITUDES

The attitudes you bring with you affect the outcome of your patient contact. Bermosk (1964) cites as essential the professional attitudes of warmth, acceptance, objectivity, and compassion. As a professional student you are responsible for what you do with your patients and families. You learn your limits and stay within these limits, and seek assistance when it is needed. Appearance is also important when you meet your patient. A neat, well-groomed appearance may be appropriate for gaining the confidence of your patient. The odor of cigarettes about the nurse negates the impact of health teaching about giving up smoking. The overweight nurse carries little impact in attempts to teach patients to lose weight. Being as natural as you can aids development of rapport; sit back in your chair. Inattention, boredom, constantly checking the time, talking about one's self without refocusing on the patient, notetaking, and other distracting behavior may indicate a lack of interest in the patient. Talking with others who may be within earshot instead of with your patient may increase his anxiety.

PRIVACY

Always do whatever you can to assure privacy when interviewing your patients. If you are in a hospital ward, pull the curtains and speak in a low voice to him when the other patients in the room are occupied. If in a busy dayroom, pull two chairs off to a corner. In a home when others are around, you may want to go outside into a garden or ask the person to come with you into the kitchen for a few minutes. In a mental hospital, you could go out with your patient for a walk or use a conference room.

CONTRACT

Early in the interaction the nurse should request from the patient his view of the reason for the meeting. Unless there is agreement about the starting point, the interview could end without the participants ever understanding what it is all about. It is also necessary to agree on the end point with respect to time as well as objective. This agreement, whose purpose is role clarification, is called the *contract*. Secured *verbally*, it is not a written piece of paper, as some students are inclined to think. Be careful not to use *jargon* with your patients. You are asked to transpose what you have learned in theory to other expressions, much like the musician takes a page of music and transposes it into another key. The melody will be the same but it comes through with different sounds.

OBSERVATION AND APPRAISAL

In the establishing phase there are mutual observation and appraisal. One of the most important skills of the nurse is observation. What is perceived?

Demeanor is my patient sad, serious, happy, smiling, or unsmiling?
Mood gay, melancholy, angry
Anxiety level mild, moderate, severe
Psychomotor activity
  Speech—talkative, overtalkative, pressure of speech, clear, slurred, foreign language, accent
  Body movement—slow, quick, smooth, jerky, immobile, agitated, wringing hands
     Gait—walks with a cane, limps, fast, slow, akathisia
     Posture—erect, slumped, horizontal, seated
Dress colors, adequacy, appropriateness, jewelry, makeup
Hygiene neat, clean, skin oily, hair oily, unshaven, body odor, halitosis
Scars and other marks birthmarks, warts, operative scars, freckles, wounds
Prostheses eyeglasses, cane, dentures, hearing aid, contact lenses
Skin color, condition

The patient appraises the motives and sincerity of the nurse, and the nurse appraises the patient. In observing the patient, the nurse should look directly at him but avoid staring. The uninitiated may tend to think that locking gazes is intended; however, this intensity makes people uncomfortable. Relinquishing one's gaze to focus on other objects for a few moments and returning to the patient is desirable.

In the process of relating to patients students often have difficulty perceiving the phases of the nurse-patient relationship. It must be understood that there is no clear line separating the phases; they are interrelated.

RAPPORT
Rapport may be quickly and easily established, or it may never be achieved. It may be easier for the student to accept the patient than it is for the patient to accept the student. One paranoid and rejecting patient who had been hospitalized for years kept the student at a distance during the whole period of the 2 months' assignment. The student, however, was able to sit outside her open door and in the adjacent day room where she could see and be heard by the patient.

RIVALRY
In your contacts with patients, there is social give and take. There is also rivalry. Rivalry may be encountered by the nurse whose patient or family takes the initiative in each contact, thereby keeping the nurse from achieving goals previously set for the contact. A bold but unaggressive direct manner by the nurse may be necessary to effect goal achievement. One nurse in a situation

where the patient's mother arrived every day to visit her son, against orders of the physician, found herself bypassed by the mother as she met her at the doorway of the psychiatric unit. Finally, screwing up her courage, the nurse took the initiative before the mother could say anything and got her point over. It took a lot of role playing for the nurse to take the initiative.

TECHNIQUES

If the nurse remembers that, in the establishing phase, the primary task is to learn what the patient has on his mind, it will be easier to assist him. The ideas and affects expressed by the patient may evoke similar reactions in the nurse, who must curb these reactions if helping the patient is to be accomplished. It is one thing for nurses to help patients discuss what is on their minds and another for patients to be told what is on the nurses' minds. The reciprocal relationship involves some giving of self on the part of the helping person but not a complete history of one's own life.

Techniques within the interview are adapted to the purpose of the interview. The use of open-ended questions, nonverbal techniques, and other reflective and restatement responses requires practice. Premature reassurance is insincere, does not meet the need of the patient, and closes off communication.

Questions Direct questions can be liberally used where necessary. However, interviewing is much more than mere probing. There are other techniques. Some nursing students who are anxious themselves may handle their anxiety by asking one question after another. Think of someone you know who does this. If you have this reaction, try another approach in your next patient contact and evaluate its success.

For example, if your patient is in pain, you can be very direct, as follows:

Where is your pain?
Describe your pain.
Show me where it hurts.
When did it begin?
Have you had it before?
How long did it last?

Or, if you find your patient with his wrists cut, your first questions may be: "What did you use to cut your wrists? Where is it?"

Such questions, words, and phrases as who, what, where, when, why, how, describe, show me, tell me, are indispensable to the nurse. If you are interviewing a patient for information, as in a screening process for determination of his emotional problem or for hospital admission, specific questions will be asked and data sought as in the following interview schedule used by a nurse in a community mental health center: [3]

A suggested outline for admission or intake interview

Date   **Name**   **Age**

Individual or conjoint interview?
    (and if conjoint, what is their relationship to the patient?)
Brief description of the patient
Presenting problem (as the patient sees it)
    Why did he come to the clinic?
Dynamic-genetic background (include birth to family of orientation, procreation, and up to the present):
    Points to discuss:
        a. Birth—normal?
        b. Siblings? Patient's order in family, relationships with siblings, sexual experimentation?
        c. Relationship with mother, father, husband, children, friends?
        d. Severe illnesses, accidents?
        e. Description of childhood, school
        f. Religion?
        g. Marriage in general, previous marriages, sexual relationship?
        h. Habits, activities in leisure time?
        i. General feelings and attitudes
Behavior during the interview, relevant quotes
Previous mental disorder and treatment? Where?
Brief mental status examination:
        a. Affect
        b. Thinking
        c. Speech
        d. Orientation (time and place)
        e. Suicidal ideation
        f. Mathematical ability
        g. Abstraction (using proverbs)
        h. Delusions? Hallucinations? Ideas of reference?
Diagnostic impression (using the diagnostic categories of the American Psychiatric Association)
Summary, recommendations
Set a fee (discuss with the patient the sliding fee scale)
Set up a time to take the MMPI (Minnesota Multiphasic Personality Inventory)

---

[3] Nancy Crow: "The Functions of the Community Mental Health Nurse," notes taken from a paper presented at the Californian Nurses Assn. Convention, San Francisco, 1969.

It is important that patients who ask questions also be given accurate information. The following nurse-patient interaction provides an example:

Patient   I feel so much better now that I've taken my shower and you changed my bed for me.

Nurse   A shower is always relaxing, don't you think? Will you please take this pill now, and just a little water?

Patient   I can't have any breakfast today. Why give me the pill?

Nurse   No, no breakfast today, since you're going to surgery. And the pill is to make you relaxed and kind of sleepy. It's good to sleep before you go up.

Patient   Do you ever see them when they cut the people? Is it messy? I watch the doctors on the T.V., but they never show when they cut the people—too bloody, I guess.

Nurse   Yes, I've been in surgery when there have been operations. And I've seen the doctors make what we call the initial incision, but it really isn't as messy as one might guess. You see, the patient is well covered with sheets, and when the doctor does make the incision, he uses many different instruments to control the bleeding.

Patient   How many people are there all together—on the T.V., they have six or seven at the same time.

Nurse   That's pretty close to right.

Patient   Oh, I feel so sleepy. I think I'll be asleep when you come to take me to surgery. Are you going to stay with me?

Nurse   You just sleep all you want and don't try to stay awake 'til it's time to go. I won't be able to stay with you during the operation, but I will go up with you, and stay until it's time to go into the operating room. You'll be in good hands.

Patient   You have to give me a shot now? I'm not afraid, you go right ahead.

Nurse   That's just fine. You are ready now, and I'm going to leave you for awhile.

Patient   You have no class tomorrow?

Nurse   No, on Saturdays we don't.

Patient   But will you come to see me? I be all done with the operation.

Nurse   Of course, I'll come see you tomorrow.

Patient   That's a good girl. I pray now and you pray for me too, today.

Nurse   I won't forget.

The open-ended question is useful in determining how a patient thinks and feels. It gives the patient a more relaxed framework within which to reply and provides for freer responses. Some examples of open-ended questions are as follows:

Tell me about yourself. . . .
Tell me about your family. . . .
Tell me about. . . .
What do you think about that?
I'm not sure I understand what you mean.
Is there anything else?

On the other hand, closed questions usually elicit a rather terse response. For example, asking, "How many children do you have?" and "How old are you?" runs the risk of stopping the patient at the numerical answer. Closed questions may give you valuable information, but you will get little if any elaboration.

Nonverbal Communication   Therapeutic communication involves both verbal and nonverbal interaction. Being there, pausing now and then to allow both you and the patient to collect your thoughts, leaning forward, and showing an alert expression of interest and concern communicate to the patient that you care for him as a person. Maintaining some eye contact and sitting near the patient are also helpful. The nurse who observes a teen-age patient pacing up and down and who quietly brings two chairs and two cups of coffee provides an example of nonverbal communication through the use of body language. The tone and inflection of your voice communicate many messages to the patient. For the patient who does not verbalize, activities may be the medium of communication.

Nondirective technique

A nondirective technique in therapeutic communication may be required occasionally to enable some patients to express themselves better. Some nurses tend to think of this technique as devious, and others cling to it as the only approach. Both tendencies can be avoided. The nondirective technique, originated by Rogers (1942, 1951), refers to an interaction in which the interviewer does not decide the subjects to be discussed or the goals or solutions of the client.

In using the nondirective technique, paraphrasing the content (the restatement response) of what the patient says and employing the reflective response are dominant. Paraphrasing aids in the establishment of feedback; you can also clarify what you do not understand. The restatement response lets the patient know that he has been understood.

> **Patient**   I have finally found a darling apartment to move to.
>
> **Nurse**   You are moving. . . .
>
> **Patient**   I get only $124 per month, and I have had my furniture stacked up in two rooms since I have been in San Francisco. I'm going to Santa Clara to be near my niece and where I can pay the rent. Wall-to-wall carpeting, a patio, a little kitchen all electric, with a counter to hand over the food. My bedroom overlooks the patio. Oh, how I will enjoy having a bedroom again! Thank God I kept my bedroom furniture. I'll miss all my friends at Dutton's where I have worked as receptionist to pay my bills in San Francisco. Now I'll be so glad to just be able to do the things I want to do. My daughter lives in Colorado, and I'm seventy, you know.
>
> **Nurse**   You're seventy. . . .
>
> **Patient**   Seventy this year. Oh, I've had so much to get ready to move. I couldn't do it myself, and movers cost so much, you know. I don't know what I would do if my nephew didn't help.

The reflective response tells the patient you understand his feelings and encourages him to elaborate on them. In using this response, the nurse paraphrases feelings that the patient is expressing. This technique immediately coordinates your perceptions with those of your patient. An example is as follows:

Patient (observed by the nurse to be sitting alone with a slumped posture and sad expression) They wouldn't let me go to conference.

Nurse You look unhappy.

Patient I'm disappointed and I'm angry. (The patient and the nurse continue to discuss disappointment and anger and ways of handling these feelings.)

A tangential response may be evoked in the nurse who is anxious or has not thought through what to say to the patient. Nontherapeutic, it is a response to be avoided.

Patient Nurse, I'm so-o-o melancholy.

Nurse Look at the pretty flowers you have. Aren't they cheery? And the sun is shining (opens the window shade).

Such a response cuts the patient off from the human communication that he is crying for and does not know how to get. The patient's cue to his feelings has been ignored, and his need to discuss his feelings has not been met. He may feel further isolated from human contact, and a deeper melancholia could ensue. A reflective response would be more therapeutic in this case.

Premature or false reassurance is a response often assumed by the uninitiated nurse. Patients who are fearful of medical procedures and surgical interventions may seek reassurances from the nurse. The nurse can acknowledge the seriousness of such events and help the patient prepare for them by giving accurate information about the procedures and outlining some of the things the patient can do to help. It is useless to tell the patient that the surgery she is having is very simple when she will wake up to find that her breast has been removed.

Nurses in their contacts with patients hear many complaints, fears, and uncertainties expressed by patients of their physicians and the institutions to which they are attached. It is not helpful to the patient for a nurse to react by defending them, but it will help to sit down and listen to what he has to say and indicate that you understand his feelings. The reportorial approach here would be of value. Reportorial refers to relating to the patient experiences the nurse has observed other patients undergo in similar situations. It is an important aspect of nursing practice; it helps the patient to know that many other patients have gone through similar experiences and reassures him that he, too, will make it. It also fills in for the patient what to anticipate and what may be expected of him in his particular situation. In using this technique, the experienced nurse may say to the patient, "Before this kind of procedure, patients often feel like you do. I have seen many patients take this safely. Now you can do this and help." The student can, for example, say to the patient something of what has just been learned about the improvements in medical care and recent diagnostic procedures.

In talking with patients it is often easy to veer from the main topics, especially if the patient "turns the tables" and focuses on the nurse. The nurse then finds a way to quickly and definitely refocus on the patient.

MAINTAINING PHASE

In the *maintaining phase* or middle phase, the stage has been set by the initial agreement or contract about goals, structure, and end-point. This phase is the period of problem solving, where the most work is accomplished. All nurse-patient relationships are not problem solving but they have the potential of being so. Of all the conditions, circumstances, and situations found by the nurse, it is in this phase that she focuses on specifics. The nurse and the patient find out what they can accomplish. If the student can be assigned to a patient and family over a long period of time, the longitudinal view itself can be valuable in learning about problems that people face, how they cope with them, and how to help them cope. The student has a better opportunity to carry out long-term goals, and the patient may also have more of a chance for interpersonal growth through the experience. As long as nursing schools rapidly rotate students through a merry-go-round of experiences and transitory contacts with people, nurses will probably continue to be complacent about work situations where the nurse-patient relationship is technical, administrative, and task- rather than person-oriented.[4]

In this phase of the helping relationship the patient will most likely feel secure and will quite openly discuss topics that he was unwilling to communicate in the earlier phase of the relationship. On the other hand, if rapport has not been established, much restatement of the purpose of the relationship may be necessary.

It is in this phase that the gratification or psychological reward of communication will be at its peak. Satisfactory communication leads to growth in interpersonal relationships for both student and patient.

TERMINATING PHASE

The ending of a nurse's relationship with patients and families may occur after a long period of time, or it may come abruptly. Until changes are made in the provision of health care which will make it possible to follow patients and families until their basic needs are met or until it is politic to withdraw

---

[4] R. S. Duff and August Hollingshead: *Sickness and Society*. New York: Harper & Row, 1968, p. 374.

and refer them to someone else, short-lived relationships between the nurse and the patient are likely to continue. Students' relationships with patients and families end with the dates set by the curriculum.

Although sociologists term this an era of transitory relationships, I have observed patients, upon subsequent admissions to the same hospital, request the same unit and room in order to be around nursing staff they know and with whom they feel secure. One patient with multiple admissions to a mental hospital preferred the staff of the "disturbed" unit and therefore in order to get the admitting personnel to send her to the disturbed unit, threw her coffee onto the floor during the admission procedures! The opposite occurs with patients who have had unsatisfactory relationships with nurses known to be in a certain unit.

Termination begins at the first contact with patients as the nurse clarifies professional role and the duration of the nurse-patient-family contact. Naturally, production-line care or curb-service nursing does not lend itself to the therapeutic use of self. However, even when the nurse functions as a steady, secure, and constant person to the patient, distorted reactions of fear, hate, and guilt may be encountered. When the patient loses the person upon whom he has learned to depend he may be hit with the impact of his own emotional needs for that person, unless he has been adequately prepared for termination of the relationship.

At the time of termination, if the patient feels insecure and unloved, he may regress. Since termination may provoke stress, knowledge of coping behavior and defense mechanisms and sensitivity to the individual needs of patients are all important at that time. Feelings of guilt and depression may occur. The patient may act out the crisis, run away, or attempt suicide. "Forgetting" appointments, destroying objects, and physically attacking others may be expected, particularly in younger patients. Other losses the patient has experienced come into play. It is a time for the nurse to help the patient with unfinished grief work and to complete it. Deaths that have occurred years before may be discussed or more recent deaths of significant others mentioned. The patient may discuss departure of previous professionals as well as other separations that he has experienced. If he has had contacts similar to the one that is ending, he may be better prepared for what to expect. Patients wonder what the next nurse will be like, and they may verbalize wishes that the next one will be "just like you."

Tapering off the amount of contact is one approach to termination. However, for a patient whose anxiety level is high at termination, intensive contact will be necessary to help him work through his feelings. Hostility and anger may also be expressed before or after the terminating date; much depends on the intensity and quality of the transference. Physical symptoms may develop during the last few contacts, or the patient may catalogue the old ones as though they might indicate to the nurse that he cannot be left in this bad condition. Giving the patient a way to contact you, even though you are transferring him to another therapist, is often all that is necessary. Patients most often do not contact the departing professional but feel secure with the knowledge that they can. Unless the patient is prepared for termination and can adapt to giving up the nurse, he may continue to mention this person repeatedly to the professional who takes over.

Gifts   In spite of rules made to the contrary in some institutions, gifts make their appearance. Although the temptation may be strong to take a gift, the motivation behind the offer must be considered in each case. Students sometimes feel that refusing a gift from a patient will hurt the patient; they accept it to avoid causing pain. It is wise not to accept an expensive item, a family heirloom (other family members may covet the item), or a present that is intimate. The need of the patient to be remembered can be met by your saying, "I'll think of you when. . . ." Although gifts are unnecessary as tokens of remembrance, students and their patients often exchange small gifts or cards at termination.

Summarizing with the patient the events of the relationship is part of the technique of termination. Verbalizing feelings of loss is one approach in preparation for termination—e.g., "I am sorry we will not be seeing each other after next week." Identification of your own feelings about termination is another important aspect of the process. Relating to the patient some of your gains from the relationship may enable the patient to do the same. Problems encountered in the relationship can be handled in like fashion. Reviewing the time span of the relationship is one way to begin; for example, start the conversation by saying, "We've been meeting now for a year . . ." and go on to review what you talked about and accomplished. Termination is like a "little death" and the dynamics involved in grief and mourning apply. You may now wish to read the sections in this book on grief and mourning and depression (see Chapter 7).

The nurse's reactions   A nurse's reactions to termination generally fall into one of the following categories: (1) anger, (2) relief, or (3) grief. Students may be especially angry with the agency staff, the instructor, or the university. Recognition of the source of the anger usually enables one to handle one's feelings. If students are angry, they may say that it is not right to get involved with a person and then to leave him, that it is unethical and not their idea of what nursing consists of.

Relief may be freely expressed by the student leaving the patient. It is my opinion that those who feel relieved usually have not gained much depth in their nurse-patient relationship, have been highly uncomfortable with their patients, or have reached an impasse in the relationship.

Students have termed grief reactions "termination pangs." They are usually of short duration, the intensity of the grief depending on the intensity of the relationship. Those who have moved frequently have experienced previous separations and may take termination in their stride. If the student is prepared to expect some personal reaction to termination and can talk freely to the instructor and peers about the relationship that is ending, it is usually easily understood. Group support from peers who may also be experiencing similar reactions can be of help to the sufferer. There may be an intense wish to continue seeing the patient past the time set by the curriculum. Students need help in accepting the reality of termination themselves—to perceive that they do move on to other experiences, that their patients survive quite well and find other relationships, and that life itself is a series of goodbyes.

The use of holidays and semester breaks as "little terminations" or "little separations" helps both student and patient prepare for ending the relationship. Although the student may wish to prolong it, acknowledgement to the patient of this feeling and that it is impossible to do so may help the patient in subsequent relationships to perceive that his world does not collapse and that there is something to be gained from every person.

Both students and patients grow and learn from each other during their contact. Focusing on what each of you has gained from the relationship is helpful in your terminating phase. In long-term relationships following which patients and/or nurses will leave the area, the emotional relationship may end before the actual terminating date. The work of termination therefore should precede the last nurse-patient contact. Patients who have been assigned students in the past often request reassignment the next year. After termination is accomplished and the pain is gone, both the patient and the nurse have places in their memories for each other.

Psychodynamics: therapeutic use of self

Self-awareness

A healthy awareness of the impact that the nursing student has on a patient is imperative. Willingness to see our patients through the vicissitudes of life with a constant awareness of the effects that other people's problems have on us can lead to objectivity in human relations. No one person can be everything to everybody. Self-awareness helps each professional become cognizant of his own limitations in addition to his strengths. There is no easy path to self-awareness. Students who have just been through adolescence may still be painfully self-conscious; they can quickly pick up and respond to feelings of patients such as loneliness, joy, grief, and despair.

Identification of feelings within yourself and others is the first step. Use of introspection, diaries, and sharing feelings in group and individual conferences can also aid in the development of self-awareness. These processes, as necessary for the experienced as for the uninitiated, continue throughout one's professional life. In the development of self-understanding, it is comforting to share thoughts with others and find that they too are experiencing similar feelings.

For beginning professionals to be able to assist their patients in fulfillment of their psychosocial needs, a healthy self-awareness is essential. One way to increase one's sensitivity to patients is through discussion of thoughts and feelings with peers and instructors. Meeting regularly throughout the year in small groups can aid the student to make the transition from student role to professional role and to be more effective as a professional person.

Small group work can increase self-understanding, the understanding of other persons, and awareness of one's impact upon them and the influence of the group on the individual. It also aids in understanding group behavior and in being a more effective group member. An increase in learning and the development of skill in carrying out role functions in other situations occur. In this kind of work these learnings can best be accomplished by analyzing whatever happens in the group sessions themselves. Situations encountered by nursing students in all aspects of clinical work and in the social system in which they receive their education are often stressful. The following are examples of incidents encountered by students:

> A student was assigned a patient, Mrs. Kent, to become acquainted with and to follow through surgery and postsurgery. Although the patient's surgery was a common operation, the surgeon's spectacles fell into the open wound. A stormy recovery ensued in which the patient had a severe infection necessitating transfer to a special precautions unit and a longer hospital stay.

Discussion with others helped relieve guilt feelings related to the possession of information about the patient which the patient did not know and anger toward the surgeon for permitting it to happen, thereby causing the patient further anguish and expense. The information was ultimately taken to a member of the hospital infection committee.

> Another student visited the home of a patient who was in psychiatric treatment in a day care center. The patient was a young woman, Miss Uhl, who was from a remote northern California county without adequate psychiatric facilities. She was staying with an aunt and uncle, both of whom worked. Their five children were in school during the day, and the grandmother was at home. All lived in a four-room

bungalow out on the flats near the river. The patient slept in a crowded room with the grandmother and was expected to do all the housework for the family, including the washing, ironing, and cleaning.

Following discussion with peers about the findings in the home, the student conveyed this information to the psychiatric team. As a result, a different long-term plan of care was made for this patient—a plan for an independent, self-supporting living situation.

Feelings of inadequacy in all clinical areas are expressed by students even up to the last day of classes in the senior year. The thirst for information and the search for perfection are real to the student. There are also feelings of imposition upon the patient in which students perceive themselves as intruders until they gain enough self-confidence to feel comfortable in the myriad roles in which they find themselves.

At periods throughout their education, nursing students feel imposed upon or overloaded in their curriculum. So much giving of self to others often leaves students feeling drained and sometimes a bit angry. The impact of space age technology has resulted in so much information and so many complexities in nursing that students desire to know and learn more about many subjects but feel themselves "bogged down" with assignments. Group discussions aid them to perceive how others are handling the input overload; methods and shortcuts in the learning process are frequently shared. Conflicts between participation in university activities and the ability to participate fully and adequately in the professional curriculum have to be faced by all students. Peers assist each other in setting up priorities for development of the broader aspects of life, getting rest and relaxation, and being effective as emerging professionals.

Contact with people of all ages and social strata in the crises of life helps mature the student. The intimate contact with life and death and the internal workings of the human body and mind together with other new experiences often result in a student's feeling alienated from friends at home and in other fields. This separation is felt very keenly. Patients begin depending on the student for help, and students express excitement and joy at finding their goal in life; a simultaneous dampening of spirits may occur because there is not time to do everything. Students begin to feel isolated from old friends when they share confidences and find that the old friends cannot understand why their thoughts are on anatomy and physiology or on what they plan to do for their patient the next week, for example. Discussion with peers aids students to view what they are gaining as emerging professionals in addition to what they are giving up.

Students dread changes in self. Requirements of coiffed hair, short finger-nails, and wristwatches with big faces and second hands have been mentioned as contributing to a loss of femininity by women students. Perhaps the opposite effect occurs with male students, who are likely to have an overdose of feminine contact both with peers and instructors. Students fear getting "hardhearted" and "hard-boiled" and comment on behavior of other professionals around them—e.g., the loud voices of nurses in the recovery room, the anesthetist who writes out his bills during an operation, and the physician in a clinic who matter-of-factly informs a mother that her child is probably mentally retarded. Discussing behavior of others in their milieu helps them to think of ways they themselves might behave as professionals in similar situations. Students realize they are in the vulnerable age group for mental problems and express fear of "cracking up" under the pressures.

An opportunity to meet in a small group over a year's time affords students the chance to observe changes and growth within members of the group. Fears and complaints that patients have are usually expressed to students, who ordinarily spend more time with their patients than do professionals. Daily contact with people who are lonely, fear death, and are helpless, who have financial problems, and who look to them for sustenance gives students a feeling of responsibility that aids in achieving the professional role. Recognition of frustration and anxiety in patients leads students to identify their own reactions such as confusion, worry, anger, fear, and resentment. For example, students who are in contact with patients who have debilitating diseases often feel that the same thing will occur to them. Focusing on identification of anxiety in patients and ways to help resolve anxiety helps students handle their own feelings and use themselves therapeutically.

In small group work, stress clues in fellow students can be identified and dealt with so that members learn something about their own limitations and ways to handle stress. Students are then better able to respond to the needs of patients and families. Instructors and other students demonstrate ways to weather and surmount anxiety and the stresses of life. There are some students who feel that small group work itself is depressing because of its emphasis on problems; others comment on the strength gained from knowing that others feel the same way about things. Other comments relate to the benefit gained in the discussion of nurse-patient relationships and assisting each other to solve problems. Students often feel closer to one another after discussing mutual problems.

Cathartic listening

"Catharsis" comes from the Greek word for purification and was introduced to psychiatry by Freud. It is also called "ventilation." Cathartic listening refers to the attitude of the nurse; it means availability to hear what the patient has to say in an endeavor to understand what is going on with him and his situation without interrupting, arguing, or telling him what to do. There is an inborn need to share information, and a person feels uncomfortable when he has to keep a secret. Usually he does not keep it too long. The best thing about a secret is that it can be told to someone else! Most people like to talk, particularly about themselves, and a concerned, persistent person will eventually get through to the most nontalkative person. It is quite common for a patient on first contact with a nurse to get everything off his chest in one session and then he may feel guilty about revealing himself so fully and frankly and avoid the next contact. The nurse may ask the patient, "Are you certain that you want to tell me all this today?" thereby making it clear that there are subsequent possibilities for contact. The problem of being present one day and gone the next and the condition of the patient may influence your decision.

Listening, not just for the words but for what the patient is really saying, requires great concentration on the part of the listener. Although beginning students may at first think that listening is passive, as listening skills improve they will find that this is not true. Like the symphony conductor, you hear all instruments separately but also in combination. Verbalizing acts as catharsis for most Anglo-Americans. However, if your patient is Yaqui, you may not expect much verbalization! Ask yourself when you are working with your patient, "Of everything that I know about my patient and his family, what is he telling me now?" This may be a most useful mnemonic device to ensure better nursing.

There is a tendency for nurses to be oriented toward physiological needs of their patients in general hospital settings. In psychiatric settings it is also easy to think that all complaints of patients result from anxiety. However, nurses in both settings should be aware of the holistic needs of their patients. Physicians may also have this tendency, as was noted in the study which showed that underdiagnosis of mental problems and overdiagnosis of physiological problems of patients in a general hospital were sometimes made when a patient's problems were actually linked to his mental status (Duff and Hollingshead, 1968, p. 162). As more patients with clearly designated mental problems are admitted to general hospitals, perhaps some changes in these misperceptions will occur.

If you as a nursing student incorporate into your role concept and professional identification the holistic view of your patients and families, you will listen more effectively to the complaints of your patients. Stop now and think of a patient and his family that you know well and identify all the needs that they have, which you met, which others on the health team met, what needs were left unmet, and what you could have done better in the same situation.

Leverage

The leverage of the therapist can be exerted through three fundamental processes: understanding, acknowledging, and agreeing (Ruesch, 1961). Understanding involves establishing an accurate idea of the patient's behavior in your mind. Acknowledging refers to the specific responses to the patient's messages. Staying with pediatric patients who have no visitors during visiting hours is an example of nonverbal acknowledgment or, if you are in a psychiatric unit, helping to plan a Sunday outing for those unable to spend the weekend at home. If you ascertain that your patient is bothered by some-thing, a direct question—e.g., "What's bugging you?"—acknowledges his nonverbal message. Agreeing implies the identification of certain aspects in the human experiences and establishment of similar views or opinions. These are three pleasurable responses and result in gratification. Once the patient experiences the gratification of the interaction, he will be moved toward more communication and can begin to help solve his own problems.

Touch

Tactile communication is transitory, lasting only while it is being done. It is also reciprocal: nurse and patient touch each other. Touch, when used judiciously, can be very reassuring to patients. The right of the nurse to the "laying on of hands" carries with it a status hierarchy that should be understood both for its responsibilities and for its limitations. The idea of the "laying on of hands" comes from the touch of the king to cure illness and also from the medicine man's power in the healing process.

The tactile sense, most primitive of the senses, serves in the lower animals as a method for exploration of their world. The antennae of butterflies, crabs, and fish as well as the whiskers of the cat give information necessary for life. In man, the receptors for touch are in the skin. People who are easily hurt are often referred to as "thin-skinned." The importance of tactile com-munication in everyday life is clearly stated in such commonly used expres-sions as "I *feel*," "I am so *touched*," "She is a *warm* person," and *"tender, loving care."*

SIGNALS, SIGNS, AND SYMBOLS

When a person touches a hot, cold, or rough object, there may be a signal for withdrawal because of pain. When he learns to associate these uncomfortable objects as *signs* of pain, he avoids them; in responding to the words "hot," "cold," "tender," and "rough" by protecting himself, he is acting symbolically. If a patient perceives roughness in nurse-patient interactions, he may refuse to talk to the next nurse, who symbolizes pain, even though the nurse may not be rough at all. If the patient perceives the nurse as cold in the interaction with him, the approach of the nurse may be the *signal* for him to turn his face to the wall. The appearance of any nurse might then act as a sign for the patient to avoid contact.

The contact comfort and motion stimulation so loved by Harlow's (1962) monkeys also applies to the human animals who run to mother for comfort or who in later years may buy "vibrator machines."

Transference

Transference is a term borrowed from psychoanalysis which refers to the phenomenon of the unconscious attribution to the therapist of characteristics of significant others in the patient's early life. It occurs in all significant relationships to some degree and may be a transitory identification that the patient makes with the nurse. The intimacy of a nurse with patients affects and colors the intensity of the relationships. The nurse's experiences with the patient's bodily functions may easily arouse the transference relationship to parent. It is very common for patients to reply to nurses, "O.K., Mother" when asked to do something. Or a child may ask, "Will you be my mother while I am here?" Likewise, the patient may also attribute to the nurse the parental role of authority usually ascribed to fathers. Transference transcends age and sex. Although your patient may be a 40-year-old executive, he may react toward you as if you were the parent. Older patients may say to you, "You remind me of my granddaughter" (or grandson, as the case may be).

Although the examples given are conscious attributions, they are signals to the importance of unconscious behavior and clues to the attachments felt by patients for nurses. Transference can either be positive or negative. A positive transference is affectionate, and a negative transference usually involves hostility. It is important to differentiate between the negative transference and other uncomfortable situations. If the patient is hostile because his call light is out of reach, this is not negative transference. If transference is positive, the "working through" phase of the relationship is facilitated; if it is negative, the work may be more difficult but can still lead to growth.

Transference may frequently take on aspects of sibling relationships. A nurse may perceive and act toward all older women patients as though they were sisters. Although the life-space, face-to-face encounters in nurse-patient relationships tend to minimize distortions, they are, nevertheless, still present.

In a general hospital setting students were assigned to patients within a three-bed ward during their stay on this particular unit. One patient was not assigned to students for care because students were not studying her particular condition at that time. When the students were present, she became more and more demanding of their attention, asking for little things. It was noted, however, that the patient was able and willing to do the same things for herself when the students were absent. The patient had regressed to the role of child at the times when students, the mothering figures, were present.

USE OF TRANSFERENCE

The transference relationship is very powerful and must be held in trust and considered with great seriousness. The patient has placed himself in the hands of the nurse and is therefore in a most vulnerable position. Feelings of every kind are displayed in the nurse-patient relationship. Feelings which have not been previously expressed may arise, for example, the need for love from a mother who did not express feelings to her child. If the transference is negative, the nurse may be required to show the patient different aspects from those of the person who elicited these feelings in the patient originally.

Nurse-patient relationships involve more than just encouraging your patient to tell you all about himself. Theoretical knowledge helps you to understand the significance of what your patients confide in you. When a patient tells you upon first contact of "the cruel nurses" who took care of her father you may be fairly sure that she needs to work through her feelings about his death.

The transference relationship is used in nursing to help the patient work through problems he has on his mind. The nurse recognizes the role of the unconscious without necessarily interpreting unconscious material to her patient. To deny and ignore the existence and functioning of the unconscious in modern nursing is to negate attention to the whole person. You are not a sponge or ink blotter merely soaking up the dependency needs of your patients; you help them and their families deal with reality situations, socialize, groom themselves, problem-solve, and move toward their highest potential.

Experienced psychotherapists are more skilled in interpersonal relationships than the beginning nurse. However, it is important for the beginner to develop skills to recognize the dynamic forces within interpersonal relationships that foster effective communication.

Countertransference

Countertransference refers to the conscious or unconscious emotional reaction of the nurse toward the patient. It is the attribution of characteristics of the patient to a significant person in the early life of the nurse. Here, it is discussed as the total emotional reaction of the nurse to the patient (Kernberg, 1965). A partial identification with the patient, it usually does not last long (Reich, 1951).

In nursing, countertransference is often paraded under the guise of personality clash. It is unrealistic to think that all professional relationships will be 100 percent compatible; however, a personality clash between a patient and nurse requires study and self-understanding, not a change of assignments. Other expressions which may indicate countertransference are "involvement," "overidentification," and "uptight." In many instances, countertransference has been thought of as not particularly helpful; however, it can enable you to further understand the patient as well as your own behavior. With nursing students who are in the process of breaking away from parents, the intense emotions of childhood and adolescence may be very near the surface and color their relationship with patients, particularly those in the age group of their parents. Students who are in their teens therefore may find it easier to relate to patients in age groups other than the parental ones. Kloes and Weinberg (1968) describe some aspects of countertransference as being related to willingness to accept a rejecting role, anger, and also loss of interest in the patient.

If you are obviously upset and crying when your patient undergoes painful procedures or experiences, you abdicate your expressive role. In such a case, each injection that you prepare and give to your patient or each limit that you have to set with him is painful to you and clearly visible to the patient.

One nurse found it very difficult to work with geriatric patients when, in fact, she was transferring to her geriatric patients, as a group, the undesirable attributes of her own grandmother. Subsequent conferences with her supervisor resulted in a change in her attitude toward her patients. Other situations involving older patients may evoke the same responses as if the patients were grandparents. Students taught to revere and respect their elders may find themselves immobilized in the presence of older patients and temporarily be unable to take the necessary initiative in providing care. A young patient, Mr. Dong, resembled the estranged husband of the nurse caring for him on the psychiatric unit. The nurse avoided and feared this patient. When she became conscious of the triggering mechanism, she was able to work with him.

An older patient, Mr. Friedenberg, whom the student visited in his home, reminded her of her grandfather. The nurse visited too frequently and, at the time of termination, was in tears.

Situations where nurses become romantically involved with patients may demonstrate transference and countertransference. One student and a patient on the psychiatric service became inseparable. The patient was an attractive young man, meticulous in appearance, who had a wife and two children. He was given special privileges by the unit staff, e.g., visits to their homes. The patient confided in the student the story of his life's difficulties and his rebellion against the establishment. They attended the evening dances together as a couple. When confronted with her behavior, the student perceived that she had become overly sympathetic with her patient in her quest to help him.

Another patient, a handsome young man and the president of the patients' council on the unit, had a history of failures in coping with the demands of society. Observed to be the favorite of one of the older nurses, he also managed to get special privileges and appeared nattily dressed for events where he presided. Sometime later the patient and the nurse eloped to Mexico.

A mentally retarded young adult with a long history of disrupted family relationships was unable to adapt to rules within the psychiatric unit. He was perceived by one of the nurses as having had a life like his own. The nurse became very protective of him regardless of his behavior.

A word of caution must be given with regard to erroneously labeling all strong emotional reactions in the nurse-patient relationship as attributable to transference or countertransference. Each complaint of a patient should be duly considered by the team involved in his care. Cold meals, cold rooms, cold bedpans, and coldness from the staff do not necessarily result from countertransference.

Cognitive dissonance

Festinger (1957) in his theory of cognitive dissonance purports that new cognitions that make individuals vulnerable to illness, infirmity, and changes in body image that are dissonant with their self-cognitions (being whole, well, and strong) may result in anxiety until new adaptations have occurred.

For example, an older person who has just decided, on the basis of being robbed several times in his neighborhood while going to the store, to sell his house and move into an apartment with a doorman may be consumed with afterthoughts about the decision and enumerate in great detail to you on every home visit the unattractive aspects of the move. Although the decision has already been made, doubts about it persist. The tension can be reduced in at least two ways. To reverse the decision and remain in the house, since apartment living seems so unattractive, is one way. If this path is taken, however, the original tension for initiation of the move continues, i.e., the possibility of being subjected to robberies. Another path is to change the cognition or information about the move. This may be done in several ways. One is for the nurse to point out the positive aspects of the move—that there is less worry about taxes, upkeep, proximity to transportation, and neighbors. Another is to use the reportorial approach that "this is what happens to some people when they make important decisions."

If a younger person is encountering a similar experience, you can point out the process of making a big decision and validate with the patient whether he thinks this is what is happening to him. It may be helpful to the person who is experiencing cognitive dissonances to discuss what is happening to him with someone else who has experienced a similar situation. It is often a comfort for one to perceive that others have survived quite admirably what one is experiencing himself.

Interviewing as a method of measurement

In nursing, precise objectives cannot consistently be made before the patient is encountered. Only general purposes can be made from which more precise objectives will emerge during the interview itself, depending in turn on what happens in the interview. It is during the interaction with the patient that hypotheses develop about nursing interventions which can subsequently be acted upon. In interviewing, there is appraisal and, after the interaction, comparison and contrast with previous experiences with patients. Behaviors observed are translated into theoretical knowledge and compared with the observations of others. The interviewer is the measuring device in nursing; there is no slide rule, pH paper, or centigrade thermometer to measure the inner man. It is the hunch you have that leads you to explore the thoughts, feelings, and perceptions of another human being. The nurse who compares the patient with textbook cases and who assesses the whole situation in relation to situations of others is using data gathered from interviewing.

Observational ability includes affective, cognitive, and sensory aspects of the person. Some people observe more than others. Is it related to personality? If we try to protect our own image, are we likely to see ways in which people we dislike resemble us? If you dislike obese people or hairy people, how does this affect your nurse-patient relationship?

In the process of nurse-patient interaction, some of the practical problems need to be understood. Knowledge of the sources and kinds of biases[5] will help you to be a better practitioner of therapeutic communication. Errors common to any interaction may occur in the nurse-patient relationship: errors of observation, in the kinds of questions asked, in recording, and in recall. Some of these are discussed on the following pages. Random errors are chance variations; however, they are canceled out over a large number of contacts.

Halo effect

Awareness of the possibility of the *halo effect*[6] is important; you must be able to look at different qualities of persons and rate them individually, instead of forming general impressions dominating the specific qualities.

The halo effect can either be positive or negative. It can be positive in the sense of, for example, a patient's being very complimentary and generous, a fact which overshadows any other behavior of his, e.g., chronic alcoholism. In a negative sense, when a patient is irritable and demanding one morning he may subsequently be labeled by the nursing personnel as irritable and demanding during his entire hospital stay.

Stereotype

A stereotype is a supposed appearance or behavior of a certain ethnic, class, occupational, or social group. Some common stereotypes of certain groups include: all Italians eat spaghetti every day, all boys with long hair or beards are hippies. The stereotype may also be referred to as a group halo.

Some other factors affecting our relationships with patients are (1) *logical error*, (2) *variable error*, (3) *constant error*, and (4) *recall*. Logical error is intellectual; it is cognitive confusion. You think rather than feel that something is true when it actually is not. Combining the halo effect and the logical error results in *constant error*.

---

[5] *Bias* is the systematic piling of errors in one direction only.
[6] Halo effect refers to the inability to isolate a trait of an individual and form an opinion about it without being influenced by knowledge of the person as a whole.

Constant error

Constant error occurs when desirable traits in individuals are given undue importance in assessment and are overestimated; less desirable ones are more or less ignored and therefore underestimated. For example, so long as a patient awaiting surgery makes few demands of you you may overlook the fact that he spends 2 hours every day in the bathroom without bothering to learn the motivation underlying his behavior. It is important to separate facts *observed* from inferences resulting from observation. Confirming your observations with the patient or others may be especially helpful.

Variable error

Variable error represents a divergence of opinion held by different persons in regard to a characteristic in an individual. The frame of reference from which a person thinks, speaks, and acts greatly influences variable error. The following is an example:

> A psychiatric nurse stopped by the adjacent surgical unit of the general hospital in which she worked to pick up her friend, a surgical nurse, to go to dinner. As she arrived on the surgical unit, she noticed her friend going into the room of a patient she had been consulted about the previous evening. A nurse's aide had preceded them into the room. The patient, Mr. Holly, complained of feeling chilly, at which time the psychiatric nurse reached for the patient's hand to comfort him, the surgical nurse clamped off the intravenous fluid, and the aide closed the window.

Errors of recording and recall

Because recall changes quite rapidly, some method of recording immediately after contact with the patient is important. Written verbatim reconstructions of the nurse-patient interaction are useful tools in teaching and learning. However, they are helpful only if written openly and honestly immediately after contact, and if omissions are indicated with "...." where memory fails. A tendency to complete patient's sentences is therefore avoided. The interaction put aside and returned to for rereading and evaluation can be very useful to the student in the application of interviewing principles and in the improvement of communication skills. It also provides a record for the student to observe growth in self as well as the interpersonal growth or change in behavior of the patient. Tape recording or video tape or handwritten process recordings are sometimes used by nurses in learning interviewing techniques. However, I do not advocate the use of taped material because of the amount of time one may have to spend on it. Process recordings, by their very nature of being written during the nurse-patient contact, remove spontaneity. Taping interviews is also expensive and omits some nonverbal communication. Films or videotapes record more completely than other methods after individuals become accustomed to the fact that they are performing.

If it is impossible to reconstruct an interview immediately after holding it, then jot down skeletal notes which, at a later date, will aid you by *recognition* to reconstruct the nurse-patient interaction. You should take care that the analysis of a nurse-patient interaction records what was said and done, not what ideally should have occurred or what could happen if one had it to do over again. After recording interactions with patients and families, the process through which one goes in thoughts and in discussions with instructors, supervisors, consultants, and others is an essential part of learning to evaluate one's interviewing techniques.

Some common problems expressed by students

Common problems expressed by students in the helping process are as follows: (1) inability to evaluate the effects of therapeutic use of self; (2) misperception of use of indirect interviewing methods as being devious, with subsequent feelings of guilt; and (3) resistance to analysis of nurse-patient interactions. Students may feel that they are invading the privacy of their patients as they assume their professional role. In the transition from nonprofessional student to professional, they may express frustration, despondency, and anger and feel it is unethical to look into the private life of their patients. Emphasis in nursing on the inner life of man may evoke anxiety and defensive reactions in the student. The helping relationship, however, cannot be learned entirely from a book.

Summary

The rites of passage from student to professional occur as nursing students enter their major field. In this chapter attention is given to aspects of therapeutic communication that aid in professional role identification. An ability to view the mirror-image self as it is reflected from the culture of the nurse is emphasized, and phases of the helping relationship in nursing with component parts are discussed.

Psychodynamic concepts of therapeutic use of self are presented. Interviewing as a method of measurement with discussion of halo effect, stereotype, constant error, variable error, and errors of recording and recall are also included. The chapter concludes with some common problems in interviewing expressed by nursing students.

References

American Psychiatric Association: *A Psychiatric Glossary*. Washington, D.C.: American Psychiatric Association, 1969.

Bermosk, Loretta, and Mordan, Mary Jane: *Interviewing in Nursing*. New York: Macmillan, 1964.

Bingham, Walter Van Dyke, and Moore, Bruce Victor: *How to Interview*. New York: Harper and Brothers, 1959.

Bird, Brian: *Talking with Patients*. Philadelphia: Lippincott, 1955.

Crow, Nancy: "The Functions of the Community Mental Health Nurse," notes taken from a paper given at the California Nurses Association Convention, San Francisco, 1969.

De Grazia, Sebastian: *Of Time, Work and Leisure*. New York: Twentieth Century, 1962.

Doane, Leona: "The Therapeutic Termination of Interpersonal Relationships," unpublished Master's Study, Boston University, August, 1963.

Duff, Raymond S., and Hollingshead, August: *Sickness and Society*. New York: Harper and Row, 1968.

Ferard, Margaret L., and Hunnybun, Noel K.: *The Caseworker's Use of Relationships*. Springfield, Ill.: Charles C Thomas, 1962.

Festinger, Leon: *A Theory of Cognitive Dissonance.* Evanston, Ill.: Row Peterson, 1957.

Flesch, Regina: *Treatment Considerations in the Reassignment of Clients.* New York: Family Service Association, 1948.

Frank, L. K.: "Tactile Communication," *ETC,* **16**:1:31–79, Autumn, 1958.

Freud, Sigmund: *The Collected Papers.* London: The Hogarth Press, Vol. XI, pp. 144–45, 1957.

———— *The Collected Papers.* London: The Hogarth Press, Vol. XII, pp. 159–71, 1958.

Garrett, Annette: *Interviewing, Its Principles and Methods.* New York: Family Service Association, 1942.

———— "Transference in Casework," in Kasins, Cora, ed.: *Principles and Techniques in Social Casework.* New York: Family Service Association of America, 1950.

Greenhill, Maurice H.: "Interviewing with a Purpose," *American Journal of Nursing,* **56**:10:1259–62.

Hall, Edward T.: *The Silent Language.* New York: Premier Book, 1959.

———— *The Hidden Dimension.* Garden City, N.Y.: Doubleday and Co., Inc., 1966.

Harlow, Margaret Kuenne, and Harry F.: "Social Deprivation in Monkeys," *Scientific American,* **207**:5:137–46, November, 1962.

Harrington, Michael: *The Other America.* Baltimore: Penguin Books, 1963.

Jourard, Sidney: *The Transparent Self.* New York: D. Van Nostrand Co., Inc., 1964.

Kahn, Robert L., and Cannell, Charles F.: *The Dynamics of Interviewing.* New York: John Wiley and Sons, Inc., 1957.

Kalkman, Marian: *Psychiatric Nursing.* New York: McGraw-Hill Book Co., 1967.

Kernberg, Otto: "Notes on Countertransference," *Journal American Psychoanalysis Association,* **13**:1:38–56, January, 1965.

Kloes, Karen B., and Weinberg, Ann: "Countertransference," *Perspectives in Psychiatric Care,* **VI**:4:152–62, 1968.

Lawrence, Douglas H., and Festinger, Leon: *Deterrents and Reinforcement.* Stanford: Stanford University Press, 1962.

Lidz, Theodore: *The Person.* New York: Basic Books, Inc., 1968.

Phillips, Lorraine W.: "Language in Disguise: Non-verbal Communication with Patients," *Perspectives in Psychiatric Care,* **4**:4:18–21, 1966.

Reich, Annie: "On Countertransference," *International Journal of Psychoanalysis,* **32**:25, 1951.

Reik, Theodor: *Listening with the Third Ear.* New York: Grove Press, 1956.

Rogers, Carl: *Counseling and Psychotherapy.* Boston: Houghton Mifflin, 1942.

———— *Client-Centered Therapy.* Boston: Houghton Mifflin, 1951.

Roth, Julius A.: *Timetables*. New York: The Bobbs-Merrill Co., Inc., 1963.
Ruesch, Jurgen, and Bateson, Gregory: *Communication, The Social Matrix of Psychiatry*. New York: W. W. Norton and Co., Inc., 1951.
——— and Kees, Weldon: *Non-verbal Communication*. Berkeley: University of California Press, 1956.
——— *Disturbed Communication*. New York: W. W. Norton and Co., Inc., 1957.
——— *Therapeutic Communication*. New York: W. W. Norton and Co., Inc., 1961.
———Brodsky, Carroll M., and Fischer, Ames: *Psychiatric Care*. New York: Grune and Stratton, 1964.
Thorndike, E.: "Constant Error in Psychological Ratings," *Journal Applied Psychology*, **4**:25–29, 1920.
Ujhely, Gertrud: *Determinants of the Nurse-Patient Relationship*. New York: Springer Publishing Company, Inc., 1968.
Weissman, Isabel G.: "Make Interviewing a Creative Process," *California's Health*, **22**:22:201–203, May 15, 1965.

Suggested readings

Benedict, Ruth: *Patterns of Culture*. Boston: Houghton Mifflin Co., 1934.
——— *The Chrysanthemum and the Sword*. Boston: Houghton Mifflin Co., 1946.
Berlo, Davis K.: *The Process of Communication*. New York: Holt, Rinehart and Winston, Inc., 1960.
Bettelheim, Bruno: *The Informed Heart: Autonomy in a Mass Age*. New York: The Free Press of Glencoe, 1960.
Brehm, Jack W., and Cohen, Arthur R.: *Explorations in Cognitive Dissonance*. New York: John Wiley and Sons, Inc., 1962.
Buber, Martin: *I and Thou*. New York: Charles Scribner's Sons, 1958.
Coleman, Arthur D.: "Territoriality in Man: A Comparison of Behavior in Home and Hospital," *American Journal of Orthopsychiatry*, **38**:464–68, 1968.
Hayakawa, S. I., ed.: *Language, Meaning and Maturity*. New York: Harper and Row, 1954.
Jourard, Sidney M.: *Disclosing Man to Himself*. Princeton: Van Nostrand, 1968.
Sene, Barbara Stankiewicz: "Termination in the Student-Patient Relationship," *Perspectives in Psychiatric Care*, **7**:1:39–45, 1969.
Travelbee, Joyce: *Intervention in Psychiatric Nursing: Process in the One-to-One Relationship*. Philadelphia: F. A. Davis Co., 1969.

6 Patients under stress

It is necessary to understand that there are many theories about the life process and its effects upon the human being. The intangible effects on the human condition of experiences in living are still only imperfectly understood. The study of human behavior is a relatively new science that is destined to have a great impact on the nursing profession, inasmuch as nurses are concerned with behavior brought about by the exigencies of life and are in a position to be of assistance during stress periods in the life arc.

Engel defined stress as follows: [1]

> *Psychological stress refers to all processes, whether originating in the external environment or within the person, which impose a demand or requirement upon the organism, the resolution or handling of which requires work or activity of the mental apparatus before any other system is involved or activated.*

Thus, stress is the introducer, not the effect of an action. Engel also states that for a situation or process to constitute psychological stress, it must be perceived, in whole or in part, and it must also be capable of some type of psychic representation or expression, whether conscious or unconscious. In contrast, physical stress is brought about by such factors as poisons, physical trauma, and the like; it affects, first of all, the operation and function of the physiological systems in man. For example, the action of *Treponema pallidum* does not meet the criterion of psychological stress, but the *idea* of syphilis does. A physical injury may be felt simultaneously as both psychological stress and physical stress.

The essence of nursing lies in recognizing the areas in individuals and families where coping mechanisms no longer work and using this knowledge to help them handle successfully the problems resulting from life. Since the nurse is in constant proximity to the inner man, the more the student learns about human behavior, the more she will be in a position to provide help where it is needed. The nurse should (1) assist those who are well toward high level wellness; (2) aid those newly in crisis to an early recovery; and (3) assist those who are mentally disordered to restoration of health.

---

[1] G. L. Engel: *Psychological Development in Health and Disease*. Philadelphia: N. B. Saunders Co., 1962, p. 264.

Conflict, tension, and anxiety

Conflict, tension, and anxiety are constructs basic to the understanding of intrapsychic human behavior, therefore, some emphasis is placed here upon understanding their origins, effects, and interrelationships. These constructs cannot be measured precisely; rather, they are inferred from behavior. They may go unnoticed unless the nurse is alert to the phenomenological approach to patients. [2] Nurses who are task-centered rather than person-oriented will probably not ascertain the inner lives of their patients. On the other hand, the relevance to nursing practice of the emotional temperature of the patient and his family, the psychic pulse, the affect, the psychic wounds, as well as the condition of the skin and the newly made surgical wound, cannot be over-emphasized.

In the process of living one thing must always be given up for another. Therefore, conflict is an integral part of human life. The ways in which human beings resolve their conflicts may determine the difference between mental health and mental disorder.

Conflict

Conflict is the clash, largely determined by unconscious factors, between opposing emotions. Conflicts create intrapsychic tension which can be reduced if the conflicts are resolved. When there is unresolved conflict, tension continues within the psyche and coping behavior is demanded of the person; repression may also occur. Experiences evoking shame, guilt, anger, or lowering of self-esteem are likely to be repressed. From repression, anxiety arises, and continued repression may lead to further problems. Indirect outlets of anxiety may result in the use of defense mechanisms. Repressed impulses maintain their intensity, are further reinforced daily beneath façades, and may emerge later in neurotic, psychophysiologic, or psychotic symptoms (see *Figure 4*).

For example, in a patient with an hysterical neurosis, the paralysis of an

---

[2] "Patient" here refers to an individual under the care of a nurse, whether in a hospital, outpatient, or home setting. This term includes the person under care and his family, regardless of absence or presence of mental disorder.

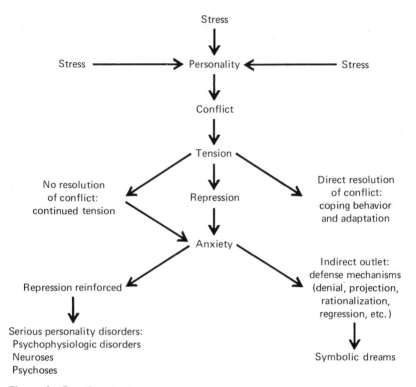

Figure 4   Reactions to stress.

arm may represent a conflict between the desire to masturbate and the prohibition against it (English and Finch, 1957). On the other hand, the principal problem of the patient with psychophysiologic cardiovascular disorder (hypertension) is that he unconsciously remains angry, which keeps his blood pressure up. The symptoms of a manic-depressive are thought by the psychoanalytic school to result from repressed trauma and unconscious wishes (Ayd, 1961).

Tension and coping behavior

Tension is a restlessness, a vague feeling that something needs to be done. The coping behavior of tension resolution is well known to most individuals, but it must be remembered that behaviors have more than a single purpose; those acceptable in some cultures may not be applicable to others. Coping behavior relieves stress, restores or maintains self-esteem, and assists the person under stress to solve the problems connected with the stress. What is acceptable to your society, culture, and age group? How do you cope with tension? The following list of coping behaviors is adapted from Menninger (1963).

1. Reassurance of touch, rhythm, and sound. (These all recall the early comfortings of infancy—lullabies, rocking, and patting).
2. Eating and other oral behavior, such as smoking and chewing gum.
3. Use of alcohol and drugs.
4. Laughing, singing, crying, and swearing.
5. "Goofing off."
6. Sleeping.
7. Thinking it through.
8. Talking it out—discussing one's problems with a sympathetic listener or even excessive verbalization.
9. Working it off in direct physical exercise; for example, running, cleaning, dancing, or working harder and later.
10. Pointless activity, such as walking up and down, pacing, scratching, finger-tapping, and hand-rubbing.
11. Retreating into fantasy and day dreaming, especially fantasies in which one's problems are solved or do not exist.
12. Boasting.
13. Asking questions.
14. Seeking new information and using it.

Anxiety

Anxiety is primarily of intrapsychic origin in distinction from fear, which is the emotional response to a consciously recognized and usually external threat or danger. It is the apprehension or uneasiness which stems from the anticipation of danger; the source of the threat is largely unknown or unrecognized. Anxiety becomes pathologic when it occurs to such an extent that it interferes with effective living, the achievement of desired goals or satisfaction, or reasonable emotional comfort. Anxiety and fear are accompanied by similar physiologic changes (American Psychiatric Association, 1969).

Anxiety has also been described as a group phenomenon which can result in riots, revolutions, and wars. Artists and writers have made it a main theme of their work, in content as well as style. The paintings and woodcuts of Edvard Munch, the ballet *The Burrow* of Kenneth Macmillan, Jean Paul Sartre's play *No Exit*, the writings of Albert Camus, the opera *Wozzeck* by Alban Berg, and *Peter Grimes* by Benjamin Britten are all dramatic portrayals of anxiety. The effect of this permeating theme has been to make the public quite conscious of the ideas and symbols of anxiety. It is a truism to call our time "the age of anxiety." This observation is as true for Europe as for America and perhaps holds for all countries with developing technologies.

Anxiety expresses itself in the loss of direction, the anomie of Durkheim (1951), and the feelings of alienation dealt with by the existentialists. Paul Tillich (1952) describes three major forms of anxiety, those of death, meaninglessness, and condemnation. Anxiety is always communicated interpersonally. It has been called existence by some theorists; others have said it is a threat to values—a threat of nonbeing, a threat of nonbelonging, or what one feels when suddenly confronted with freedom and the opportunity to do things previously forbidden.

PHYSIOLOGIC CHANGES

Any threat to the ego causes anxiety. It is now known that anxiety, like fear, releases epinephrine; but because the threat is invisible in the former state, the results are in the nature of biochemical scarring and impairment of the physiological functioning. These effects depend upon the degree of anxiety; in general, mild and moderate anxiety heighten the use of an individual's capacities, whereas severe anxiety and panic paralyze or overwork the person. Increased heart rate, increased rate and depth of respiration, rise in arterial pressure, rapid and extreme shifts in body temperature and blood pressure occur. The blood is diverted from the stomach and intestines to the heart, the central nervous system, and the muscles; processes in the alimentary canal cease; the spleen contracts and discharges corpuscles; and the adrenal medulla secretes its hormone. Symptoms ensue of "cold sweat," disturbances of menstrual flow, urinary urgency and frequency, dryness of mouth, anorexia, loss of appetite, dilation of pupils, abdominal cramps, and release of sugar by the liver. An anxious person may feel weak in the knees, may have nausea and vomiting, vertigo, headache, insomnia, syncope; he may feel tight around the collar, be tense and silent, complain of butterflies in his stomach, sigh, have diarrhea, turn pale, be unable to talk, tremble, say the same thing repeatedly, and have an urge to do something. Cannon was the first to pinpoint the significance of the physiological effects of intense feelings.[3]

---

[3] Walter Cannon: *The Wisdom of the Body*. New York: W. W. Norton Co., 1932, p. 227.

Fear has become associated with the instinct to run, to escape; and anger or aggressive feeling, with the instinct to attack. These are fundamental emotions and instincts which have resulted from the experience of multitudes of generations in the fierce struggle for existence and which have their values in that struggle.

He also noted that the responses of the body to intense emotions are designed to prepare the person for "fight or flight." The brain cortex sends a stimulus via the sympathetic branch of the autonomic nervous system to the adrenal glands. Epinephrine is secreted and induces deep respirations and accelerated heartbeats. The body is prepared to use the released energy or to act. Later workers found that the parasympathetic system is also involved during emotional stress; i.e., slowing of the heart rate and lowered blood pressure may also result from anxiety (Grinker, 1945). Selye (1956) described the *general adaptation syndrome*, focusing attention on the role of the pituitary-adrenocortical axis in the body's response to stress. He identified three stages: (1) the alarm reaction, (2) the stage of resistance, and (3) the stage of exhaustion. According to Selye, the general adaptation syndrome comprises adrenal stimulation, shrinkage of lymphatic organs, gastro-intestinal ulcers, loss of body weight, alterations in the body chemicals, and related changes. A *local adaptation syndrome* may occur—for example, at the point that microorganisms enter the body. Both of these syndromes are closely interconnected and work together to combat wear and tear within the body.

The reader should note that Selye's stress theory applies to a biologic unit and does not refer to the psychodynamic processes brought into play by specific intrapsychic threats to the ego. Psychological constructs are inferred from behaviors of individuals, and there is as yet no known way to predict which of the coping behaviors and/or defense mechanisms will be brought into action when the ego is threatened. There are no microorganisms to observe for paths of entry to the human psyche or for triggering psychological defenses.

LEVELS OF ANXIETY

Anxiety occurs at different levels, ranging from mild forms to panic. You may feel mild anxiety before taking an examination, making a speech, or meeting a new patient. It is also felt by people making changes in their lives, e.g., entering a hospital, meeting a new physician or nurse, or undergoing a new diagnostic procedure. Visits of anxious friends and relatives to a sick person may engender mild anxiety in the patient. In the mild to moderate levels, a person may have heightened perception which gradually lessens. His ability to learn and to grasp ideas may be increased, only to be interfered with as anxiety mounts. It is imperative for nurses to be aware of the anxiety level of a patient in order to assess more accurately what he can absorb and what protective actions must be instituted by the helping person.

Persons in severe anxiety states are panicky—they may be immobilized so that they cannot walk or talk. This kind of reaction may keep a person in a burning house or in the path of a flood. It must certainly have been one of the reasons that many Jews in Nazi Germany were unable to leave that country. There is a kind of emotional paralysis that leaves the victim unable to fight or to take flight, the final process of which is catatonia.[4] Others, however, may run over women and children to get into the lifeboat or fight those who are hospitalizing them.

A panicky person may shoot a gun if he has one, jump off a high building, attack others, or beat himself. He may yell at the top of his voice, run away, or wander about aimlessly. Persons in panic may be observed at the scene of an accident, in the emergency room, at suicide prevention centers, or in their own homes. Operations and treatments may precipitate panic, as may life encounters such as robberies, attempted rapes, and homosexual overtures. Role-transition points may also bring on panic, such as leaving one job for another, going to college, marriage, and childbirth. Role-transition points in life are those in which changes are made in what others expect or demand of a person. Change of role may result in high levels of anxiety. Leaving familiar people, institutions, and patterns of behavior may present overwhelming conflicts to some individuals. Anxiety highly affects the individual's adaptation to new roles; each new role that a person has in life may demand different skills and new defenses.

Following is an example of an interaction with a very panicky patient in a psychiatric unit. The patient-nurse contact lasted for a period of $1\frac{1}{2}$ hours, but the critical time for assessment of the situation occurred during the first few minutes of contact.

Ecological unit   The room of a patient in the psychiatric unit of a neuro-psychiatric institute. The time is 4:00 A.M., and all the other patients on the unit are asleep.

The patient   She is a nurse, a very frail, pale young woman who is tall and thin. Her brown, closely cropped hair is tousled, she is barefoot, and she is wearing hospital flannelette pajamas. Her hands grasp the nurse's arm in a viselike grip. She is breathing heavily, her pupils are dilated, and there is an expression of terror on her face.

---

[4] Here catatonia refers to immovable posture, inability to express feeling, and a lack of affective facial expression.

Nurse   Hello, Miss Carr.

Patient   Nurse, nurse, I'm so afraid. Something unusual is going on on this ward. That Tommy is going to surgery. (Peeks out from the door down the hallway.) They're going to do surgery on me too, I know. I want to see Dr. Sams and the O.D. (officer of the day) right now. There is something funny going on around here. (She returns to her bed, closes her eyes, and rocks back and forth in a sitting position, moving her hands in bizarre gestures.) Are you a Catholic? (All of this is said with a great rush of words, some stammering, and quick, jerky movements as though very tense.)

Nurse   No, I am not Catholic. You remember me from last week? I'm Miss Norton. I work only part time. Dr. Sams arrives at 8:30 A.M., and the O.D. is asleep. You are not going to surgery. You can talk with me.

Patient   I'm so afraid I'm pregnant, but Dr. Sams says that I am not. But I've missed six periods. I have faith in this place and the nurses and the doctors, but I'm the sickest patient on the ward. You know what my trouble is? I take on too much, even here; I see too much of the other patients' symptoms. I'm worse since I got here. I don't like them (refers with gesture to other patients). I can't stand Mary and Horace. Don't you think I'm the sickest patient here? (Her voice is calmer now.)

Nurse   Oh, Mary and Horace are okay (matter-of-factly). I don't think of patients as being sick or sickest. Why do you think you're the sickest? (This is a statement of fact, plus an indication of interest in her feelings.)

Patient   (Ignores question.) Well, I guess all of us are sick sometimes. I'm so upset. Look at me. (Trembles all over.) I'm a psych patient. I think I'm the center of the world (assumes a rather histrionic stance). But I don't hear voices. (She covers her face with her hands and counts to six on her outstretched fingers.) Nurse, you're not listening. (I had glanced away to look through the doorway at another patient who had gotten up.)

Nurse   Yes, I *am* listening. I just looked out at Mr. Jorge so he would know where I am if he needs anything. My name is Miss Norton. I will go make my rounds now and be right back.

How the patient felt   She was very tense, anxious, full of conflicts. She was suspicious of the hospital surroundings, although at the same time she said that she had faith in the hospital staff. She was probably trying to reassure herself; she had made the decision herself to come to the hospital. She verbalized this and also indicated it in her manner and movements. She had been acutely psychotic for 2 days. At this encounter, she was preoccupied with the thought of pregnancy and with sex in general. The patient was also testing me out to see if I would ring the O.D., call the supervisor, give her more sedation, or talk with her. She was also claiming my full attention, except for the time I left her room to make rounds. In order to alleviate her conflict "that something funny was going on," I asked her to walk with me up and down the hall, into the day room, and to help me wash the coffee cups. She could see for herself that the day was like any other day, that the other patients were asleep, that the morning routine was the same, and that there was no preparation for surgery. My role was primarily one of listening and of reassurance.

Evaluation   The patient had a frightened facial expression, pressure of speech, and tense muscles, all of which attested to her anxious, suspicious, and conflicted feelings. She verbalized her concern and watched every move I made to see if I was getting ready to give her preoperative medications. Because the other patients were asleep, I was able to devote my entire attention to her. I repeated my name in an attempt to make her contact with me more realistic and personalized.

I encouraged ventilation, used verbal reassurance, and listened. Exploration of the unit with Miss Carr relieved her anxiety about the pending surgery (as a nurse herself she knew what preoperative procedures would need to be done). Directing her motor activity into such a routine thing as washing coffee cups was helpful. Being present as a nonanxious person involved a fortuitous use of the concept of negative feedback.

I was, however, unable to understand the bizarre hand movements of the patient and did not question her as to their meaning because our relationship had not developed to the point where I felt comfortable about asking for meanings that might be heavily laden with emotion. My glancing out of the doorway while she was speaking to me was a mistake which I immediately tried to rectify; otherwise, she probably would not have trusted me. A need that was not met was an understanding of the source of her anxiety.

Defenses against anxiety

Although some psychiatric nurses advocate steering clear of unconscious material in their patients, I do not see how they can avoid it. The mental mechanisms are largely unconscious mechanisms and, since the time of Sigmund Freud, they have been central to the study of human behavior.

In human beings, behavior is integrated and indivisible. No behavior stands in isolation; all behavior is part of a developmental series; and all behavior is meaningful, multipurposeful, and multidetermined. Behavior includes manifest actions and the psychological processes or activities of the mind: learning, perception, dreams, moods, fantasies, and affects. Psychological defenses are constructs and therefore intangible. Their existence is synthesized from observations of behavior and assessment of the personality. Constructs explain observable behavior but have no clear physical existence of their own. Although Freud thought of the defenses as irrational ways of dealing with anxiety, current psychiatry views them as necessary to existence and ego management. They may be viewed as reactions to the emotional pain of anxiety. When the defenses are no longer in operation for the defense of the ego, psychoses may occur.

Tension management is conscious, but mental mechanisms are largely unconscious. However, one may *become* conscious of one's own defense mechanisms. The level of intensity of use of defense mechanisms may be viewed as a continuum in which such things as hyperrepression, and hyperprojection are progressively severe developments of mere repression or the use of coping behavior. If the ego is unable to overcome the punitive superego, depression results; or if the id behavior overcomes the superego, acting out behavior may follow, culminating in asocial acts.

It is assumed in modern psychiatry that every person has his breaking point and that particularly stressful events may not be managed by the ego as adequately as the ordinary events of everyday life. Crisis theory relates to this concept and hypothesizes that there is a point at which the person requires help to defend the ego and thereby to adapt successfully to the stressful event. Intervention at this point may prevent serious mental disorder. If help is given at the critical point, healthy adaptation and growth may occur. If it is not given, however, the result may be maladaptive behavior. Nurses are in a particularly important position to help people in periods of difficulty; however, this aspect of their professional role has not yet been fully exploited in nursing practice (Evans, 1968).

The emphasis on the psychological needs of persons in this chapter does not negate the holistic approach to the assessment of each individual, by means of which his biological, socioeconomic, and cultural needs are also given due attention. *Figure 5* is a mnemonic device to help nurses place the patient in his social environment, with four key questions that help place him in his mental environment as well.

Since Freud proposed the original list of defense mechanisms, many others have been added. In this book, consideration is given to those reactions most commonly observed in nursing practice, particularly those which nursing students need help in identifying. Unless a student is able to recognize defense mechanisms in her patient, she will be of little assistance to him in anxiety-producing situations. Outstanding is the mechanism of denial, which is discussed in many of its forms in the following pages.

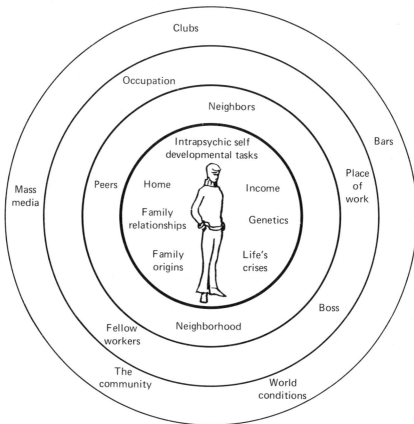

1. What kind of person is this?
2. What precipitated his condition?
3. Why is he behaving the way he is?
4. How can I be of help?

Figure 5   The patient in his social environment.

DENIAL OF REALITY

Denial is an intrapsychic defense mechanism by means of which consciously untenable wishes, needs, ideas, deeds, or reality factors are disowned by an unconscious refusal to admit their existence. What is consciously untenable is unconsciously rejected by a protective mechanism of unawareness. Reality is regarded as nonexistent, or it is transformed so that it is no longer threatening. The term "denial" as used in a psychiatric sense does not include a conscious attempt to repudiate or disown, as in malingering or lying (Noyes,

1968). The attitude of denial of a disorder is probably a lifelong pattern. Psychodynamically, denial of illness is probably determined in part by an inability to accept changes in body image or in role perception. Such a reaction to illness is also called anosognosia (when first used, this term referred mostly to paralysis). The function of denial is to defend the ego. When the defense is used by people with minor disorders such as the common cold, it does not receive much attention; when, however, it is evident in people who have major disorders, it assumes a much greater importance. Denial, one of the most common mental mechanisms evidenced when people are under the stress of diagnosis and illness, is almost a universal reaction to the diagnosis of cancer. It may be revealed either verbally or symbolically. Some patients may refuse to admit that they are ill or affected in any way. Verbal denials most commonly heard by nurses are, "I am not a mental patient" and "I am just here for a rest." Other patients may refuse to admit to a major disability but will complain of minor discomforts.

Following is a list of five types of denial:

1. Nonverbal denial   Some patients may refuse to admit that they are ill in any respect; others may deny illness through being overly compliant with therapeutic personnel but not making any references to their illness. Only close questioning will get them to verbalize that they are ill.

A patient with skin cancer, Mrs. Horner, was close to death but refused to accept her diagnosis although she had been transported from another state to the cancer-treatment unit. Every day when Miss Baldwin changed the dressing over her entire back, Mrs. Horner asked how the area looked and latched onto any observation by the nurse that could be interpreted as a hopeful improvement. Mrs. Horner kept making plans to return to her home state. She was unable to verbalize that she had cancer to anyone.

2. Postponement   The almost universal denial that accompanies the diagnosis of cancer may continue for long periods, or it may be transitory. The affected individual's philosophy of life may greatly influence his psychological reactions. How his parents and other significant members of his family have reacted to stresses in their lives may also be an influencing factor. One of the most common forms of denial is seen when patients develop symptoms that make them suspect cancer.

A patient, Mrs. Bocaccio, married, with two children and expecting a third, observed a lump in her breast for two months before mentioning it to anybody. Finally, she told her priest who immediately sent her to her physician. A biopsy showed it to be a cyst.

Mrs. Kent had been noticing some bleeding with her stool and finally, after months had passed, went to her physician for a check-up. He sent her into the hospital, where a G.I. series showed polyps in her colon. Exploratory surgery revealed carcinoma that had already extended to her liver. The surgeon informed her that it was cancer. In subsequent discussions, she said that the cancer had been removed and made plans for returning to work.

Another patient with newly diagnosed cancer of the G.I. tract said that she would wait and ask her physician back in the Midwest about her condition when she returned there from the West Coast, although immediate surgery had been recommended to her.

3. Due to harmless cause   The third type is one in which the changes are said to be due to rather harmless causes; for example, the person who says that he was admitted to the mental hospital because of fatigue or the paralyzed person who says that he is just too lazy to move his legs.

Although a patient's arm or leg may be paralyzed, he will complain only of minor things such as headaches and constipation. (This phenomenon closely approximates "la belle indifférence"[5] of the patient with an hysterical neurosis.) A patient who has had a massive coronary may say that his "ticker" slowed down a bit and that he will be back in his office the next month; or he will tell his nurse that he is glad his friends call so he can cheer them up.

4. Attributed to someone else   The fourth type of denial is that in which the disorder of the patient is attributed to someone else. For example, a patient in an acute psychotic episode refuses to leave her home for treatment, saying that there is nothing wrong with her, that it is her husband who is ill. Another aspect is that of displacement in time in which the patient who is obviously mentally disordered states that he was ill some years ago but made a full recovery. This type of denial may also resemble the mental mechanism of projection.

An example of projection is shown in the case of Mr. Brown, whose injured leg required amputation. Subsequently he placed the blame for the loss of his limb on his surgeon. By blaming another, the patient rid himself of unacceptable ideas, especially when neglect on his part resulted in the condition; his ego, therefore, was defended.

One patient, Mrs. Davis, who had been hospitalized for 15 years with a diagnosis of schizophrenia, paranoid type, was now in her retirement years. In the hospital, she managed the kitchen and the feeding of 80 to 90 patients on the unit. Her maladaptive behavior evidenced itself in the writing of voluminous letters to the superintendent of the hospital and to the governor of the state denying that she was a mental patient or had ever been one and, furthermore, casting serious aspersions as to their characters.

---

[5] An inappropriate lack of concern.

5. Ignoring disability   The fifth type of denial refers to ignoring or paying little attention to the severity of major disability. An example is the diabetic patient who refuses to adhere to his therapeutic regime, who eats what he pleases when he pleases and adjusts his insulin accordingly, or who skips doses.

Mr. Watkins, retired and living alone, without any family left, was in the hospital for surgical removal of his ulcer. Although he also had a severe heart condition, he defied the physician's instructions with regard to bed rest and climbed out over the bed rails at night to go to the bathroom, in spite of admonishment from his roommates.

Ignoring the affected part of the body, such as a devastating scar or a particularly unwanted wound from an ileostomy or breast amputation, is another variant. The patient who does not look at his wound may be using denial; he may wish to have his eyes covered or will look in the opposite direction while his wound is being dressed; or he may joke about the wound so as to belittle its existence. Men who have suffered facial injuries may avoid shaving and thus the necessity to look into the mirror. Adolescents may particularly ignore changes within themselves in order to meet long-awaited events; for example, they may pay no heed to the fever and malaise of mono-nucleosis in order to graduate with peers.

Therapeutic tasks

Since denial of disorder is a defense, if the situation is such that denial is the best solution for the individual patient and his family, the mechanism should be supported. Relatives may consider it providential, especially when the patient has cancer and it is uncomfortable for them to talk about it. Denial can help a patient cope with his situation in a way that otherwise would not be possible for him. Some nurses may feel that patients should face up to reality even though, psychologically, the patient's use of denial may be saving him from a more serious personality disorder or from suicide. Forcing the conflict to consciousness may be harmful. A sense of the right time to talk about what is happening to the patient is necessary in the art of nursing. Denial may be a momentary attempt to avoid reality. The need for time for the patient to work through the shock of a serious or a fatal diagnosis should be recognized by the nurse, along with the fact that not everyone accepts illness and trouble in the same ways.

The use of denial is more than a function of experience, knowledge, or intelligence. Just because your patient is a prominent "heart man" in the community does not mean that he does not use mental mechanisms when it comes to dealing with his own heart attack. Now that many patients spend less time in hospitals, it is even more imperative that nurses avoid jumping to conclusions that patients have bad attitudes simply because they are still denying aspects of their disorder upon discharge, after being hospitalized for 2 weeks. Denial will most likely continue until the patient has accepted the change in body image or in role. The nurse can (1) learn what part denial plays in the patient's patterns of adaptation—e.g., how he has previously reacted to stressful situations; (2) assess the underlying motivation of the patient (interventions to alter denial may not be appropriate); (3) assess the patient's particular level of anxiety and mental state at many points in time since the nurse is in continuous contact with the patient; and (4) act as a representation of reality to the patient through which he can "check out" his perceptions. Nurses can also learn more about the ways that people express denial and therefore be in a better position to help patients under stress.

If denial is manifestly harmful to the patient, as when he refuses to follow the therapeutic regime or runs away from the mental hospital, it is important to find out the exact motivation for his behavior. This usually requires the efforts of all members of the health team. If, for example, a previously described patient, Mr. Watkins, who denied his severe heart disease and prescription for bed rest by climbing over the bed rails to go to the bathroom, dies soon thereafter (as he did), a psychological autopsy may diagnose cause of death as a subintentioned suicide.[6] Preventive techniques could perhaps have been employed with him had his motivation been known to the health team.

When the motivation of the patient is a wish to be admired for his strength and virtuosity, the task of the nurse and the health team is to help him adapt to other ways of winning approval—to help him develop ego-strength that does not require such extremes of self-sacrifice. When fear is the motivation for the use of denial, the least effective intervention is to frighten the patient into adherence to the therapeutic regime. Helping him review his assets so as to discover what he can do within the limits of his disability can be the first step to acceptance of his altered self-image. The nurse has an important role to play in encouraging the patient to accept help, whether it be vocational rehabilitation after a bout with schizophrenia or arranging for some other family member to go out and work until convalescence is complete. Giving accurate information to the patient about his condition, without forcing the conflict of self-destruction, is of primary importance in the healthy recovery of the patient.

---

[6] The individual has played some role in hastening his own demise.

There is much psychic energy used up in the maintenance of mental mechanisms that can be used in more constructive ways once the ego is well defended and the patient can accept the changes in body image or role. Helping him identify with a friend or another patient who has successfully dealt with a similar problem can be supportive. The therapeutic potential of another person who has undergone a similar event and who has recovered should be tapped. It is vital that nurses in all areas of practice should be familiar with the various patients' organizations and the ways to put people in touch with each other who have adapted in healthy fashion to similar afflictions. Various clubs are now in existence in this country for patients and families of patients to help each other. The Lost Chord Club for patients with laryngectomies has helped many persons through the despair of this surgery; Recovery, Inc., has a large number of clubs for mental patients in many states. The international office of the United Ostomy Association, Inc., claims many branches. All attest to the therapeutic potential of one person for the other.

Stress of sensory deprivation

Under the rubric of sensory deprivation are found other concepts: sensory restriction, sensory reduction, sensory isolation, and perceptual isolation. Research with regard to sensory deprivation deals with experimental conditions aimed at reducing, altering, or by some means interfering with a person's normal stimulation from and interaction with his environment.

Brainwashing techniques and the isolation of individuals with mental disorder in seclusion rooms and in large remote public mental hospitals have some aspects of sensory deprivation and are therefore relevant to the field of psychiatric nursing. Seclusion was used by professionals when other techniques failed and at other times because of administrative failure to meet staffing standards. Helping patients to achieve internal controls of acceptable behavior was rarely aided by the use of seclusion rooms.

Several developments have been related to the topic of sensory deprivation.

The theoretical development in psychoanalysis of ego psychology— particularly the primary and secondary drives—and ego autonomy (memory, reasoning, and reality testing)

The study of the arousal system in the reticular formation of the brain; the work in neurophysiology demonstrating that electrical changes in the central nervous system follow reduced sensory input

Adding the "exploratory drive" to the primary drives list

The study of the hallucinogenic drugs

The concern with the many problems connected with the security of the
country. Examples are the brainwashing techniques used on prisoners
of war during the Korean conflict, space flight, military duty in isolated
regions, and maintaining vigilance for certain night operations, such
as radar and night nursing. (Remember that the *Scharnhorst* went up
the English Channel during World War II undetected by English radar
watchers.)

With the increased use of machinery and new techniques in surgery, such
as monitored intensive care cardiac units and heart and kidney transplants, a
new emphasis is required in nursing for application of principles derived from
research on sensory deprivation. The hyperbaric unit and also the Life Island
Isolator (Lunceford, 1965) for treating patients who are especially vulnerable
to severe infection have implications for application of findings from sensory
deprivation experiments.

Much of the research on sensory deprivation was done at McGill University
by Bexton, Heron, and Scott (1954). They began by studying how human
beings react in situations where nothing at all is happening. Male students
were offered $20 per day to stay in bed in a lighted cubicle with time out
only for meals and toilet. They wore translucent plastic visors, cotton gloves,
and cardboard cuffs to reduce tactile input. All sounds were masked with
ear plugs and the constant whir of the air conditioner. Each subject was hooked
up to an EEG machine. They soon found themselves unable to think clearly
although they had planned to use the time to prepare lectures. Some
reminisced, reviewed their lives and trips, became irritable, and had hallucinations. The hallucinations consisted of dots of light, rows of yellow men with
black caps on and their mouths open, squirrels marching down a field,
processions of eyeglasses marching down a street, and a choir singing in
stereophonic sound. The results showed impairment of thinking, childish
emotional responses, disturbances of visual perception, hallucinations, and
changes in brain-wave patterns.

Vernon (1956) at Princeton University used a soundproof underground
room with bed, toilet, and a well-stocked refrigerator, placing the observer
in an adjacent room. University students volunteered to remain in the chamber
for 48 hours. Other experimenters used a reclining chair in a small, dark soundproof room without giving out prior information about the purposes of the
experiment. Lilly (1961) at the National Institute of Mental Health and Shurley
(1960) developed the immersion technique in a hydrohypodynamic environment: a soundproof tank of tepid, slowly flowing water and total darkness.
Subjects remained immobile, floating in the tank and breathing through
oxygenated face masks. A monitor was constantly available just outside the

tank, and a subject could leave the tank by signaling. Dr. Shurley reports that no subjects panicked.

Another group of experimenters (Wexler *et al.*, 1958), psychiatrists at Harvard, used the polio tank type of respirator for confining their subjects. While in the respirator their visual fields were confined to the front of the respirator and the blank walls of a screen. Arms and legs of the subjects were encased in cardboard splints, and a masking of sound was provided. Thus, an environment of perceptual monotony was created, rather than one of total deprivation.

Although all these techniques have certain similarities, the use of the polio tank type of respirator probably presents the severest form of confinement. Fortunately, the control of polio has drastically reduced the need for this type of respirator in treatment. Other types of apparatus, institutions, and processes used in the treatment of patients which necessitate changes in sensory input and output are as follows: institutionalization, oxygen tents, complete bed rest, respiratory treatment units, intensive care units, body-splinting and immobilization of body parts, and isolation of patients (special precautions unit for communicable disease; seclusion).

The reticular activating system

The concept of homeostasis refers mostly to the vegetative actions in our bodies and does not credit the influences of the psyche, the brain, and the central nervous system in motivation.

Recent work in neurophysiology cites the importance of sensory input and output via the reticular activating system. The reticular formation is the lower brain stem, where the brain connects to the spinal cord. It is a "dense neurone network forming a central core which extends from the medullary of the lower brain stem to the thalamus of the diencephalon." [7] It contributes impulses upward to the cortex and downward with the autonomic nervous system and the muscles. It receives a collateral branch from every channel or nerve connection between a sense organ and the cortex and interconnects extensively with systems of motor nerves. The reticular activating system can be thought of as a kind of control center for sensory input and output.

The two major sources of stimulation for the reticular activating system are considered to be sensory stimulation and cortical impulses. Stimulation from somatic, visual, auditory, olfactory, and visual sources can act somewhat

---

[7] D. P. Schultz: *Sensory Restriction*. New York: Academic Press, 1965, p. 15.

interchangeably in activating the system. Excessive interaction may lead to complete blocking of the reticular activation of the cortex, resulting in disturbances in awareness and attention (Duffy, 1962). There are also marked behavioral disturbances under the opposing conditions of sensory restriction and sensory distortion. Behavioral effects can be explained in terms of the ascending reticular activating system (ARAS). Located where it can monitor the incoming and outgoing messages, it can influence alertness and attention, as well as serve a balancing function. It regulates sensory input and also provides a connection between the cortex and the reticular formation. Continued and persistent sensory variances may result in disrupted perception, distractibility, and boredom. Resulting behaviors may be stereotyped or maladaptive.

The need for experience

The need for sensory variation, exploration, and expatiation of curiosity appears to have been added to the list of drives (Meerloo, 1964). Psychoanalytic and neurophysiologic research have indicated that the human organism requires a varied sensory input. Conclusions from current research show that *meaningful sensory input is necessary for psychic adjustment and that immediately unmeaningful stimuli often produce intense fear.*

Either too much sensory input or too little can lead to devastating mental states in man. Both the ego and the reticular formation are credited with being monitors of sensory input. This need for experience seems similar to the concept of heterostasis, moving away from the old and moving toward the new. The story is told of an animal experimenter who put a small monkey into an empty room in order to observe what he would do. The experimenter hastily closed the door on the monkey, then peered through the keyhole to see what it was doing, only to find a bright, brown eye staring right back at him.

The need for expansion or expansive creativity has been described by Buhler (1962) as reaching toward the realization of one's own potentialities. For example, at the age of 8 months or so, a child chooses a toy that he can do the most with. In the older age group, the need may also be expressed as the wish to influence others as well as the desire to be remembered after death, a yearning for immortality that contributes concretely to the founding of institutions as personal memorials. The need for experience is observed in the activities of explorers, including astronauts and cosmonauts. In comparing the need for experience with that of homeostasis, it can perhaps be said that experience is a goal of the human organism, whereas homeostasis is a condition to which the organism attempts to return after disruptive events. Viktor Frankl has made one of the most relevant statements in defense of this reasoning.[8]

> Thus it can be seen that mental health is based on a certain degree of tension, the tension between what one has already achieved and what one still ought to accomplish, or the gap between what one is and what one should become. Such a tension is inherent in the human being and therefore indispensable to mental well-being. We should not, then, be hesitant about challenging man with a potential meaning for him to fulfill. It is only thus that we evoke his will to meaning from its state of latency. I consider it a dangerous misconception of mental hygiene to assume that what man needs in the first place is equilibrium or, as it is called in biology, "homeostasis," i.e., a tensionless state. What man needs is not a tensionless state but rather the striving and struggling for some goal worthy of him.

Sensoristasis

A state in the human being in which there is optimum sensory input is called sensoristasis. It can be defined as a drive, "a state of cortical arousal which impels the organism (in a waking state) to strive to maintain an optimal level of sensory variation."[9] The reticular formation acts as a monitor in service to the sensoristatic balance. Other theorists, however, purport that the exploratory drive is nonhomeostatic in character (Buhler, 1962).

Stress of confinement and immobilization

Confinement refers to restraint or restriction of freedom on the activities of an individual or group by command, fear, or physical enclosure. It calls for adjustment to physical and temporal limits and adaptation to the changes perceived by self.

---

[8] V. E. Frankl: *Man's Search for Meaning.* Boston, Mass.: Beacon Press, Copyright © 1959, 1962, by Viktor Frankl, pp. 106–107. (Also London: Hodder and Stoughton, Ltd.)
[9] Schultz, *op. cit.*, p. 30.

There is much in literature that deals with confinement and these poems or stories are of value to the nursing student as a means of deepening her understanding of and empathy with the conditions of confinement and the feelings of patients.

The "little tent of blue which prisoners call the sky" in the *Ballad of Reading Gaol*, written by Oscar Wilde [9a] who was jailed for homosexuality, is a particularly poignant and vivid description of imprisonment. The feelings of Hans Castorp in Thomas Mann's *The Magic Mountain* are also expressive of the conditions of confinement to a sanitarium for the treatment of tuberculosis. Two poems by Robert Louis Stevenson, who had tuberculosis, describe a reaction to sickness and the use of play and a confinement by command of parent.

The Land of the Counterpane

When I was sick and lay abed
I had two pillows at my head
And all my toys beside me lay
To keep me happy all the day.

And sometimes for an hour or so
I watched my leaden soldiers go
With different uniforms and drills
Among the bed-clothes, through the hills;

And sometimes sent my ships in fleets
All up and down among the sheets
Or brought my trees and houses out
And planted cities all about.

I was the giant great and still
That sits upon the pillow-hill,
And sees before him, dale and plain,
The pleasant Land of Counterpane.[10]

Bed in Summer

In winter I get up at night
And dress by yellow candlelight
In summer, quite the other way
I have to go to bed by day.

[9a] Oscar Wilde: "The Ballad of Reading Gaol," in Maine, G. F., ed.: *The Works of Oscar Wilde*. London: Wm. Collins Sons & Co. Ltd., 1948, p. 822.
[10] R. L. Stevenson: *A Child's Garden of Verses*. New York: Charles Scribner's Sons, 1901, p. 5.

> I have to go to bed and see
> The birds still hopping on the tree
> Or hear the grown-up people's feet
> Still going past me in the street.
>
> And does it not seem hard to you
> When all the sky is clear and blue
> And I should like so much to play
> To have to go to bed by day?[11]

Drug users often confine themselves to coffins while "firing up." The coffin without the drug might have a similar effect!

Factors of considerable import in affecting tolerance of confinement have been described by Ruff, Levy, and Thaler (1959) as follows:

Activities undertaken by the subject
Circumstances surrounding the confinement
Factors with the subject: personality, motivation, education, and experience
Extent of enclosure or restraint
Sensory input (quantity, modality, and pattern)
Degree of intercommunication
Extent of "aloneness"
Time
> Duration of confinement
> Degree of subject's control over confinement
> Subject's knowledge of expected duration of confinement
> Presence or absence of methods of measuring time

Confinement requires adjustment and adaptation of the individual. Adjustment is the establishment of a relationship between an individual and his meaningful environment. The stability of the mental state of man depends on his perception of the outside world. Adjustment criteria are external to the self-system. The patient, confined to a state hospital, can be adjusted to his role as a psychiatric patient, go to bed and get up at the expected hours, devote himself to industrial therapy (which has been called "institutional peonage" by Bartlett [1964]), and carry on in the manner expected and remain mentally disordered. A patient admitted postsurgery to an intensive care unit who similarly goes along with the plan of the health team may never verbalize his longing for his loved ones or his abandonment of hope for lack

---

[11] R. L. Stevenson, *op. cit.*, p. 21.

of their emotional support. Likewise, a patient who has been newly admitted to a convalescent center, having given up hearth and home for institutional life, may go to meals as requested, be present when the physician makes his rounds, have all his physical needs adequately cared for, and give all appearances of adjustment to the change in ecological unit; but he will die because he has not really adapted himself.

Real adaptation requires intrapsychic changes that people must make to the social and cultural milieu in which they exist. Adaptation, learning to live in a particular way, involves coming to terms with one's inner self. A confined person must reorganize his territory in order to maintain control over his personal self, he also must seek alternative sources for satisfying his needs. Perhaps fantasies and dreams fulfill some needs not immediately gratifiable. The person must establish a new identity. He does this as a patient and through his desire to be known by personnel. Patients being readmitted ask for familiar staff members by name; they also ask if they themselves are remembered in order to establish identity. Sometimes gifts are given to nurses by departing patients as a way of being remembered. Patients who have formerly visited relatives and friends in a certain unit of an institution will often, when it is their turn to be admitted, request the same room.

The following vignette is an example of what effect confinement had upon one patient. I was unable to verify by personal observation the described conditions.

> A patient, now past the acute phase of mental disorder and attending a fellowship club, told the group at one of its meetings about being placed in a seclusion room at his local county hospital. Since this hospital had no treatment facilities whatsoever for patients with mental problems, they were placed in some locked rooms just off the medical ward. Each room contained a bed and a toilet. The door had a window for observation of the patient and a slot for passing food and other necessities to him. He stated that since people were looking in at him as a "crazy" man, he decided to fulfill their expectations. He wrapped himself up in his sheets because he felt strange just wearing a hospital gown and started singing and dancing every time somebody came to the door. (At this meeting, other patients from the same county described similar experiences to such effect that the fellowship club decided to act as a group to try to remedy these poor conditions.)

The effect of confinement itself is profound, and in the cited instance it was probably influential in contributing to the patient's mounting anxiety.

Relationships formed within institutions, hospitals, and outpatient departments and other care-giving agencies are not put to their best therapeutic use by nurses.

In one large medical center cancer patients receive chemotherapy as part of a multiple-states research project; patients returning to outpatient status are greeted by their former nursing staff, who assume responsibility for remembering names, faces, and individual situations of their former patients. This remembrance may be most supportive for a patient holding on to the thread of life, as well as for his family. A more formal commitment to continuity of relationships with the same nursing staff can take the form of a fellowship club with definite meeting times and places.

Biographies of mental patients are of particular value to nursing students in contact with patients and families with mental disorder. Over a century ago a patient in an autobiography described his experiences with mental disorder. With respect to his confinement to an asylum, he wrote that "it is in the busy haunts of men, not in the comparative solitude of the asylum, that the cure must be perfected."[12]

There does seem to be some correlation between the ability to endure pain and the ability to endure confinement. The possibility of synergistic effects of confinement plus other conditions must be considered in the care of patients. Confinement produces stress of a different type from that evident in experiments of perceptual and social isolation. In addition to psychological stress, there are also physiological effects, such as cardiac deconditioning, which result from reduction of physical exercise.

Prometheus eternally bound to the rock by Zeus suffered both social isolation and confinement. One of the most stressful situations for an organism to endure is to be tied down literally. The impact of immobility upon a child is rather severe and may lead to a pervasive and persistent *immobility fear.* It is now commonly seen in patients who had poliomyelitis in their childhood and who may suffer from reactivation of the immobility fear if they have to be reconfined. Patients with fractures or who are confined to bed for other reasons may have periods of anxiety due to earlier experiences. The nurse's primary aim is toward prevention. If your patient is an immobilized child, meaningful input from all the other sensory modalities aids in preventing immobility fear. For the adult, in addition to meaningful sensory input from you, your patient needs to ventilate about the earlier immobilizing event as well as the present ones. Immobilization is in conflict with our life style. We live in a technological society that is in constant motion. To be immobilized is truly to be put out of action. Think for a moment of the implications of the stress imposed upon patients by the use of physical restraints.

---

[12] A Late Inmate of the Glasgow Royal Asylum for Lunatics at Gartnavel, 1847 (no other publication data available).

A patient, Miss Dawson, now in her late seventies, was in a convalescent center. She had come from a distant state for retirement; all of her family had died, and her friends of 40 years' standing lived in a far distant state. Now in the convalescent center after a stroke, she refused to get out of bed. Instead, she turned from side to side in bed, constantly displacing her covers so that her body under the short hospital gown was fully exposed. In order to cover her up, the aide tucked a sheet snugly over her body, tying it tightly to the bed, and tied another sheet over the bed rails in a tentlike covering. The result was that the patient could not move from side to side and immediately began to cry, complaining that the nurses thought she had lost her mind because they tied her down. Hearing the crying, the aide came in and reprimanded the patient. The use of pajamas by the patient would have been a solution; she could then have moved back and forth in bed without exposing her body. For this patient, restraint symbolized a loss of mental control and resulted in an increase of regressive behavior.

The adaptation of patients to surgeries and to intensive coronary care units involves many changes in sensory modalities. In these units, only brief visiting may be permitted to relatives, and at times even this is done through a glass partition, without benefit of touch or smell, as in the case of heart-transplant patients. Some surgical intensive care units are designed to exclude all visitors in the striving toward surgical asepsis. Aside from the visiting and care of the staff, the patient's visual field may be restricted to the white acoustical tile ceiling which is punched full of holes, arranged in symmetrical monotony, and viewed through the oxygen tent. There may also be other restrictions, especially of movement.

Visual illusions may first occur as patterns on the ceiling. Hallucinations may follow. Patients in intensive care units may also experience the opposite of sensory deprivation; they may have a greatly increased sensory input, almost amounting to sensory bombardment. Body orifices may hold uncomfortable catheters, nasogastric tubes, and rectal tubes; patients may be receiving intravenous therapy, or they may have a tracheotomy and be unable to talk. Noise, continuous light, frequent examinations, many injections, conversations of staff, and constant awareness of patients all around them and what is happening to them may impinge upon the individual and contribute to his sensory input. Patients may also watch the cardiac monitors of other patients and vicariously suffer others' attacks. As intensive care units use private rooms, some of the sensory input will be exchanged for isolation. However, at this time, in some units little privacy is afforded, men and women patients may occupy adjacent beds, and there is inadequate provision for private care of natural body functions or for conversations with significant others about oneself.

Sensory deprivation is a new era of inquiry in nursing. Through literature, accounts of adventurers, and tales of recent experiences of prisoners of war in the Far East, the concept has become familiar to us. Investigations in sensory deprivation date from the decade of the Fifties and are now given an important place both in space flight programs and the care of patients. For the nursing student, a new area in clinical nursing has been opened in which she can explore practical approaches to problems presented by her patients. Mental aberrations reported by patients with sensory deprivations of various kinds may be due in fact to their sensory deprivations. Preventive techniques should be adopted by the nurse in caring for these patients. Implications for nursing practice are described below.

The nursing task: prevention

The importance of establishing a specific nurse-patient relationship aimed at preventive intervention cannot be overestimated in the clinical nursing care of patients who are experiencing sensory deprivation. The attachment of nurses to the practice of physicians or to a psychiatric team would greatly facilitate their ability to effect this needed relationship with patients and their families. In the practices of some obstetricians, general practitioners, and psychiatrists, this has occurred. Few physicians would now think of sitting with their patients through the first night of reduced sensory input as did Dr. Greenwood (1928) with his cataract patients four decades ago.

Where there is limited sensory input through one modality because of restriction of its usual function—such as in the use of eye patches, institutionalization, immobility resulting from the casting of broken bones, or central nervous system defects—consider how to substitute *meaningful* sensory input by means of the other senses and teach the patient and his family these modes of input. For example, for your older patient whose hearing and eyesight are failing, teach him and someone in the family the importance of touch and movement. Senior centers that are organized for sitting exercises and folk dancing provide this touch and movement and other sensory stimulation. Meaningful stimuli reduce the disruptive effects of sensory deprivation upon the human psyche. Strangeness and unfamiliarity contribute to the development of confusion in patients.

Think of the blind person whose senses of hearing and touch become very acute. The modality of the input is not as important as that the input be meaningful to the patient. This factor must therefore be assessed carefully with each person. Merely flooding the room with sound or perfume is not the answer, but taking a bouquet of roses to a rose gardener is meaningful. If your patient, for example, is a musician with multiple sclerosis or Parkinsonism, taking him to a concert would be appropriate. For patients with broken bones, other limbs or areas of the body can be exercised. Reactions to sensory deprivation may be most severe at night and may occur with greatest intensity in those who are old and who have already suffered some degree of sensory impairment. Stress susceptibility is particularly high with foreign patients, whose reality testing may be verbally impaired. You may have to remind your patient of your identity, where he is, what day it is, and what has happened to him.

Getting something familiar for the patient, such as special foods to which he is accustomed at home, repeating the fact that he is in your care, showing yourself as an ally, inquiring about his thoughts, feelings, and fears—these acts of primary prevention will help him adapt more readily to his situation. It is pertinent to remain with your patient as long as possible or to get some other person or family member to stay with him. If you can, try to introduce him to others who may have recently been through what he is experiencing. To explain and describe to the patient what is happening to him, using the reportorial approach, can also be helpful. Although patients can in many instances relate examples of cases like their own, accounts may be embroidered or exaggerated. There is an authenticity of reporting by the professional who has a broader experience and the scientific knowledge of what happens to patients, and this is listened to quite carefully by the patient. One might inform the patient as follows: "Patients who have their eyes covered may have different visual images. If you have them, tell me about them." Be specific about the significant and available person, who may be a family member, the physician, or the night nurse. Other examples are: "Sometimes people lose their sense of time when they have been very anxious and have gone through a lot in making a decision to get psychiatric care"; or, "Many people find that having their eyes covered is associated with considerable difficulty. We try to help you here by giving you some roommates to talk with who also have their eyes covered. We have found this to be very helpful to patients."

Patients with eye patches may awaken at night and, unaware of the hour, start talking merrily away to each other, perhaps disturbing the sleep of others before they learn to take their cues from the rhythm of the day and the sounds that tell them the time. Leaving the door open to the room of an eye-patched patient gives him more access to the sounds that aid in orientation. Although the hospital has a hard-and-fast rule against smoking in bed, I have found that a ward of eye-patched patients will monitor those who smoke at all times of the day and night and that these patients are more careful about extinguishing their cigarettes than those who can see. Sleeping patterns of these patients may be disrupted because they sleep off and on during the 24 hours; few of them sleep through the whole night without awakening. If the nurse is aware and vigilant, she will be on hand to do her preventive work. The preventive work emphasized throughout this section is the establishment of a specific nurse-patient relationship and provision of meaningful sensory input through the unaffected modalities.

One of the problems in hospital nursing is the number of nurses and levels of nursing that come into contact with the patient without fully understanding what is happening to him. It is the responsibility of the nurse in charge to see to it that all staff under her supervision are adequately informed of the needs of all her patients and of the ways to meet those needs. The use of familiar objects, articles, and routines is helpful to the patient. It is therefore recommended that the patient use his own clothes (if he is in a hospital), his own radio and the like, and that he follow his usual newspaper and morning routine insofar as this is possible. Darkness, silence, solitude, and interruption of usual habits and ways of meeting psychological needs may all be significant factors of stress. In a study of 78 patients with eye surgery, averaging 63 years of age, the conclusion was made that "orientation, reassurance, and support which the nurse can provide can help the patient to cope with experiences that occur" (Ellis, 1968). Much more investigation is needed about the different reactions of people and the appropriate nursing interventions for the particular patient who is undergoing the experience.

Nursing students want to know positive ways to meet the needs of their patients. We also learn from mistakes if we are able to analyze what went wrong and what should have been done to prevent the negative consequences. I am therefore including the following case, which clearly delineates the effects of verbal confinement. As you read it, think of all the nursing actions that you could have initiated on a preventive basis. Discuss your suggestions with your peers.

> Mr. Fior d'Italia, a patient in his sixties who speaks and understands little English, is now in his second postoperative day for eye surgery. He has both eyes covered and is in a ward with three other patients who have other kinds of surgical problems. He awakens early in the morning while the aide is taking TPR's and asks for a cheroot. Since it is hospital policy that patients cannot smoke in bed unless attended by a staff member, the aide refuses permission because she cannot spare the time to attend him. When informed of this, the patient becomes increasingly excited, tears off his eye bandages, gets out of bed, and gropes around for his clothes and cigars, announcing that he is leaving the hospital. Six people are required to put him back to bed and to hold him there.

When the day shift nurse, who came ahead of time, arrived, she gave the patient his cheroot, sent all the other staff out of the room, held his hand, stayed with him, and spoke comfortingly to him. By the time his physician came, he was able to carry on a calmer conversation with him in Italian.

Stress of social isolation

Social isolation is a condition resulting from few contacts with family, community, and significant others. All of the experiments and situations discussed in the section on sensory deprivation also involve social isolation to an extent. Social isolation or solitude refers to the separation in time and space from human contact. Hermits endure this kind of environment, as do subjects confined in a normal sensory environment either alone or with a small group of people. Servicemen in remote posts—in the Aleutian Islands during World War II, in submarines, and at the South Pole stations—have been and are familiar with the monotonous environment of small groups, as well as some degree of confinement. The early flyers who carried the mail from continent to continent, desert travelers, truck drivers, concentration camp victims, astronauts, and night nurses encounter this experience. Feelings of detachment from the usual rhythms of life that result from working at night and attempting to sleep during the day have implications for those nurses who work the night shift. Being out of tune with the opportunity to attend social events that those working the day hours can participate in or going to such events anyway and having to leave early, for instance, demand special adaptation and adjustment by the nurse assigned to night duty.

The Department of Psychiatry at the University of Oklahoma is conducting an experiment at the Amundsen-Scott Station to study the role of motivation in adaptation to the effects of the perpetually monotonous environment upon the men engaged there. This is done in support of the hypothesis that those who are highly motivated will adapt easier than those who are not. Navy men provide the logistics or back-up for the experimental work as part of their tour of duty. The navy program associated with the research project is called Operation Deep Freeze.

Albert T. Joern, a medical student studying for his M.D. and Ph.D. in psychophysiology who wintered at that station, described his situation as an "old Arctic explorer." While there, he felt he had reversed roles with his fiancée, so that he had become the dependent partner. He found himself relying on her for emotional support and understanding; before his adventure to the South Pole, he had been the dominant partner in the relationship.

In addition, his sense of the time lost due to the adventure was strong. Deprivations at the South Pole were lack of sexual experience; an environment without stimulation, sterile, and always white and cold; loss of contact with current events, newspapers, T.V., and sports; and separation from family and other loved ones. He noted that many of these changes and deprivations are quite similar to those experienced by the hospitalized or institutionalized individual. It is certainly of interest that the pin-ups at the South Pole are not pictures of girls but travel posters and landscapes.

The question arises as to whether the sexual drive is really as strong under the stressful conditions of social isolation as is commonly believed. There was uniform agreement on the disappearance of sexual feeling among the ordinary prisoners of the Nazi concentration camps—not among the privileged prisoners, however (Luchterhand, 1967). Pairing within groups without reference to sex was ubiquitous and so necessary to the survival behavior of the camp inmates that those who failed to make such alliances were the most likely not to survive.[13]

> . . . *Much of the strength for survival—psychic and physical—seems to have come from "stable" pairing. With all of the raging conflicts in the camps, it was in the pairs, repeatedly disrupted by transports and death paradoxically restored in the general bereavement, that the prisoner kept alive the semblance of humanity. The pairs gave relief from the shame of acts of acquiescence and surrender. The pairs produced expertness in the survival skills known as "organizing."*

Although the foregoing is an example of extreme isolation complicated by many other factors, it can also serve to guide us in nursing. People who are socially isolated by reason of accident or against their wishes may have the most difficulty in adapting. For example, the old person who lives alone may experience various degrees of social isolation. If he has a confidante with whom he can share his thoughts and feelings about the little things that happen every day, he may be able to cope better with the crises of aging. If his social relationships have narrowed to the point that he knows no one by name and his acquaintances are merely familiar faces in cafeterias, outpatient clinics, and church, his reduced sensory input from social relationships may result in fantasies, delusions, and hallucinations. It has become increasingly evident that the isolation of the aging in our culture contributes to the beginnings of mental disorder.

---

[13] Elmer Luchterhand: "Prisoner Behavior and Social System in the Nazi Concentration Camps," *International Journal of Social Psychiatry*, **13**:259–60, 1967.

Isolation and aging

The following situation is an example of an isolated older individual who has been visited by nursing students in successive classes for several years. The situation also includes nursing intervention.[14]

> *Mr. Houlihan, now retired for several years, left Ireland several decades ago and has never returned. Although he says that he has brothers, they do not correspond. He worked for many years as an orderly and now lives in a boarding house with 10 to 12 others in a neighborhood close to a hospital and the outpatient department where he gets his medical care. He is also very near the church and the bus line. Mr. Houlihan spends his days and some of his nights in church, helping to do whatever needs to be done. He has no hobbies. In one church, his favorite, which is in the central part of the city, he ushers people out at night, locks up, cleans, and spends the night there to avoid the dangers of being on the bus late at night. He seems to have no significant others in life. However, he knows the people in the churches, the hospital cafeteria where he takes his meals, and the outpatient department where he gets his medical care by their faces but not by name. He feels secure in these places and seldom ventures outside them unless accompanied by his nursing student. He is a bachelor and an octogenarian.*

> *Mr. Houlihan expresses much prejudice and at times borders on having somatic delusions and hallucinations. At one time he thought that an organ in his body had burst, creating a bad odor in his nose which could be detected by those around him. When the student visited, they met in the hospital cafeteria over coffee. She aided him in reality testing by meeting him in his usual environment, commenting on the everyday occurrences as she saw them, listening to his thoughts and feelings, and stating that she did not detect any bad odors about him (when he brought up the subject). She would then go on to discuss subjects that were more reality-oriented. She did not push discussion of odors and prejudice (which he expressed quite pointedly), thereby using negative feedback to lessen their importance. Instead, she focused on other events.*

---

[14] F. M. C. Evans: "Visiting Older People: A Learning Experience," *Nursing Outlook,* **17**:3:20–23, March, 1969. Copyright, The American Journal of Nursing Co.

The student aided Mr. Houlihan in reality-testing by her presence, calling him by name, and being a person herself with a name and interests to be remembered and with whom interaction was required. The memory requirement made of Mr. Houlihan by the student to note the time, place, and date of the visits was another aspect of reality-testing. A young person with whom he could relate over a continuing period of time gave him contact with the upcoming genera- tion and a sense of connection with the present which he otherwise would not have experienced. With the student, he was able to sit down and check out his perceptions on different topics, which may have been one of the most important facets of reality-testing. Because he had worked as an orderly for a great part of his life, he felt free to discuss these former times with the nursing student, who, in turn, encouraged him to do so. The anticipation of the student's visit, the visit itself, and thinking about it afterward all required relating to the world outside of himself.

During the third year of visits by the nursing student, Mr. Houlihan agreed to visit a senior center, but only if the student accompanied him. Because the center is located in a maritime museum, they also visited the latter, where Mr. Houlihan grandly pointed out the type of ship that brought him to this country. The student was amazed to learn that he had never been in the museum before and, in fact, had not known of its existence.

For Mr. Houlihan, the contact with the student provides a sense of connection with the present. She aids him in reality-testing because she is one of the few persons he knows by name, and she attempts to expand his sphere of social relationships. By her presence and thera- peutic use of self, she interacts in the relationship, which reduces his need for defensive reactions.

Although there could have certainly been other factors in the disappearance of Mr. Houlihan's symptoms, it is my view that the human influences of the nursing student were of central importance.

Institutional isolation

Patients with communicable diseases who are socially isolated often com- plain of the monotony of their restricted environment, and especially about the few visitors encountered or permitted and the hasty entrances and exits of the staff. Nurses are often wrapped up so securely that all that is evident to the patient are their eyes and their hands. In remote mental institutions or infrequently visited units within institutions, the envelopment of the visitor by the patients may be evidence of the monotony of their environment; someone new and different is being sought out by the group. A similar phenomenon may be observed in the staff in these units, who often show a great need to verbalize.

When elderly patients are admitted to psychiatric institutions, programs organized on the model of the resocialization program at Napa State Hospital in California would certainly prevent further social isolation (California's Office of Public Information, 1970). This program, which was set up by Wrenshall A. Oliver for geriatric patients, has now expanded to include other age groups who have been hospitalized for many years; patients are selected by a screening committee from the hospital population. Four steps are followed. First, the patient is assisted to relate to another person within the unit. The second step begins when he can show warmth toward this person; he is then brought together with another patient and they become buddies. Subsequently, he is brought into group discussion. After progress in group discussion, he is ready for the fourth step—becoming reacquainted with life outside the institution. Trips are made into the community, and patients become familiar with things they may not have ever seen before in their preparation for discharge.

Social isolation is one component of alienation, the others having been described as powerlessness, normlessness, meaninglessness, and self-estrangement (Seeman, 1959). While lifelong extreme isolation (i.e., the life of a hermit) is not in itself conducive to personality breakdown, because of adaptation patterns, lifelong *marginal* social adjustment very often contributes to the development of mental disorder (Lowenthal, 1968). Each of us has a social identity in addition to our personal identity, a sense of our own situation, a kind of continuity of character that is developed as a result of our various social experiences. Stresses affecting individuals can be both within and without the person. In the case of social isolation, the influence on the human organism may be directly damaging unless they are reversed.

Loss of personal liberty, imprisonment, solitary confinement, being lost at sea, or cast adrift constitute highly stressful experiences. The film *King Rat* gives a realistic picture of life in a Japanese prisoner-of-war camp during World War II and should be seen by every student of human behavior. The classic film on war, *Grand Illusion*, shows Eric von Stroheim as the manager of a war prison for officers in World War I, located in a remote castle. He becomes highly interested in a living plant, a lone geranium on the windowsill of the castle's turret.

Stop now and think of examples of isolation that you may have experienced.

Put yourself in a quiet room for a few hours away from others and study the effects upon yourself.

Components common to all experiences of isolation involve separation from familiar surroundings, objects, and persons, danger to life and health, severe restriction of quantity and variety of sensory experience, and limitations on the range of motor activity. There may be monotony, little opportunity to exercise, and a limited environment to explore, and one may be at the mercy of those in charge. If the person is lost at sea or in a snowstorm, he is helpless in the face of nature. In all individuals there is the need for sensory input and motor activity for psychic adjustment. In solitary confinement, the hunger for human contact is so great that prisoners welcome even interrogation by their captors.

The process of social isolation involves a difficulty in maintaining contact with reality, the emergence of vivid imagery, visual or auditory hallucinations, a tendency to misinterpret environmental stimuli, and depersonalization[15] and a decrease in rational thinking. Individuals may fight it by systematically reviewing their past experiences or making contact with animals. Patients in remote mental institutions or people who are otherwise socially isolated may feed stray cats and rats and become agitated when exterminators appear. If contact can be made with a lower animal, the isolation can perhaps be made more bearable. Sometimes a very isolated person can make such contact when he is unable to relate to available persons. The money spent yearly on pet food in this country attests to the importance of animals to people. I have observed long-stay patients in mental hospitals save parts of their dinners to feed the rats that gathered together at the proper time for their surreptitious handouts. Others gathered food and daily fed the cats that had gradually accumulated around the institution.

In every city park are socially isolated people who feed squirrels, pigeons, and other animals as a daily ritual, in spite of the admonished dangers of adding to the rat population. At least one person in a Nazi concentration camp kept his sanity through his interests in a rat. Other isolates become interested in insects, invent elaborate mathematical equations, recite poetry or the multiplication table, write, improvise games with pebbles or other materials, and count the features of the cell or room. Sergeant Daniel Lee Pitzer (1969), a prisoner of war of the Viet Cong, described the effect of having a cage mate:[16]

---

[15] Depersonalization refers to the feelings of unreality or strangeness concerning the environment, the self, or both.

[16] Sgt. Daniel Lee Pitzer: "The Animal Called POW: My Four Years in a Vietcong Prison," *Look*, Feb. 18, 1969, p. 48.

For eight months, I had only animals for companions. There was a squirrel—I called him Cyrano de Bergerac because he had an unusually long nose—who was hilarious. I fed him whatever I had, usually shrimp shells. On hot sunny days, he would perch on one of the logs of my cage and doze, batting his eyes and slumping, and finally toppling over in dead sleep. There was a cat, the only rice-eating cat I ever saw. . . .

A game one person played was what she called the "mostest game." She was a university dean confined to her bed by a stroke. Although living with friends, she was far across the country from her place of work and many friends and acquaintances. She asked herself, "Of all the places I have been, what did I enjoy the most?" and went on down the line with different places and events. Persons who do not have the capacity, experience, or opportunity to engage in mental play of this nature may become profoundly depressed or withdrawn, often experiencing periods of disorganized panic and dying prematurely.

The extraordinarily high death rate of American prisoners of war in the Korean conflict focused attention on the lack of inner resources in otherwise healthy young men. Under the same conditions of imprisonment the Turks did not lose one soldier. As a consequence, the Armed Services now have a program in which the men are instructed, as part of the indoctrination program, in what to do in case of capture. The recent release and the escapes of American prisoners of war in Vietnam give evidence of survival tactics. Major James N. Rowe (1969), who escaped after 5 years in a Viet Cong cage, explained his survival to a newspaper reporter: [17]

You do anything you can to keep your mind occupied. Your mental attitude—the psychological aspect of the entire thing—is what determines whether you live or die. Physically, you can survive if your mind will allow you to do so.

The behaviors of individuals under circumstances over which they have little or no control give pertinent data for the study of human behavior and suggest possibilities for application of concepts learned in nursing.

The age of the person undergoing social isolation may be a factor in his ability to withstand the isolation. If the aging process changes the nature and strength of the individual's attachment to the social system and the bonds are weakened, social isolation may ensue. For example, with a work-oriented

[17] Maj. James N. Rowe: *The New York Times*. Jan. 4, 1969, p. 10.

generation of older persons such as we have today, retirement brings about a significant change in contacts with a familiar social system. In a youth-oriented society, where values are vastly different, the older person may be alienated from the larger social system and feel separated from his milieu. Decreased income upon retirement may result in a change in living arrangements that, in effect, greatly alters the contact with previous social systems. Illness decreases the person's ability to maintain his pattern of action and the life style of his social system, as does poverty or the sudden stoppage of income. These catastrophes are most severe for an elderly person who lives alone. If the aging person's relatives cannot provide care for him, social isolation may occur rapidly, accompanied by mental changes.

With respect to those in other age groups, it should be noted that adaptation and adjustment *to confinement and social isolation* has been found to be easier than adapting and adjusting to the usual or normal environment *after confinement.* Awareness of the patient's problems when he returns home after hospitalization may help the health team to be of assistance to him. As one patient after a long hospitalization expressed it, "Convalescence is the most difficult part of getting well—it's so lonely and painful." The increased readmission rate to mental hospitals and its relation to the decline in the long-term mental hospital population require close examination. Obviously, more attention must be given to the needs of people who are returning to their communities.

Silverstein (1968) notes that of 10,786 releases of patients from 18 state mental hospitals in Pennsylvania within the year 1962–63, services most frequently requested were medications, counseling, and psychotherapy. There was, however, a low frequency of recommendations for vocational rehabilitation, resocialization, and related services. One of every four patients did not plan to live in the community with a spouse or relative. This group of released patients would especially need services to overcome social isolation.

The return to the home is as much of a crisis to the patient and family as the upset which originally led to his hospitalization. The nurse can determine whether the patient is welcome to return home, in the first place, at this particular time. More suitable arrangements for aftercare may then be made if the home situation is not conducive to the patient's recovery. Or, if the conditions at home are worse than at the hospital, the patient will naturally find a way to return to the hospital. One can also be certain that if the patient is not wanted at home, he will soon be readmitted to the hospital. If the patient is to remain at home, the nurse can inform the relatives of what to expect from him. For example, will he require aid in taking his medication, in bathing, grooming, and other aspects of personal care? How much can he be left alone? How much should he be expected to help with the household chores? The nurse can discuss with the family their feelings about the re-entry of the patient to the home setting.

Where other community agencies may be involved in the care of the patient, the nurse can tell both the family and patient how to make the best use of them. Patients who have been in a hospital where most social activities and decisions are made for them often find it extremely difficult to resume these responsibilities for themselves upon discharge. Use of the local fellowship club, church group, or other established organization can be encouraged by the nurse.

In a study of mental patients returning to the community, Silverstein (1968) noted that three out of four would live with a spouse or relative. In the same study, it was determined that 35.5 percent of the patients who returned to the hospital during the period of the study did not use available aftercare facilities. There is no doubt from the humanistic point of view that a supportive human relationship helps the returning patient reintegrate himself into society. The nurse can help the patient keep his outpatient appointment, for example, by going with him for the first time if necessary. The family may even need to be convinced that psychiatry might be of benefit, before follow-up outpatient care is accepted. The parents of one returning patient, their daughter, had no trust in psychiatry or the medical profession in general. The patient herself stated that every time she went to a doctor he sent her back to the mental hospital. A nurse could have been of assistance to the following patient, who had no available family: [18]

> *A patient discharged to his home in a big city was trying to find his way to his first out-patient appointment. His account of getting to his first appointment is as follows: "I told a man I'd pay him to go with me. Somehow we missed connections and I had to go alone. I got on the first streetcar that came along. After I'd ridden a long time, I found out I was going the wrong way. Later, when I had to change street cars, I didn't want to ask for a piece of paper, so I just kept putting money in the box. Must have spent two dollars."*

The accepting attitude of the nurse toward the patient can aid the family to realize and adapt to the fact that mental disorder has occurred to one of them.

Nurses in the homes of discharged patients can assist in the research efforts to learn about the failure syndrome of patients who are unable to cope with stressful situations encountered in the home. The nurse who is familiar with

---

[18] Max Silverstein: *Psychiatric Aftercare.* Philadelphia: University of Pennsylvania Press, 1968, p. 55.

the patient and his situation can aid in the resolution of crises and other stress points which have been documented as causes of rehospitalization. (The reader is referred to F. M. C. Evans: *The Role of the Nurse in Community Mental Health.* New York: Macmillan, 1968, for further discussion of the nurse's role.) Nurses need to be in the home with the patient and family to assess the particular situation and to assist the patient's re-entry into his usual environment.

Preventive tasks

An isolated patient should have visits from the nurse as often as is feasible for that particular patient. In addition to regular visits during meals and at the times for medication and treatment of hospitalized patients, who anticipate them eagerly, unscheduled visits are highly valued. Intercommunication systems are of great assistance here and should be used more effectively in hospitals in this age during which, it seems, communication is more easily accomplished between the earth and the moon than between the nursing station and the patient. Machines can be put to excellent use to improve human relations.

Ways to keep in touch with *time* are necessary. Every good convalescent center and nursing home should have a wall calendar with the date of the month in bold black letters easily visible to old eyes. A clock is also essential, and radio and television will help. Institutional walls are often monotonous; the nurse can see to it that patients place some of their favorite objects around the walls. The nurse should also give her attention to prompt delivery of mail and favorite foods to the patient.

Ways to overcome boredom may be found for the individual patient; what works for one may not work for the other. A thorough explanation should be made to the patient as to what is happening to him. For example, if a patient has contracted an infection during his stay in the hospital, he should be informed about the nursing preparations being made for a change in his care. Status hierarchies have no place in these interventions. However, if they are present, tact and skill are required in interpersonal relations. A nurse may feel guilty when her patient develops an infection when, in fact, she may not have had anything at all to do with it. If a patient is to be transferred to an isolation unit, now euphemistically called "special precautions" in some hospitals, the physical layout of the isolation unit should be described to him. Informing him of the name of the chief nurse and of the special rules observed in the new unit may help him adjust to the change of environment. In short, he should be prepared in every way possible for the change.

If the patient is in a ward, some explanation should be made to the other patients. They have a right to know, and some may even be enlisted to aid the patient being transferred by continuing communication with him afterward via the telephone.

To assist the patient's orientation to his new surroundings in an isolation unit, nurses can do the following: give him his new floor and room numbers and inform the visitor's desk so that all visitors, messages, and telephone calls will be transferred promptly to his new location. A patient will wonder whether the new nurse will understand what medications he is to take. How will his physician find him? Will the nurses in the new unit know that he likes to have a bath at a certain time, and so forth. It is a simple matter, but often forgotten in the hustle of transfer, to inform the patient that you will alert the nursing staff on the new unit of his needs and predilections and that the kitchen will send his special diet to the new room. Patients should be fore-warned of the restrictions on visitors in the isolation unit.

Because isolation is stressful and anxiety-producing and can be potentially detrimental to the mental health of individuals, all actions for preventive care should be carried out after an assessment has been made of the needs of the particular individual who is being isolated.

In the isolation unit itself, the nurse informs the patient of the particulars in this special environment and the purpose of what she does. Provision of an aesthetically pleasing environment is the responsibility of the nurse; for example, she can see that room equipment is arranged so that an ambulatory patient can move around freely and provide disposable decorations to break the monotony of the four walls. Seeing to it that the patient's room is clean is essential, particularly if the unit does not have a unit manager and/or a housekeeping department prepared for doing this work in isolation units. Solitary games and reading material should be made available. The preventive, restorative, and supportive potentials of the family members should be tapped if the patient has an available family.

Preventive potentials of families for isolated members center around ful-fillment of the need to belong to a group. If an isolated patient feels that he is truly still part of a family, he is more likely to be motivated to withstand the stresses of isolation. Therefore, the nurse can mobilize the family to show their concern, if they are not already doing so, with letters, cards, telephone calls, visits, and other signs and symbols of caring. Encouraging the family to talk about what is going on in the family itself can be restorative action to the isolated patient who temporarily loses his family role. The nurse can aid the family in supportive action toward the patient by keeping them informed of his condition and asking them to be helpful. Explanation can be given to them for the necessity of isolation, and they can be told ways to protect themselves so that they may be able to conquer their own fears and therefore be more accepting of the isolated member. If the isolation of the patient is to continue on a long-term basis, the need for catharsis may be met through talks with family members, telephone conversations with significant others, and venting feelings to the nurse and others who are available. The concerned nurse tries to elicit thoughts and feelings from her patient as an aid to him in adapting to the environment of isolation.

The opportunity to express thoughts, feelings, and perceptions about the experience of isolation itself can be helpful to the patient, along with reflection of feelings and restatement of responses by the nurse. Once they are shared, they become less of an emotional burden and the patient can be more objective about the question, "Why did it happen to me?" The nurse can also help the patient think through what he will do when he is released and has recovered by asking leading questions. When periods of isolation are known, the nurse can also assist the patient to note the midpoint and to celebrate that day and the day the isolation ends.

Stress of changes in body image

The body image refers to the picture a person has of himself, his inner sense of identity, where he belongs, what he can do, and his assets and liabilities. It includes sensations from muscles and their innervations. Concerned with whatever originates within—voice, breath, odors, body discharges, and hair—it is a composite of feelings and perceptions each person has of his own body, its characteristics, functions, and limits.

Development of the body image

The body image is intimately related to the development of ego functions with particular reference to reality-testing and perception. The perceptions of sight and touch in the development of the ego are differentiated as follows: [19]

[19] Willie Hoffer: "Development of the Body Ego," *Psychoanalytic Study of the Child*, Vol. 5. New York: International Universities Press, 1950, p. 19.

Coming in touch with its own body elicits two sensations of the same quality and these lead to the distinction between the self and the not-self, between body and what subsequently becomes environment. In consequence this factor contributes to the processes of structural differentiation. Delimitation between the self-body and the outer world, the world where the objects are found, is thus initiated.

In infants, the first perceptions are tactile. The ability to differentiate between the "me" and the "not me" is achieved through tactile experiences (Frank, 1958). The differentiation between the "me" and the "not me" by the infant is probably related to recognizing objects within his very specific environment. Objects experienced through tactile communication such as *my* rattle, *my* bottle, and *my* mother are recognized quite early. Later, the child replaces his specific world of "not me" objects with the concepts and symbols of the world in general. Auditory and visual cues and language add to the growth of concept formation. Therefore, transition is gradually made from the highly specific world of the child's "not me" to the world of symbols and adult concepts.

The postural model of the body plays a part in the building up of knowledge about the body (Schilder, 1950). Movement and dance change the postural model, as do sickness or maldevelopment. The horizontal patient has a different feeling about himself from having to stay in bed. The depressed patient feels differently about his body because of psychomotor changes and the older person because of sensory and motor changes. Kinesthetic stimuli are connected with a high level of cortical activity. The kinesthetic receptors are in the muscles, tendons, and joints. The labyrinthine receptors, which keep one informed as to his position in space, are in the inner ear.

There seems to be a human need to build up some idea of the wholeness of a person, whether it be accurate or not, even if we use a medium that leaves out everything but that which can be observed during a single moment of perception. Draw a circle and the human mind completes it. We can see a photograph of someone just fleetingly and feel that we know something about that person. A T.V. performer may be a familiar visitor in our home, even though he is only a picture on a screen. We often feel disappointed when we meet a person whom we have previously known only through an intervening medium. When we read a book and later see a play or a film based on it, we are frequently disappointed because our imaginings and fantasies are more satisfying to us than the interpretation projected by others. This also is true of our acquaintances, who can disappoint us because we have built up fantasies about them from the limited ways in which they appear to us; only through later experiences do we discover that they are more human and therefore more fallible than our original concept. We often feel that "they have let us down." Nursing students often experience these feelings with regard to both the profession of nursing and to physicians, if they have not had members of these professions in their families.

Parents do something similar with their children, as do teachers with pupils and nurses with patients. Nurses may judge their patients by an image that they themselves created of the "ideal patient" or the "good patient." There is a tendency to have a mental image of patients and to place them into categories. The moment you are aware that this process is going on within you, get rid of the image and find the real patient, *not what you think the patient should be.* Nurses sometimes take it as a personal affront whenever they are forced to alter the first mental picture they have of a patient. This also applies to engaged couples, whose ideas of each other often change as they become better acquainted. The "halo effect" is real. All observations have some distortions. The tendency to give to the image of oneself should also be recognized; for example, parents often force on their children goods or experiences that they themselves would have liked.

In hospital nursing, we make our patients very much aware of their bodies by constantly asking what goes in and out of them. Innumerable questions must be answered by the patient with regard to his body. The examination by the physician which may have preceded entrance to the hospital has already alerted the patient to high body concern, and further examination by the interns and residents may have occurred. Determination of the temperature, pulse, and respiration, securing urine and blood for analysis, and the routine chest x-ray may contribute to the patient's mounting body concern. In the medical history the patient has to recall all the illnesses and operations he has ever had as well as the significant diseases of his ancestors to which he might be susceptible. Inasmuch as the event of hospitalization is itself a crisis, the patient should not be asked the same questions repeatedly by different nurses. One means of avoiding repetition is to have one nurse write up the patient's history and place it on his record for all to see.

Body image is also derived from those around us, our family and our society. It may be transformed by clothes, jewelry, wigs, makeup, and false eyelashes. Some peoples put holes in their ear lobes; others put them into their noses and lips and insert wood or metal into different parts of their bodies. Body image refers to the postural model of the body and to the emotions, attitudes, and sociocultural implications.

In some hospital environments patients are estranged from contact with family members and significant others; they are cared for totally by personnel dressed in white, the symbol of sickness, dependency, and death to many patients. Those with mental problems sometimes joke about being ready for the "men in the white coats." A movement is now current to eliminate the distressing symbolism of white uniforms in favor of wearing ordinary street clothes in nursing.[20] Nurses are now beginning to doff the traditional white in some hospitals where patients stay for long-term illnesses other than psychiatric problems. At the Loeb Center, which is connected with Montefiore Hospital in New York City, all direct patient care is given by registered nurses who decide how to dress for duty. One who wore street clothes on duty stated that her dress created an association with home and wellness (Alfano, 1964). The resulting influence on the patients is a worthwhile subject for further investigation.

Stigma

Stigma[21] is a Greek term for the brand that was cut or burned into the body to advertise that the bearer was a slave. Later, in Christian times, stigma referred to bodily signs of physical disorder. Hawthorne, in the *Scarlet Letter*, records its use by the Puritans in this country to brand an adulteress. More recently, the Nazis used this method to identify Jews, criminals, and traitors.

Disease, mental disorder, and body imperfections may create in the individual the sense of bearing a stigma (whether immediately observable or not), with consequent feelings of shame and guilt. Whole families may be ashamed that one of their members has mental disorder or some debilitating disease. Huntington's chorea and other genetically determined diseases still stigmatize a family line.

Mental retardation is a classic example of stigma within families in this culture; however, Pearl Buck and the family of former President Kennedy, among others, have helped people in this country to perceive that it is no disgrace by talking freely about their own mentally retarded family members. The Mental Retardation Facilities and Community Mental Health Centers Act of 1963 (Public Law 88–164) attests to President Kennedy's concern.

---

[20] It is of interest to note that in the Soviet Union, where uniforms are otherwise quite prevalent, nurses and physicians wear street clothes over which they put on a kind of smock.

[21] Body signs designed to expose something unusual or undesirable about a person's moral status.

Impaired body image

"Imperception of body impairment" refers to a frequently observed behavior in patients who do not seem to recognize the impairment. In major disability, such unawareness takes the form of denial, as discussed earlier. It may occur with some hemiplegic patients who insist that a paralyzed arm is as good as the unparalyzed limb. Others pay no attention to their paralyzed arms, acting as if they do not belong to them. This behavior may also be an hysterical reaction, an unconscious wish which leads to changed perception and function of the body. It has also been found that obese individuals increasingly overestimated their own body size during and following weight loss. This has been referred to as "phantom body size" (Glucksman, 1969).

The phantom experience of the person who has undergone an amputation can occur with loss of arms, legs, breasts, and other external body parts. It is chiefly represented by tactile, thermal, optic, and kinesthetic sensations although it has been reported in blind persons. There may be sensations of itching, pain in a part of the limb (heel or fingernail), burning, and throbbing of an amputated part. These sensations may show the wish to maintain the body's integrity.

Occurrence of the phantom is best explained as ". . . the patient's enduring concept of his total body image after the loss of a part through amputation." [22] It does not occur in individuals who have lost internal organs. The phantom limb experience is one of the most dramatic examples of existence of a body image. Endocrine imbalances may also produce disturbances of body image. The psychiatric significance of the phantom represents an attempt at restitution of the missing part, a denial of its absence, or a somatic substitute for mourning over its loss (Gorman, 1969).

Surgical wounds may not be accepted by the patient as part of himself. Some patients may avoid looking at their wounds or washing them. Nurses can determine whether or not the patient has inspected his wound and instruct him to wash it just as he would any other part of the body, once the wound has healed.

---

[22] L. C. Kolb: *The Painful Phantom*. Springfield, Ill.: Charles C Thomas, 1954, p. 8.

Therapeutic tasks

In reference to patients with impaired body image, nurses may make such comments as: "He doesn't admit that his leg is gone"; or "She will not admit that she is fat." It must be recognized that such reactions are defenses. Tell the patient with phantom experience that you understand that he feels he still has his arm or leg and refer to the date of amputation and the reality of the situation. When the time is right, inform him of the availability of prostheses and talk it over with him several times. With a paralytic patient, acknowledge the affected limb while bathing him, feeding him, and carrying out other nursing activities. Get him to touch the affected limb and use the senses of sight and movement to aid in reorienting his body.

A main objective to remember is to aid the patient in the defense of his ego. One of the most ego-strengthening devices for the patient is to have available all the materials necessary for the body arts.

Perception of change in body image

Examples of recognition of change in body image are discussed under this heading, together with some of the implications for the nurse. No attempt will be made to cite all possible changes in body image, because it is an impossible task. However, some examples from the literature and actual nursing practice may be of help to students.

> When I got up at last . . . and had learned to walk again, one day I took a hand glass and went to a long mirror to look at myself, and I went alone. I didn't want anyone . . . to know how I felt when I saw myself for the first time. But there was no noise, no outcry: I didn't scream with rage when I saw myself. I just felt numb. That person in the mirror couldn't be me. I felt inside like a healthy, ordinary, lucky person — oh, not like the one in the mirror. Yet, when I turned my face to the mirror there were my own eyes looking back, hot with shame. When I did not cry or make a sound, it became impossible that I should speak of it to anyone, and the confusion and the panic of my discovery were

> *locked inside me then and there, to be faced alone, for a very long time to come.*[23]

A similar feeling of shame must have been felt by a patient, Mrs. Doherty, who was in a general hospital for a medical check-up and was so successful in hiding her deformed arm that the nursing staff did not notice it. An older woman, Mrs. Lloyd, now in her ninetieth year, said of her own changing body image:

> I'm looking older and uglier. I used to be so pretty. Now, look at me. I'm getting so old and ugly. My hair was so pretty and thick and now it is thin and gray and my arms are so thin.

Consider all the changes in body image of an octogenarian from birth to death and what they must have meant to the individual during the transitions. The developmental changes of infancy, childhood, and latency are well known and looked forward to by most children, who marvel at growing older and moving closer to the adults whom they admire. The infant moves from a horizontal to a crawling and then to a vertical position in this growth. At puberty there are hormonal changes with subsequent changes in body contour, hair growth, and sexual urges. Adulthood may be a kind of leveling-off period, and then comes the climacteric with decreased hormonal activity as well as other physiological changes. Continuing maturity and old age are usually accompanied by gradual changes in body image.

CHANGE IN BODY IMAGE DUE TO CANCER OF THE BREAST

If a member of your family has had a mastectomy, you may be keenly aware of the psychological impact upon her. Since cancer of the breast occurs more in middle-aged and older women who, at the same time, may be undergoing other changes, the nurse has much preventive work to do.

Teaching regular breast self-examination is done by the American Cancer Society through the use of films and brochures. All women should be taught this simple technique and urged to perform it regularly. Ninety-five percent of all breast cancers are first discovered by the women themselves. Eighty-two percent of all patients with cancer of the breast will be free of any evidence of the disease after five years—if it is discovered while still localized and if it is treated properly (American Cancer Society, 1970). Patients who have radical mastectomies will have regular and frequent check-ups and should be urged to make periodic examinations of the remaining breast. If a woman discovers

---

[23] K. B. Hathaway: *The Little Locksmith*. New York: Coward-McCann, 1943, p. 41. Copyright 1943, Coward-McCann Co.

a lump in her breast or elsewhere, she should go at once to her physician. *The lump should not be manipulated.*

After discovery of the lump, fantasies of body mutilation may be set in motion. The appointment with the physician, mammography, and the long wait for results often lead the patient to spend her waking hours thinking:

> Will the cancer have already spread? If so, how long will I have to live? Should I make my will and otherwise prepare to die? What effect will my having cancer have upon my family? What will the scar look like? Or will it heal? Will my husband ever look at me again?

The patient may review her life, looking at what she should and should not have done. She may have already prepared for death when the nurse arrives at her bedside with the preoperative medication. Waking up after surgery, the patient will instinctively examine the operative area to determine whether her breast is still there. Heavy dressings tightly taped omit some of the usual tactile clues to body image. Relaying "good news" to a patient is always a joy for the nurse, but informing a patient that her breast has been removed is painful. If the lump was benign, the patient's relief is immediate. If a radical mastectomy has been performed, the nurse prepares to assist the patient in adapting to the stress of diagnosis and to the change in body image.

The affects of guilt, shame, and depression occur. Depression is the most common (see Chapter 7 for therapeutic tasks). Patients with amputated breasts need time and privacy to sort out their thoughts and feelings. In a ward setting, patients are usually supportive of each other and respect each other's needs. If this is not the case, the nurse should enable patients to transfer to more suitable arrangements during this crisis.

Although the patient may be quite aged, widowed, or a great-grandmother with withered breasts, it is still her breast and body image. Nursing students are sometimes amazed to perceive that women in their seventies, eighties, and nineties whose breasts have served their function, so to speak, are greatly affected by a mastectomy.

For younger patients, it is difficult for the patient and her husband to take the first look at the scar. Since there is a wide variety in patient management by physicians, nurses need to be thoroughly acquainted with the style of each doctor. Some surgeons give a great deal of attention to the psychological needs of their patients; others, with busy practices, may have different priorities. The nurse should be aware of whether the patient and her husband have looked at the scar. If they have not, she should encourage them to talk about it and make a plan to do so.

Some equipment companies will send emissaries to the hospital with an assortment of prostheses. More often, with the rapid recovery rate common today, patients are returned to their homes before being fitted. Nurses can do a great deal while the patient is in the hospital to help her get ready for returning to her family and facing friends. Giving accurate information about the price of the prosthesis, the kinds available, and adjustments to be made in clothing are all necessary, but, for the patient, the actual purchase of the prosthesis is another kind of problem. If you have ever bought a "falsie" or known anyone who bought one, you understand the doubts, fears, and trepidation about approaching a saleswoman for the first time to make such a purchase, even *without* a big ugly scar.

The following is an account of the work of a student visiting an older person in her home following mastectomy.

> Mrs. Broughton had a radical mastectomy a few weeks previously. She lives with her daughter in the central city and is a member of a nearby senior center. The student learned that the patient had not been instructed about a prosthesis and did not know where to purchase one or how much it would cost. The student gave this item priority in her care; she telephoned the Social Security Office and asked if Medicare paid for it, which it did. She also did telephone shopping to determine which store had the best buy and accompanied her patient to purchase it. She learned through the surgeon that the patient had asked him to give her breast back. The student informed the surgeon and his office personnel that Medicare paid for the prosthesis (it can really be a big item in a monthly income under $120). Later, Mrs. Broughton returned to her senior center. She proudly told others "my little nurse helped me to get a breast." The student, in addition to her instrumental role (as described above), also encouraged Mrs. Broughton to discuss her thoughts and feelings concerning the loss of her breast.

The prosthesis enables the patient with a radical mastectomy partially to restore her body image. Upon seeing family and friends for the first time, after removal of a breast, she is aware that their gazes drop immediately to the breast area. Consequently, some patients may not wish to receive visitors until they are "whole again." Psychological support by the nurse to the patient and her family is one of the most important aspects of the care of those with breast cancer.

OTHER EXAMPLES

Cancer patients who have multisurgery may suffer many changes in body image. It is not uncommon for some patients to have had hysterectomy, oophorectomy, mastectomy, and adrenalectomy (see *Figure 6*). Note that the figure is neither male nor female. This diagram is used in a cancer research center to mark the sites of the cancer. Like the sexless diagram in *Figure 6* the patient may feel like an "it" instead of a man or a woman. Patients may

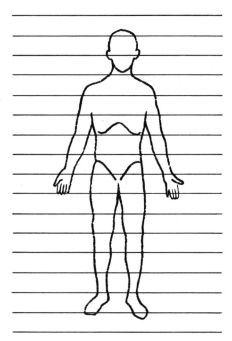

Figure 6   Diagram to mark the sites of cancer.

state that they feel "cleaned out" and as if "there isn't much left." Depending on the site of the cancer, patients may require paracentesis, thoracenteses, bone marrow studies, lymphangiograms, or other tests, all of which necessitate entry into the body. Women patients who receive androgens may develop masculine characteristics, e.g., facial hirsutism and a deep voice. Men who receive estrogens, on the other hand, may be highly embarrassed at the development of their breast tissue. Discussion with the nurse of how the patient feels about himself can help him toward adaptation to the changes within himself.

Depersonalization may also occur. It is of interest to note here that in a sensory deprivation experiment (Schulman *et al.*, 1967), 4 percent of the subjects reported changes in body image. One person reported that several times his body felt heavy and numb; another subject had the feeling that he had two heads, the second separated from the first. Still another subject had the feeling of being out of his body, above it, where he could watch it lying on the bed. He also had the feeling that he and the room were rising and floating in space.

Nursing students may often think and feel that the study of psychological man deals only with negative feelings. However, think of the changes in body image made possible by plastic reconstructive surgery. Patients who have burns and other disfiguring traumata suffer major and sometimes permanent changes in body image unless reconstructive surgery is possible. Scars acquired early in life may result in a child's avoiding any athletic or other activity that requires uncovering the scars—e.g., wearing a gym suit—unless he is assisted to make an earlier healthy adaptation. The nurse, at the time of the traumatic event, can aid the parents to look at the pretty features of a child with disfigurement and to then make plans for reconstructive surgery, if feasible. Operations for cleft palate are known to give an improved appearance, and someone dissatisfied with the shape of his nose can easily get a new profile. Those who wish to retain a youthful appearance may have their faces "lifted." A young woman with kidney disease and regular dialyses may be sensitive about the shunt in her leg.

In a study of patients with renal transplants, it was found that eight out of eleven who died following their operations had felt a sense of abandonment by their families or had experienced a panicky state and a pessimistic feeling to a greater degree than those patients who survived (Eisendrath, 1969). It may fall to the nurse and others on the health team to motivate the patient to live. If other family members can be assisted with their feelings about what is happening to one of them, the patient will have a better chance for healthy adaptation. Deep and painful psychological wounds, on the other hand, may not be so readily manifest. The nurse's sensitivity to the interrelationships and psychodynamics of the individual and his family may elicit some of these wounds also for healing and reconstruction at the same time that the body is healing.

In the era of organ transplants there is an opportunity for nurses to truly *be* health team members in a new field of surgery. Patients who receive transplants have usually been ill for a long time and welcome the decision for this change in body image by transplant. Some patients, soon after receiving organ transplants, often feel jubilant and the nurse shares in this joy. Other affects are evoked during the rejection process which call for psychological sustenance for all those concerned.

PREGNANCY

Pregnancy, which evokes universal concern with self-image (Bobak, 1969), is considered a crisis by Gerald Caplan (1962) and Highley (1963). In Bobak's work with parent education classes, she found that the area of most concern to potential mothers was that of changes in body image. The following are typical complaints:

My body does not look the same and I do not like what I see in the mirror.
My breasts are so big and ugly. The veins show terribly.
I'm so out of shape! A butterball! My husband laughs at me.

A patient, Mrs. Lockridge, pregnant with her fourth child, was admitted to a mental hospital for the latter half of her pregnancy. This was a usual occurrence in her pregnancies. She had become so irritable and hostile to her husband and her family members that the situation was unbearable for them. In the hospital, she seldom verbalized her hostility but glared at the staff with such intensity that it made them very uncomfortable. After the birth of her child the hostility gradually disappeared and she was able to return home and care for her family. Some of the main points in the nursing care of Mrs. Lockridge were to help her work it off through daily walks and enable her to meet the basic needs of personal hygiene, nutrition, and rest. Psychodynamically, it was hypothesized that she had never resolved her Electra complex and adolescent identity crisis. With each pregnancy, the fact of being a woman was re-emphasized and the old unresolved conflict brought again into the forefront.

Clinical disturbances of the mothering function are more likely to occur where the new mother does not have a well-established body image and when childbirth is seen as a loss (Main, 1968). Family-centered nursing focuses around recognition of one's own impulses and therefore being better able to assist mothers to tolerate and understand impulses within themselves. Unmarried nurses and those without children may especially be faced with recognizing their conflicts and impulses.

Sharing thoughts, feelings, perceptions, and actions within the treatment team can be of benefit to all. Since interpersonal crises may be more acute to you as a student when you are working with children and families who have new babies for the first time, look to others who are more experienced in this area for guidance and for support.

Therapeutic tasks   As individuals perceive the changes in their body images, the nurse can assist them in adapting to the new status by being available, assuming the listening and sustaining role, encouraging expression of feelings, and pointing out their assets. A pregnant patient can be given ego-strengthening support by a nurse who is able to describe what is happening in such a way that the patient can accept present body changes and look forward to their ultimate reversal. Suggestions can also be made to the husband and others to refer to the time of "getting her figure back" and to offer to buy a new dress at that time.

A fractured ego is not as easily repaired as a fractured bone—patients need time to adjust to changes and to incorporate the new image into their perception. Nurses can be supportive and do a lot of anticipatory guidance by helping the patient look ahead to the probable course of his condition until its ultimate resolution or termination.

Psychophysiological aspects of stress

Stress produces different reactions in man according to the structure of his personality, his constitution, and his experience. The nature of the stress is also a factor.

The disorders to be discussed under this heading represent the visceral expression of affect. Physiological and psychological effects of stress are interrelated, and the intermediary system between them is the autonomic nervous system (Weybrew, 1967). Where coping behavior and defense mechanisms no longer work for individuals, psychophysiological disorder may emerge. These reactions are commonly described as psychosomatic.

Psychophysiologic refers to those conditions caused by the physiological expression of chronic and exaggerated emotion, much of which is unconscious. It includes those conditions in which physiological and eventually pathological dysfunction are brought about by a chronic, repressed emotional state in the individual. A functional etiology is proposed which involves a single organ system, usually under autonomic control. The psychophysiologic disorders involve suppressed or repressed emotions gaining expression through body organs and organ systems. An example of a young woman who was unable to express grief at her mother's death demonstrates the relationship. Every time her boy friend sent her roses, she had an asthmatic attack. In a psychotherapeutic session, she recalled the roses on her mother's coffin. In this case, the asthmatic attacks were symbolic expressions of grief.

Theories of specificity with regard to the etiology of psychophysiological problems are now questioned. Selye advocates the nonspecific theory (1956). We do not yet know whether the emotional constellations of patients with these problems have specific etiology. Because they are so prevalent in our society and nursing practice, some aspects of these conditions are discussed here. Students are advised to consult textbooks of medical-surgical nursing which emphasize the physiological needs of patients with these problems.

Patients with psychophysiologic gastrointestinal disorders

A study of disability claims of 13,525 persons for a one-year period (1963–64) found 14 percent were due to disorders of the digestive system, with peptic ulcer high on the list (Cunnick, 1968). Ulcers seem to be related to the vicissitudes of the middle class in our culture.

Everybody has experienced the effect of emotions on the gastrointestinal tract. Nausea before an anticipated event or diarrhea is quite common. The transposition of feelings into words related to the organ affected are many— e.g., "You make me sick to my stomach" or "He makes me want to vomit"— and the imitation of the sounds of vomiting are quite expressive in our culture. The familiar "butterflies" in the stomach before an examination or similar performance is a universal experience. The study of an infant with a gastric fistula showed that, with the appearance of food, his stomach became hyperemic, motile, and secreted juices. It did the same thing when his favorite physician arrived. The hypothesis is made that environmental events can thus either be cognized or interpreted; they can be felt and responded to as if they were "gut" processes, which thereby involve the limbic system [24] or the visceral brain.

PATIENTS WITH PEPTIC ULCERS

Probably the most frequent of the psychophysiological disorders is the peptic ulcer. Studies of patients with gastric fistulas tend to support the impression that worry about business reverses and family quarrels affect the function of the stomach. At one time peptic ulcer was prevalent in women; now it is more frequent in men. The change in sex ratio is unexplained. Psychologically, the patient has developed a superego that forbids expression and gratification of his inner feelings and attitude of dependency. He overcompensates by being or giving the impression of being self-sufficient, competent, and industrious. Underneath the façade of self-confidence, however, he is a person with strong dependency needs.

Helping the patient with a peptic ulcer   Usually the dependency needs of the patient with a peptic ulcer are met in a very direct way. Rest and relief

---

[24] The limbic system borders the part of the brain that has to do with olfaction. It consists of two rings of medially located cortex along the amygdala, hippocampus, and septal nuclei. The limbic system has several circuits; it is connected with the hypothalamus and is concerned with sex and emotions (Guyton, 1969).

of stress and anxiety are recommended by the physician. Achieving these is accomplished in various ways within different individuals. A hunting or fishing trip, a vacation, or hospitalization may be prescribed.

One of my patients, a prominent executive in high tension work, promised his physician that he would come into the hospital if he could have a telephone in his room. The compromise was made, and instead of dealing all day with his usual business, he made $1000 on the horses that week. In hospitals, the nurse-patient relationship can be strengthened by frequent contacts; sending others to make the contact for you is not the answer. Chronic psychophysiological disorders arouse dependency needs, and whether the dependency needs are present because of illness or the basis of it is not always clear. After the ulcer is healed, it may be difficult for some patients to give up their dependency gratifications.

Secondary gain[25] is sometimes a factor in delaying recovery. Fear of the unknown is of concern to all people. The nurse can educate the patient about his disorder and help eradicate fear.

The first goal to accomplish with the patient is to meet his dependency needs. If he requires a bed bath, give it to him. If he needs someone with him constantly, give him the necessary attention so he can then move gradually to independence again. Sensitivity to dependency needs of patients can be developed. In hospitals, bureaucracies and hierarchies should not interfere with your meeting the needs of your patient. Since the patient with an ulcer is likely to be on a diet of half milk and half cream together with an antiacid medication at designated and regular intervals, attention must be given to this to prevent added stress and attention. Being on this kind of diet is a symbolic return to infancy and arouses many feelings relating to the image of the "good mother" and "bad mother." The diet itself of milk and cream is a kind of symbolic return to the breast (or bottle), and the nurse therefore becomes a mother figure. The giving, loving mother figure provides the patient with the supplies he needs without his having to ask for them.

The nurse is responsible also for the milieu of the patient and must be alert to noxious stimuli from the environment. If he is in a ward with other patients, constant analysis of interaction among the patients will aid in early identification of conflicts and tension which perhaps can be handled.

Patients with peptic ulcers frequently have tests done on the G.I. tract that require fasting. Considering the patient's comfort, the thoughtful nurse arranges for him to have these tests the first thing in the morning.

With regard to "no smoking," the nurse is often caught up between the

---

[25] Secondary gain refers to the rewards derived from illness. Attention, disability benefits, and other rewards such as release from responsibility are not easily relinquished.

order of the physician and the wishes of the patient. Policing the patient is not the nurse's role. Cigarettes removed from the room of a patient who is not ready to quit will soon be replaced. An emotional contretemps between nurse and patient over the "no smoking" rule only aggravates the ulcerous condition. The nurse can reiterate the effects of smoking and perhaps help the patient give it up. Very little impact will be made on the patient if the nurse reeks of tobacco smoke.

Anticipation of needs, provision of supplies, a therapeutic environment, and meeting dependency needs add up to effective nursing care of the patient with a peptic ulcer.

PATIENTS WITH ULCERATIVE COLITIS

One of the interesting facts of history is that a medical student in the 1930's observed in his patients with ulcerative colitis a well-marked relationship between an emotional disturbance and the onset of symptoms (Murray, 1930). One of his patients had bloody diarrhea on the very day that she was secretly married. Many patients with this disorder have had humiliating rejections from their mothers. Every patient with ulcerative colitis should have a psychiatric consultation before any consideration of surgery. In the course of treatment, the protective support of a hospital setting may be necessary. The seriousness of a bleeding bowel must never be overlooked. The psychiatrist may insist on no medication for the patient, the internist may prescribe many medications, and the surgeon may recommend an ileostomy.

Helping patients with ulcerative colitis   With every patient, the principal aim of nursing care is to provide support. If the etiology of the ulcerative colitis is loss, knowledge of the process of grief and mourning will aid in helping the patient to accomplish his grief work. Sensitivity to the changes of mood and interactions with others enables the nurse to help the patient discuss his feelings. Dietary intake is important; special diets are usually provided from which the patient can make choices. Patients may be ambulatory, or complications may require bed rest. In the latter case, dependency needs take precedence. It is not uncommon for the patient with ulcerative colitis to have a psychotic breakdown, and all members of the health team should be alert to this possibility. Each person is different, and there are no easy rules to follow. It is important to avoid getting into a tug of war with the patient over what he will eat and what he can eat, just for the sake of observing limits. Mistakes made in the diet kitchen can be corrected matter-of-factly and a real attempt made to get the food the patient can eat and to make it look attractive. Since food is the "original tranquilizer," it and the attitudes of the helping persons toward providing it are of central importance in nursing care.

Patients with psychophysiologic cardiovascular disorders

The effect of emotions on the heart and the blood vessels is symbolized in our culture by such expressions as "He'll give me a heart attack yet" or "She makes my heart ache." We also admonish angry people to "watch out for your blood pressure." The attention given to the heart emphasizes the importance of this organ. Any hint of trouble in the cardiovascular system itself may increase anxiety.

Paroxysmal tachycardia, vascular spasms, and migraine also fall under this heading.

If a person is angry, one of the normal results is an increase in blood pressure. This occurs in everyone. However, the patient with psychophysiologic cardiovascular disorder—e.g., hypertension—is thought to remain constantly angry; therefore, his blood pressure remains higher than normal (see *Figure 7*). Increased epinephrine flow constricts the blood vessels and increases the heart rate. The constricted blood vessels result in a patient's being "white with anger" and having heightened blood pressure.

Following is a description of a patient with hypertension.

> The patient, now in his fifties, was the oldest child in a large family. The father died when he was 12, and he assumed the role of father and "husband" to the mother in the sense that he listened to her problems and those of the family members. During adolescence, he was not permitted the normal activities and expressions of rebellion and detachment from the family, because of heavy responsibilities—social, emotional, and work. One affect denied expression was anger. If things within the family had to be done—taking care of the pets, a stray dog, or a kitten; being sure that all the kids got their share at the table; being nice to siblings when he would prefer to give them a big wallop—he had the responsibility. This child with the highly developed sense of responsibility, not permitted to express anger, developed hypertension.

Although there is no unique personality pattern in the patient with hypertension, certain relationships are hypothesized and acted upon in treatment. Clinically one sees psychophysiologic disorders in all kinds of personalities. However, in one study the hypertensive subjects did appear to be similar in their view of life, in their evaluation of events, problems, and challenges, and the manner in which they dealt with them (Wolf, 1955).

Treatment of the patient usually centers around long-term outpatient

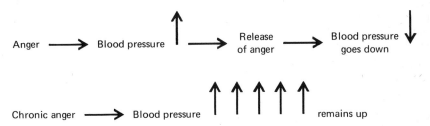

Figure 7   The relationship of anger and high blood pressure.

care in which a rapport between the patient and his physician is of utmost importance. Various drugs are used, as well as other therapeutic modalities.

THE ROLE OF THE NURSE
Denial is one of the frequent adaptive mechanisms and should be recognized by the nurse. The reader is referred to page 153 of this chapter for further discussion of this mental mechanism. Removal of the patient from the stressful environment may help. In the immediate surroundings of the patient in the hospital, a careful monitoring of his environment is necessary to assure rest and relaxation. With the numbers and kinds of personnel involved in hospital care, jurisdictional disputes often occur in a patient's room. The milieu has traditionally been the responsibility of the nurse. If the maid and the janitor have an argument in front of the patient, for example, you are not providing a therapeutic milieu.

The nurse can discuss ways of handling anger with the patient. Use of various methods to bring about self-assertion can be helpful. Physical exercise releases anger and can be encouraged by the nurse within the limits advised by the physician. The totem of sticking pins into the image of the boss is not a bad idea. Changing jobs may temporarily help relieve the stress of difficult situations. When professionals advise patients with hypertension to take it easy, they are not being very helpful. A patient with repressed and suppressed anger needs assistance in finding diversions. Peaceful walks and nature studies on a regular basis may be all that he needs. Family members may participate in provision of this diversion; enlist their aid.

Patients with psychophysiologic respiratory disorders

Respiration is the only essential bodily activity under both voluntary and involuntary control (Wittkower and White, 1967). It is the first independent action of the newborn. Breath-holding attacks, characteristic of childhood, customarily disappear spontaneously between the ages of four and six. Attacks usually occur after a frustrating event which result in rage and crying. Crying stops with expiratory apnea, and recovery is spontaneous. Nurses can gain pertinent data from family visits where determination of ways that they handle frustration and anger can be made and suggestions for improvement outlined.

Asthmatic attacks are frequently brought on by crises in life such as marriage and pregnancy. An asthmatic attack is serious and demands immediate attention. Patients are therefore likely to be seen in outpatient departments, emergency units, and intensive respiratory care centers of general hospitals. Some bronchial asthmas are due to high allergic situations. Many patients, however, do not have strong reactions to allergy tests. There may be an undercurrent deeply repressed, of a need for mother, a fear of estrangement from mother, or the mother substitute. Asthmatic attacks are tied up with the way in which the infant's cries brought mother; they can be viewed as symbolic cries for mother (French and Alexander, 1941). Other factors such as surgery, respiratory infections, or a traumatic experience with water may activate the patient's unconscious conflicts, with the respiratory tract becoming the organ for somatic expression. A constellation of factors probably accounts for the etiology of asthma (Wittkower and White, 1967).

THE ROLE OF THE NURSE
The nurse's presence helps allay anxiety. Staying with the patient during an acute asthmatic attack is important to provide security, one of the antidotes for a stressful situation. Special nonallergenic mattresses and pillows are usually available. A carefully made allergy history must be made available to all. Nurses take this history in some institutions and post it on the cover of the patient's chart in a visible spot. Listening to the patient's description of the onset of his attack may be helpful to the health team in determining etiological factors which, in turn, determine the treatment modality.

Patients with neuroses

Patients with neuroses usually receive treatment on an outpatient basis. Psychoanalysis and psychoanalytically oriented psychotherapy are the treatments of choice. Hypnosis and narcosynthesis have been used in the past, and hypnotherapy is still employed. Behavioral therapy is now advised for some patients. These patients are apt to be of more concern to the nurse as nursing practice moves beyond the walls of institutions.

Hysterical neurosis

The hysterical neurosis, conversion type,[26] differs from the psychophysiological disorders in that the anxiety is alleviated by the symptom, the symptom is expressed symbolically, and there are usually no structural changes within the body that threaten life. In a sophisticated society, conversion reactions are generally rare. This is thought to be due, in part, to the prevalence of mass media satire of these conditions. However, they still do appear in individuals. The first patient I saw with hysterical paralysis could not move her right leg. The chief of psychiatry inserted a spinal needle into the muscle, and the patient sat as if she had not been touched at all. This dramatic demonstration convinced skeptical students of the impact and importance of the unconscious life of the individual.

An hysterical neurosis is differentiated from malingering, which is a conscious simulation of disability. For example, the patient who makes up her own eye medicine and applies it to keep the pupils dilated and achieve a status of blindness does not have the same problem as the individual whose wife is killed in an accident and who becomes blind on the spot.

Hysterical neuroses are more likely to occur during catastrophes. In a highly technological society such as ours, their occurrence does not assume the importance they had in other centuries. During the time of Florence Nightingale, for instance, they were fashionable and socially acceptable.

Since one of the most anxiety-producing situations for man is severance of communication, the nurse can help the hysterical patient by maintaining a nonjudgmental attitude toward him and keeping communication channels open. If she is visiting in the home, she can, by example, influence family members to do likewise. Reassurance that function will be restored can be helpful.

In the dissociative type of hysterical neurosis, alterations in the patient's state of consciousness appear. Attempts to deal with anxiety can result in a walling off of some parts of consciousness from others. Amnesia is one result, somnambulism, fugue states, and multiple personality are others.

[26] In the conversion type, the special senses are affected, causing symptoms of blindness, deafness, anosmia, anesthesias, and paralyses.

The amnesia patient may be discovered miles away from his home and loved ones without any idea as to how he got there. The amnesia may be circumscribed (for a certain period of time), anterograde (from the traumatic situation forward), or retrograde (for all events prior to the trauma).

Although anorexia nervosa does not appear in the *Diagnostic and Statistical Manual of Mental Disorders, II* (1968), it is mentioned here because one of the principal problems of the nurse and the medical team is to get the patient to take enough food to stay alive. Anorexia nervosa occurs mostly in adolescent girls. There is marked reduction in food intake and a distaste for food. Amenorrhea is common; constipation, a slowed pulse (56–60) and respiration (12), and a subnormal temperature (one-half to one degree below normal) occur. Although the patient remains active and energetic, there is a significant weight loss. This is so marked that the skin is drawn tightly over the bones and the sufferer presents a cadaverous appearance.

The distinguishing signs from other conditions of cachexia and weight loss are: (1) it occurs mostly in teen-age girls; (2) the reduction in dietary intake is psychically determined; (3) vomiting occurs and is sometimes self-induced; and (4) amenorrhea, constipation, and cachexia are present (Thomä, 1967). The condition can lead to death. Patients with anorexia nervosa are treated out of the family environment. A variety of medications have been used in treatment as well as the biological therapies of psychiatry and psychotherapy. Thomä reports that there is no doubt that those patients under his care who receive psychotherapy have the best prospects for recovery (1967, p. 62).

One of the principal nursing problems centers around dietary intake. Forced feeding does not solve the problem and sometimes leads to suicide. Also, self-induced vomiting can reduce temporary effects of forced feedings. The patient needs attention at meal time. Sitting with him may help, or spoon feeding him if he will not feed himself; if it is possible, get him food that he will eat. It may be necessary in some cases to inform the patient that he will die if he does not eat.

The psychopathological picture of patients with anorexia nervosa is so diverse that a tabulation is meaningless (Thomä, 1967). Freud equated anorexia nervosa with melancholia and related it to undeveloped sexuality. He also advised that psychoanalysis should not be attempted in a case of hysterical anorexia (Freud, 1957, p. 264). If the patient is punishing himself by not eating, adding more punishment is not effective. Forced feeding has an element of punishment and therefore should be avoided; intravenous feeding may be necessary. Research on this psychically determined reduction of food intake will undoubtedly give further guidelines to the helping professions.

Psychological invalidism

In our culture, there is often a stigma attached to people who have psychological problems. However, it is socially acceptable to have physiological problems. Psychological invalidism may be a form of social disability, which can also appear as unemployment or crime. In France, West Germany, Austria, Italy, and other countries, people with psychological invalidism go to the "baths," which were popular in some sections of this country in the 1890's and early 1900's.

Some members of the aging population, who may already have several chronic diseases, take refuge in somaticizing. With the decline in physical health and strength, every ache and pain may be interpreted as the beginning of the final dissolution of the body. Outpatient departments and case loads of public health nurses include some of these people.

If attention is given to bodily complaints and little of it is available elsewhere, the complaints are likely to continue. Patients sometimes go to clinics and physicians' offices two to three times a week for this attention. The same type of person may seek out spurious practitioners of medicine or buy fake devices he thinks will make him feel better.

Patients with psychological invalidism may not have any concomitant physiological changes. Everybody is familiar with the milder forms, where nausea and vomiting occur when a distasteful event is in store for the individual, or a transitory headache appears if a date has been made that one would like to cancel. In individuals with psychological invalidism, secondary gain may be the central focus.

Iatrogenic (physician-induced) heart disease should be mentioned here. We all know patients who pay close attention to every aspect of a health examination. If the physician hears a slightly different heart sound and mentions it, such a patient may interpret and distort this as an indication that he has a serious problem; he will then behave as if he actually has heart damage. Another example is the patient highly anxious about going to the physician whose blood pressure increases markedly. Some physicians simply have someone else take the blood pressure of such an individual.

In caring for patients who are hypochondriacal, one of the principal aims of nursing care is directed toward giving the patient attention in areas other than those of the body complaints. One of the first reactions of students is frustration because all initial contacts with the hypochondriac person are prefaced by catalogues of body symptoms. In the development of a meaningful relationship with the patient, listening to what he has to say is imperative. Hypochondriacal patients may develop physiological problems just like anyone else; all symptoms should receive the attention of a professional. Anticipate the needs of your patient and administer to them without his having to demand this from you. This disarms the patient, allowing you to take the initiative and move forward to discuss something other than symptoms. The patient only feels further isolated, rejected, and unloved if he has no one to whom he can turn.

> A patient, Joachim, an Israeli student, far away from home on the West Coast of the United States, had an operation on his nose. After the operation his nose was heavily bandaged. Every time the nurse entered his room he recited a long list of body sensations and clung to her presence. His body complaints were determined by the staff to be due to anxiety about respiration, so a nurse was assigned to special duty to relieve the anxiety. The presence of the nurse, to whom he could turn instantaneously, relieved his anxiety. The somaticizing disappeared, and he relaxed.

Patients with obsessive compulsive neuroses

Unwelcome and unwanted thoughts, urges, and actions characterize the person with an obsessive compulsive neurosis. They are repetitive, and the patient views them as nonsensical; however, he is unable to stop them. These individuals separate an idea from its associated affect, which is repressed and expressed later as an obsession. The ritual of the compulsion negates an unacceptable urge.

Severe obsessive compulsive behavior is difficult to treat. Psychoanalysis or psychoanalytically oriented psychotherapy is preferred. A patient with this neurosis may appear for psychiatric treatment only after losing a job, alienating family members, and spending all the family money. In institutional settings, the nurse can note the compulsions and take required action to preserve life. For example, if the patient spends most of the day washing his hands, his nutritional state will suffer. If his compulsion is interfered with, his anxiety level heightens; thus it is up to the nurse to find a time to help the obsessive compulsive patient meet his basic needs. He may be ostracized by other patients if he makes them late for an outing. It is best to make individual schedules for the obsessive compulsive patient. A warm permissive nurse who does not feel threatened by the patient's rituals will usually be able to help him meet his basic needs. A lot of repair work may be called for to help the patient restore his position within his family. The nurse's attitude toward the patient influences the family members, and discussing his limitations with them can help them to better understand the behavior. I once had a patient who had a compulsion to sit on the toilet all day and another who could never wear the same set of clothes twice without their being cleaned in between wearings.

It is important to avoid adopting a perceptual set about the patient and acting as if every day is the same. Diversion is important to the patient, and a nurse with broad interests—e.g., in music, theater, art, sports, and current events—will help him find enjoyment in life.

Patients with phobias

In the case of phobias, there is an intense fear of objects or situations such as dogs or high places. Manifestations of phobias range from a mild faintness to panic. At the same time, the patient is conscious of the fact that these objects or situations are not harmful to him. His anxiety is displaced to the object or situation from some other object or situation of which he is unaware. A list of phobias includes nyctophobia, agoraphobia, claustrophobia, aerophobia, phonophobia, xenophobia, carcinomatophobia, ylophobia, syphilophobia, thanatophobia, zelophobia, and zoophobia. There are many others. Childhood is fraught with phobias of many kinds. School phobia is discussed in Chapter 2.

Psychoanalysis or psychoanalytically oriented psychotherapy is usually the treatment of choice, and nurses usually do not intervene in the phobic situation. However, collection of data relevant to the total life situation and personality of the patient can be of great importance in the treatment. Support of family members is needed. Close collaboration of all members of the psychiatric team aids in setting treatment goals if the patient is in an interdisciplinary treatment setting. Behavioral therapy with its desensitization techniques is now being used by psychologists and others in treating phobias (Susskind and Franks, 1968).

Summary

This chapter on patients under stress focuses on conflict, tension, and anxiety with emphasis on identifying the defenses against anxiety. The therapeutic tasks of the nurse are outlined. Stresses of sensory deprivation upon the individual are presented, effects described, and the concepts of confinement, immobilization, and social isolation emphasized.

Some background discussion of the development of the body image is included in this chapter. Stigma resulting from multiple causes is presented. Impaired body image is discussed with some concentration on the phantom limb. Changes of body image due to cancer of the breast, obesity, and pregnancy are discussed with reference to therapeutic and preventive nursing action. Some psychophysiological aspects of stress in patients are included in this section, which concludes with a discussion of some neurotic conditions encountered in nursing practice.

References

Alfano, Genrose, and Bernardin, Estelle: "Can Nursing Care Hasten Recovery?" *American Journal of Nursing*, **64**:80–85, June, 1964.

American Cancer Society: pamphlet on "Breast Self Examination," New York, 1970.

American Psychiatric Association: *A Psychiatric Glossary*. Washington, D.C.: American Psychiatric Association, 1969.

———— *Diagnostic and Statistical Manual of Mental Disorders, II.* Washington, D.C.: American Psychiatric Association, 1968.

Bartlett, Lewis F.: "Institutional Peonage," *Atlantic*, **214**:1:116–19, July, 1964.

Bexton, W. H., Heron, W., and Scott, T. H.: "Effects of Decreased Variation in the Sensory Environment," *Canadian Journal of Psychology*, **8**:70, June, 1954.

Bobak, Irene: "Self-image: A Universal Concern of Women Becoming Mothers," *Bulletin of the San Francisco County Nurses' Association*, **20**:2, 1969.

Bowman, Karl M.: "Group Psychotherapy—Historical Perspectives," *Proceed-

ings of 2nd Annual Western Regional Meeting, American Group Psychotherapy Association, 1957, p. 43.

Buhler, Charlotte: *Values in Psychotherapy*. New York: The Free Press of Glencoe, 1962.

California's Office of Public Information, Dept. of Mental Hygiene: "Stepping Out: A Resocialization Production," *One System Ten Services*, **1**:4:4–5, July 20, 1970.

Cannon, Walter: *The Wisdom of the Body*. New York: W. W. Norton Co., 1932.

Caplan, Gerald: *Principles of Preventive Psychiatry*. New York: Basic Books, Inc., 1964.

Cunnick, W. R., Eide, Arne, Smith, Norbert J.: "Digestive Disease as a National Problem." New York: Metropolitan Life Insurance Co., Medical Department, 1968.

Duffy, E.: *Activation and Behavior*. New York: John Wiley and Sons, 1962.

Durkheim, Emile: *Suicide*. New York: Free Press, 1951.

Eisendrath, Robert M.: "The Role of Grief and Fear in the Death of Kidney Transplant Patients," *American Journal of Psychiatry*, **123**:3:381–87, 1969.

Ellis, Rosemary, Jackson, C. Wesley, Rich, Rosemary, Hughey, George Ann, and Schlotfeldt, Rozella M.: "Suggestions for the Care of Eye Surgery Patients Who Experience Reduced Sensory Input," *ANA Regional Clinical Conferences*. New York: Appleton-Century-Crofts, 1967, pp. 131–38.

Engel, George L.: *Psychological Development in Health and Disease*. Philadelphia: W. B. Saunders Co., 1962.

English, O. Spurgeon, and Finch, Stuart M.: *Introduction to Psychiatry*. New York: W. W. Norton Co., 1961.

Evans, F. M. C.: *The Role of the Nurse in Community Mental Health*. New York: The Macmillan Co., 1968.

———— "Visiting Older People: A Learning Experience," *Nursing Outlook*, **17**:3:20–23, March, 1969.

Frank, Lawrence K.: "Tactile Communication," *ETC*, **16**:31–79, 1958.

Frankl, Viktor E.: *Man's Search for Meaning*. Boston: Beacon Press, 1959, pp. 106–107.

Fraser, T. M.: "The Effects of Confinement as a Factor in Manned Space Flight," National Aeronautics and Space Administration, Washington, D.C., 1966 (NASA CR-511).

French, T. N., and Alexander, F.: *Psychogenic Factors in Bronchial Asthma. Psychosomatic Medicine*. Monograph 4, Washington, D.C.: National Research Council, 1941.

Freud, Sigmund: *Complete Psychological Works*, Vol. 7. London: Hogarth Press, 1957.

Glucksman, Myron L., and Hirsch, Jules: "The Response of Obese Patients to Weight Reduction," *Psychosomatic Medicine*, **31**:1:1—7, January-February, 1969.

Gorman, Warren: *Body Image and the Image of the Brain*. St. Louis: Warren H. Green, Inc., 1969.

Grand Illusion, Film, by Jean Renoir, 1938.

Greenwood, Allen: "Mental Disturbances Following Operation for Cataract," *Journal of the American Medical Association*, **91**:1713—15, December 1, 1928.

Grinker, R. R., Sr., and Spiegel, J. P.: *Men Under Stress*. Philadelphia: Blakiston, 1945.

Guyton, Arthur C.: *Function of the Human Body*. Philadelphia: W. B. Saunders Co., 1969, pp. 349—54.

Hathaway, K. B.: *The Little Locksmith*. New York: Coward-McCann, 1943, p. 41.

Hawthorne, Nathaniel: *The Scarlet Letter*. Boston: Houghton Mifflin, 1883.

Heron, Woodburn: "The Pathology of Boredom," *Scientific American*, **CXCVI**: January, 1957, pp. 52—56.

Highley, Betty: "Antepartal Nursing Intervention," *Nursing Forum*, **II**:63—80, 1963.

Hoffer, Willie: "Development of the Body Ego," *Psychoanalytic Study of the Child*. Vol. 5. New York: International Universities Press, 1950, p. 19.

Joern, Albert T.: Personal communication, 1967.

King Rat, Film, Columbia, 1965.

Kolb, Lawrence C.: *Noyes' Modern Clinical Psychiatry*. Philadelphia: W. B. Saunders, 1968.

————— *The Painful Phantom*. Springfield, Ill.: Charles C Thomas, 1954.

————— "Disturbances of the Body Image," in Arieta, Silvano, ed.: *American Handbook of Psychiatry*, Vol. 1. New York: Basic Books, 1959, pp. 749—69.

————— "Phantom Sensations, Hallucinations, and the Body Image," in West, Louis Jolyn, ed.: *Hallucinations*. New York: Grune and Stratton, Inc., 1962, pp. 239—48.

A Late Inmate of the Glasgow Royal Asylum for Lunatics at Gartnavel, 1947. (No other publication data available.)

Leiderman, P. Herbert, Mendelson, Jack H., Wexler, Donald, Solomon, Philip: "Sensory Deprivation: Clinical Aspects," *Archives of Internal Medicine*, **101**:389—96, 1958.

Lilly, J. C., and Shurley, J. T.: "Experiments in Solitude on Maximum Achievable Physical Isolation with Suspension of Intact, Healthy Persons," in

Flaherty, B. E., ed.: *Psychophysiological Aspects of Space Flight*. New York: Columbia University Press, 1961.

Linn, L. *et al.*: "Patterns of Behavior Disturbance Following Cataract Extraction," *American Journal of Psychiatry*, **110**:281–89, 1953.

Lowenthal, Marjorie F.: "Social Isolation and Mental Illness in Old Age," in Newgarten, Bernice L., *Middle Age and Aging*. Chicago: University of Chicago Press, 1968.

Luchterhand, Elmer: "Prisoner Behavior and Social System in the Nazi Concentration Camps," *International Journal of Social Psychiatry*, **13**:4:245–64, 1967.

Lunceford, Janet L.: "Nursing Care of Patients in a Life Island Isolator," 1965 Regional Clinical Conference. New York: American Nurses Association.

Main, T. F.: "A Fragment on Mothering," in Barnes, Elizabeth, ed.: *Psychosocial Nursing*. London: Tavistock Publications, 1962.

Mann, Thomas: *The Magic Mountain*. New York: Knopf, 1946.

Meerloo, Joost A. M.: *Illness and Cure*. New York: Grune and Stratton, 1964.

Menninger, Karl: *The Vital Balance*. New York: The Viking Press, 1963.

Murray, Cecil D.: "Psychogenic Factors in the Etiology of Ulcerative Colitis and Bloody Diarrhea," *American Journal of the Medical Sciences*, **239**:248, 1930.

Pitzer, Sgt. Daniel Lee: "The Animal Called POW: My Four Years in a Vietcong Prison," *Look*, February 18, 1969, pp. 46–51.

Pratt, Joseph: in Bowman, op. cit.

Rowe, James: *The New York Times*. January 4, 1969, p. 10.

Ruff, G. E., and Levy, E. Z.: "Psychiatric Research in Space Medicine," *American Journal of Psychiatry*, **115**:793–97, 1959.

———— and Thaler, V. H.: "Studies of Isolation and Confinement," *Aerospace Medicine*, **30**:599, 1959.

Schilder, Paul: *The Image and Appearance of the Human Body*. New York: International Universities Press, 1950.

Schoenberg, Bernard, Pettit, Helen F., and Carr, Arthur C.: *Teaching Psychosocial Aspects of Patient Care*. New York: Columbia University Press, 1968.

Schulman, Carol A., Richlin, Milton, and Weinstein, Sidney: "Hallucinations and Disturbances of Affect, Cognition, and Physical State as a Function of Sensory Deprivation," *Perceptual and Motor Skills*, **25**:1001–24, 1967.

Schultz, Duane P.: *Sensory Restriction*. New York: Academic Press, 1965.

Seeman, Melvin: "On the Meaning of Alienation," *American Sociological Review*, **24**:783–91, 1959.

Selye, Hans: *The Stress of Life*. New York: McGraw-Hill Book Co., Inc., 1956.

Shurley, Jay T.: "Reduced Sensory Input States," in McCally, M., ed.: *Hypodynamics and Hypogravics.* New York: Academic Press, 1968.

———— "Stress and Adaptation as Related to Sensory/Perceptual Isolation Research," *Military Medicine*, **131**:254–58, March, 1966.

———— "Adaptation to Sensory Isolation," in Rhead, C., ed.: *Stress and Adaptation.* Forest Hospital Lecture Series, **4**:32–41, November, 1965.

———— "The Hydro-Hypodynamic Environment," *Proceedings of the Third World Congress of Psychiatry.* Toronto: University of Toronto Press, **3**:232–37, 1963.

———— "Problems and Methods in Experimental Sensory Input Alterations and Invariance," in Tourlentes, T. T., Pollack, S. L., and Himwich, H. E.: *Research Approaches to Psychiatric Problems.* New York: Grune and Stratton, 1962, pp. 145–60.

———— "Hallucinations in Sensory Deprivation and Sleep Deprivation," in West, L. J., ed.: *Hallucinations.* New York: Grune and Stratton, 1962, pp. 87–91.

———— "Mental Imagery in Profound Experimental Sensory Isolation," in West, *supra.*, pp. 153–57.

———— "Profound Experimental Sensory Isolation," *American Journal of Psychiatry*, **117**:539–45, 1960.

Silverstein, Max: *Psychiatric Aftercare.* Philadelphia: University of Pennsylvania Press, 1968.

Solomon, Philip, Kubzansky, Philip E., Leiderman, P. Herbert, Mendelson, Jack H., Trumbull, Richard, and Wexler, Donald: *Sensory Deprivation.* Cambridge, Mass.: Harvard University Press, 1965.

Spitz, René A.: "Hospitalism: An Inquiry into the Genesis of Psychiatric Conditions in Early Childhood," *The Psychoanalytic Study of the Child*, **1**:53–74, 1945.

Stevenson, Robert Louis: *A Child's Garden of Verses.* New York: Charles Scribner's Sons, 1901, p. 5 and p. 21.

———— *Dr. Jekyll and Mr. Hyde.* New York: Charles Scribner's Sons, 1897.

Susskind, Dorothy, and Franks, Cyril M.: Notes taken from lecture and demonstration of behavioral therapy, Kujbischeff Sanitorium, Yalta, U.S.S.R., July 30, 1968.

Thomä, Helmut: *Anorexia Nervosa.* New York: International Universities Press, 1967.

Tillich, Paul: *The Courage to Be.* New Haven: Yale University Press, 1952.

Townsend, Peter: *The Family Life of Old People.* Baltimore: Penguin Books, 1963.

Vernon, J., and Hoffman, J.: "Effects of Sensory Deprivation on Learning Rate in Human Beings," *Science*, **123**:1074–75, 1956.

Weddell, Doreen: "Family-Centered Nursing," in Barnes, Elizabeth, ed.: *Psychosocial Nursing.* London: Tavistock Publications, 1968.

Weinstein, Sidney, Richlin, Milton, Weisinger, Marvin, and Fisher, Larry: "The Effects of Sensory Deprivation in Sensory, Perceptual, Motor, Cognitive, and Physiological Functions," Washington, D.C.: National Aeronautics and Space Administration, 1967 (NASA CR-727).

Weismann, A. D., and Hackett, T. P.: "Psychosis After Eye Surgery, Establishment of a Specific Doctor-Patient Relation in the Prevention and Treatment of 'Black Patch' Delirium," *New England Journal of Medicine*, **258**:2:1284–89, 1958.

Wexler, D., Mendelson, J., Leiderman, P. H., and Solomon, P.: "Sensory Deprivation: A Technique for Studying Psychiatric Aspects of Stress," *Archives of Neurology and Psychiatry*, **79**:225, 1958.

Weybrew, Benjamin B.: "Patterns of Psychophysiological Response to Military Stress," in *Conference on Psychological Stress*, Toronto. New York: Appleton-Century-Crofts, 1967, pp. 324–62.

Wilde, Oscar: "The Ballad of Reading Gaol," in Maine, G. F., ed.: *The Works of Oscar Wilde*. London: Collins, 1948, p. 822.

Wilson, M. W.: "Nursing Care in Adult Cataract Cases," *American Journal of Nursing*, **31**:33–36, 1931.

Wittkower, Eric D., and White, Kerr L.: "Psychophysiologic Aspects of Respiratory Disorders," in Arieti, Silvano, ed.: *American Handbook of Psychiatry*, Vol. I. New York: Basic Books, Inc., 1959, pp. 690–707.

Wolf, Stewart, Cardon, Philippe, Shepard, Edward M., and Wolff, Harold G.: *Life Stress and Essential Hypertension*. Baltimore: The Williams and Wilkins Co., 1955, p. 232.

Wolff, Harold G.: "Stressors as a Cause of Disease in Man," in *Stress and Psychiatric Disorder*. Mental Health Research Fund Proceedings. Oxford: Blackwell Scientific Publications, 1961, pp. 17–31.

Suggested readings

Alvarez, Walter C.: *The Neuroses*. Philadelphia: W. B. Saunders, 1951.

Bleestone, Harvey, and McGoher, Carl L.: "Reaction to Extreme Stress; Impending Death by Execution," *American Journal of Psychiatry*, **119**:5:393–96, November, 1962.

Bruch, Hilda: "The Insignificant Difference; Discordant Incidence of Anorexia Nervosa in Monozygotic Twins," *American Journal of Psychiatry*, **119**:5:393–96, November, 1962.

Cleaver, Eldridge: *Soul on Ice*. New York: Dell Publishing Co., Inc., 1968.

Dlin, Barney M., Perlman, Abraham, and Ringold, Evelyn: "Psychosexual

Response to Ileostomy and Colostomy," *American Journal of Psychiatry,* **123**:3:374—81, September, 1969.

Engel, G. L., and Schmale, A. H.: "Psychoanalytic Theory of Somatic Disorder: Conversion, Specificity and the Disease Onset Situation," *Journal of the American Psychoanalytic Association,* **15**:334—65, 1967.

Fenichel, Otto: *The Psychoanalytic Theory of Neurosis.* New York: W. W. Norton and Co., Inc., 1945.

Franks, Cyril M., and Susskind, Dorothy J.: "Behavior Modification with Children: Rationale and Technique," *Journal of School Psychology,* **6**:2:75—88, Winter, 1968.

———— ed.: *Behavioral Therapy.* New York: McGraw-Hill Book Company, 1969.

Goffman, Erving: *Stigma.* Englewood Cliffs, N.J.: Prentice-Hall, Inc., 1965.

Greenacre, Phyllis: "Certain Relationships Between Fetishism and the Faulty Development of the Body Image," *The Psychoanalytic Study of the Child,* Vol. 8. New York: International Universities Press, 1953, pp. 879—98.

Grinker, Roy R.: "The Psychosomatic Aspects of Anxiety," in Spielberger, Charles D., ed.: *Anxiety and Behavior.* New York: Academic Press, 1966, pp. 129—42.

Guyton, Arthur C.: *Textbook of Medical Physiology.* Philadelphia: W. B. Saunders Company, 1966.

Izard, Carroll E., and Tomkins, Silvars: "Anxiety Is a Negative Affect," in Spielberger, Charles D., ed.: *Anxiety and Behavior.* New York: Academic Press, 1966.

Janis, Irving L.: *Psychological Stress.* New York: John Wiley and Sons, Inc., 1958.

Karush, Aaron, Daniels, George E., O'Connor, John F., and Stern, Lenore: "The Response to Psychotherapy in Chronic Ulcerative Colitis," *Psychosomatic Medicine,* **31**:3:201—26, May-June, 1969.

Laufer, Moses: "The Body Image, the Function of Masturbation and Adolescence," *The Psychoanalytic Study of the Child,* Vol. 23. New York: International Universities Press, 1968.

MacLean Paul D.: "Psychosomatics," in *Handbook of Physiology,* Vol. III. Washington, D.C.: American Physiological Society, 1960.

Mahler, M. S.: "Thoughts about Development and Individuation," *The Psychoanalytic Study of the Child,* Vol. 18. New York: International Universities Press, 1963.

Norris, Catherine M.: "The Professional Nurse and Body Image," in Carlson, Carolyn E., ed.: *Behavioral Concepts in Nursing Intervention.* Philadelphia: J. B. Lippincott Co., 1970, pp. 39—67.

Rubin, Reva: "Body Image and Self Esteem," *Nursing Outlook,* **16**:6:20—23, June, 1968.

Ruesch, Jurgen, and Prestwood, A. Rodney: "Anxiety—Its Initiation, Communication and Interpersonal Management," *Archives of Neurology and Psychiatry*, **62**:527–50, November, 1949.

Saint-Exupéry, Antoine de: *Night Flight*. New York: Signet Classics, 1942.

Schaefer, Halmuth H., and Martin, Patrick L.: *Behavioral Therapy*. New York: McGraw-Hill Book Co., Inc., 1969.

Slonim, A. R.: "Effects of Minimal Personal Hygiene and Related Procedures During Prolonged Confinement," Aerospace Medical Research Laboratories, Springfield, Va.: U.S. Department of Commerce, 1967.

Spitz, René A.: "Anaclitic Depression," *The Psychoanalytic Study of the Child*, Vol. II, pp. 313–42. New York: International Universities Press, 1946.

Van Sant, Genee E.: "Patients' Problems Are Not Always Obvious," *American Journal of Nursing*, **62**:4:59, April, 1962.

Vernon, Charles R.: "Psychiatric View of Cardiac Rehabilitation," *Journal of Rehabilitation*, pp. 18–19, November-December, 1958.

Walters, Cathryn, Shurley, Jay T., and Parsons, Oscar A.: "Differences in Male and Female Responses to Underwater Sensory Deprivation: An Exploratory Study," *The Journal of Nervous and Mental Disease*, **135**:4:302–309, October, 1962.

Weinstein, Sidney, Richlin, Milton, Weisinger, Marvin, and Fisher, Larry: "Adaptation to Visual and Nonvisual Rearrangement," Washington, D.C.: National Aeronautics and Space Administration, January, 1967 (NASA CR-663).

Wolf, Stewart G., and Wolff, Harold G.: *Human Gastric Function*. London: Oxford University Press, 1943.

Wolff, Harold G.: "Stressors as a Cause of Disease in Man," in *Proceedings of Mental Health Research Fund*. Oxford: Blackwell Science Publications, 1960, pp. 17–31.

Wolpe, Joseph, and Lazarus, Arnold A.: *Behavior Therapy Techniques*. New York: Pergamon Press, Inc., 1966.

World Health Organization: "Neurophysiology and Behavioral Science in Psychiatry," *WHO Chronicle*, **22**:5:204–207, May, 1968.

Zubek, John P.: "Counteracting Effects of Physical Exercises Performed During Prolonged Perceptual Deprivation," *Science*, **142**:3591:504–506, October 25, 1963.

———— *Sensory Deprivation: Fifteen Years of Research*. New York: Appleton-Century-Crofts, 1969.

7 The problem of loss[1]

Sadness and grief for the loved and lost are perhaps the most powerful emotions affecting mankind. Inability to cope with these feelings has tragic consequences that can shatter a person's life. The problem of loss is a primary focus in caring for the mental patient, who is encouraged to bring his feelings into the open and discuss them with helping persons. In general nursing, however, the feeling of loss that a patient endures because of conditions inherent in his illness and hospitalization has not been dealt with adequately.

Although young nursing students, for the most part, have not experienced great and intense losses at the time they enter the profession, they must prepare themselves to help patients and their families through crises of development, life, and illness and through the ultimate crisis of life—death. They can do so only by understanding and watching for the many ways in which feelings arise and are expressed, both verbally and nonverbally.

This chapter deals with the ways in which people handle their feelings of loss of body parts, function, capacity, or accustomed environment.

Depression and normal states

Many people say they are depressed when their usual feeling of well-being is lessened. A lowering of mood resulting from internal or external factors may influence others to comment that they are "feeling blue" or "having the blues." "Blue Monday" is a common colloquialism referring to the day following the weekend traditional time of rest and relaxation when unfinished work and responsibilities must be resumed, distasteful as they may be, and joys and pleasures be put aside. Sadness, dejection, and despondency are synonyms for "blue" feelings. Premenstrual and postpartum "blues" are well known but not fully understood. They are thought to be connected with changes in endocrine patterns. "Feeling blue" may also be a mood related to loneliness, grief and mourning, and feeling sorrow for one's self and condition.

[1] Loss refers to the lack of external and internal supplies required by the individual to satisfy his basic needs.

Other adjectives that describe this lowering of mood are gloomy, hopeless, discouraged, pessimistic, unhappy, downhearted, and low. They all describe an affect that is a normal response. It is emotional pain which can be thought of as analogous to physical pain. Just as physical pain is not illness per se, so emotional pain is not mental disorder. A deep intensity of this affect, however, is usually labeled depression.

These low spirits may be observed in the older person who has just given up hope of maintaining his independence. In persons of all ages, it is a familiar mood caused by feeling trapped in a situation from which there is no apparent escape. Broken love affairs and failures to meet goals long sought may result in an unhappy state. It may arise in students who receive a lower grade in an examination or on a term paper than they had expected. Patients admitted to the hospital for diagnostic tests or for long-term illness may become discouraged about the results or their lack of progress.

Although there is no definite line of demarcation between these affects and clinical depression, a continuum between the low mood of the normal person and the depressed person is accepted by most clinicians. A prolonged state of these affects may deepen into depression, which has a greater number of symptoms and is more difficult to reverse.

Depression

Depression, one of the most common reactions to loss, is probably experienced by all to some degree during the life span. The depths of depression are discussed at conferences of psychiatrists, psychiatric nurses, and other professionals.

Depression is "a state of feeling sad; psychoneurotic or psychotic disorder marked by sadness, inactivity, and self-depreciation; a reduction in activity, amount, quality or force; a lowering of vitality or functional activity." [2] Another definition of depression is "psychiatrically a morbid sadness, dejection, or melancholy; to be differentiated from grief, which is realistic and proportionate to what has been lost. A depression may be a symptom of any psychiatric disorder or may constitute its principal manifestation. Neurotic depressions are differentiated from psychotic depressions in that they do not involve loss of capacity for reality testing." [3]

[2] *Webster's Seventh New Collegiate Dictionary*. Springfield, Mass.: G. and C. Merriam Co., Publishers, 1965.
[3] American Psychiatric Assn. *A Psychiatric Glossary*. Washington, D.C., 1969.

In depression there is a failure to perform household and other tasks—work may mount up as the depressed person feels overwhelmed by his usual daily chores. He may cancel all household chores, which he will expect other family members to perform for him, but he will still be able to work in his public occupation. As the depression deepens, he will also be unable to do his outside work. In a deep depression, the patient is psychologically immobilized. There may be a paucity of thinking, or he may have nihilistic[4] thoughts. Preoccupation with sin, feelings of unworthiness, and concern about death may predominate. Patients may display a diurnal mood, i.e., they will feel very low early in the morning hours and cheer up later in the day.

Body symptoms

Preoccupation with the body is a common symptom, especially preoccupation with the body organs. A feeling of malfunction or other disorder of the organs will often bring the patient to the doctor or outpatient clinic for the first time. In this connection, it is worth noting that high body concern is socially acceptable, whereas "losing one's mind" is still somewhat of a stigma in this country. Other symptoms are loss of interest in one's usual pursuits—a kind of withdrawal from social contacts, family members, neighbors, and fellow employees—impotence and lack of interest in sex, weight loss, constipation, amenorrhea, insomnia, anorexia, fatigue, heightened tension, and increased restlessness. The mood is one of great sorrow, and crying spells may come without warning. Psychomotor retardation may also occur.

Depressed persons fail to maintain their personal appearance. They do not bathe, they neglect personal hygiene, and their hair and skin may appear oily. If they are menstruating, they may forget to use napkins or tampons. In severe stages, people pace up and down, wring their hands, and say they are worthless and deserve to be shot. They will even ask for electric shock, hoping that it will give them an early death. Suicidal thoughts may occupy the waking hours of the depressed person, who will attempt, often successfully, to kill himself.

---

[4] A delusion that the self or part of the self does not exist.

Occurrence of depression

Loss is one of the major causes of depression. The loss may be real or fancied; it may stem from childhood or from the immediate past. Depression may come from loss of love or the feeling of being important to others—two of the basic needs essential to positive mental health.

Individuals who become depressed are likely to be shy, oversensitive, and inclined to worry too much. Delicately balanced emotionally, they are very self-conscious. The unconscious mechanisms involved in depression are regression, oral sadism, anal traits, a primitive return to a hedonistic level of existence, a desire to return to the womb, and a sense of being wronged.

There are also elements of sadomasochism, self-depreciation, and per- fectionism in the depressed person. The patient may feel a loss of prestige, both in and out of the family, a loss of sexual love and function, and a sense of abandonment by his loved ones. A depressed person with an overpunitive superego will internalize his hostility through the process of introjection [5] and hurt himself. If externalization or projection occurs, the person hurts someone else, symbolically, actually, or both simultaneously.

Depression involves rage intended for someone else turned back onto the self. Dr. Karl Menninger (1938) wrote that with every suicide there is one of three complaints: (1) the wish to kill, (2) the wish to be killed, or (3) the wish to die. If the helping person is too nice, the depressed patient may feel unworthy and will kill himself; on the other hand, if the helping person is too harsh, the depression may deepen. The therapist, therefore, must be very sensitive to the balance between supporting the overly punitive superego and encouraging the ego functions in communication with the depressed person. For example, assets of the patient can be deservedly complimented and shortcomings realistically pointed out at the same time, with psychological support readily available from the therapist.

Perfectionistic, high-performance, and maximum-performance people who are constantly going at high rates of speed are particularly susceptible to depression when their work has been interrupted. Depressive states also occur frequently in old people who have experienced a sudden change for the worse in their lives. Enforced retirement, death of a loved one, loss of limb,

---

[5] Introjection is a primitive type of identification in which loved or hated objects are transferred to oneself symbolically. It is related to a more primitive defense mechanism— incorporation, or the figurative ingestion of a symbolic person or part of a person, e.g., the mother's breast (American Psychiatric Association, 1969).

or removal to a nursing home are serious problems to the aged. An unexpected change in health status brought on by a stroke or accident, particularly one which requires long periods of hospitalization with no prospect of return to former levels of functioning or to one's own home, may understandably precipitate depression. Very often, the patient's apathy, following upon such a personal catastrophe, is attributed to senile processes, although the cause may in fact be a reversible depression. Nurses sensitive to their patients' feelings and needs can do much to uncover the roots of the symptomatology and help in the recovery process.

Research shows that the first months of institutionalization constitute a difficult period for the aging, one in which some of the most adverse psychological effects occur (Lieberman, 1968). In addition, effects that have previously been attributed to confinement in an institution are now considered aspects of the waiting period, in which crises about separation and loss are being experienced. The fantasies and symbolic meanings of institutionalization which occupy the patient's mind during this period may be connected more to his psychological changes than to the institutionalization itself. Both concepts are of great relevance to the nurse's preventive role in dealing with feelings of separation, loss, and despair in patients.

Anaclitic depression is a syndrome of a depressive nature shown by infants who lose a love object during the latter half of the first year of life, namely, the mother or the mother substitute (Spitz, 1946). It is manifested by three phases: (1) *protest*, in which crying, apprehension, and struggling occur; (2) *despair*, a quiet stage in which the infant may refuse to eat and fall into a state of marasmus; and (3) *detachment*, in which the infant withdraws. The term "anaclitic" refers to the infant's depending on the mother for his love and security.

Depressions can occur with any abrupt change in body image, during any of life's crises, and at other stress points in the life cycle. They are evident in all age groups. Childhood depression, the "old soldier syndrome," and the "empty nest syndrome" all occur. Depression in older age groups may be characterized by loneliness and a preoccupation with physical illnesses (Schwab et al., 1968). Depressed feelings are commonly associated with certain illnesses, such as cancer of the bowel, postviral states, and intracranial problems (Motto, 1968). Other physical disabilities which give rise to depressive episodes are hysterectomies, rapid weight gain, amputations, mastectomies, pregnancy, colostomies, and strokes. Anniversary depressions are a special category; a specific date recalls to the patient the extent of a previous loss. One patient, Mrs. Potter, became depressed every year at the beginning of the deer season when her husband left her to go hunting. Severe scars on young people and mutilating operations on old people may evoke particularly strong depressive reactions. With older conditions, such as arthritis and metastatic cancer, there may be chronic depression.

The characteristics and symptoms of depression as described above may not all occur in one person at any one time, but any of them is indicative of its existence. In all cases, however, differentiation must be made between the clinical definition of depression and its lay meaning of sadness of a transitory nature that is causally related to an immediately preceding event.

The nurse's role in recognition of depression

Recognition of depression in others is of major importance in nursing. Because they spend more time with patients and families than other professionals, nurses are therefore in a particularly important position with regard to recognizing depression. A depressed patient may not present a clear-cut, easily recognized pattern. Changes in usual behavior, such as refusing to eat, bathe, or apply the other body arts, wearing dark colors, and slowing down in usual activities, may be taken as cues. A family member may say that the person does not do the things he used to do, does not seem to like to be with people, is irritable, and easily bursts into tears. One of my patients with chronic depression literally spent months building a white garden to help herself overcome her melancholia. The depressed person may have had many absences in his work record before finally reaching the point where he is unable to make the effort to get out of bed. The distressed family may ascribe such behavior to laziness or other factors. Nurses learn to consider behavioral changes as events to be probed because of their significance in regard to the patient's underlying motivation.

Constant reference to melancholy or morbid subjects may precede depression. A patient may also firmly assert, "I want to die; why don't you leave me alone?" When asked by the nurse how he is feeling, he may respond sadly, "I am no good to anybody," and begin weeping. Some patients who are depressed as a consequence of multisurgery become surgical invalids; others are repeatedly admitted to general hospitals for series of diagnostic tests. Still others become iatrogenically addicted to drugs.

Professionals often mistake depression in older persons for organic disease—cerebral arteriosclerosis, for example. Irritability in the aged, a common sign of depression, is also often confused with cerebral arteriosclerosis. I am reminded of many older patients, severely depressed, whose mood lifted dramatically after treatment for the depression. Patients and families are thereby relieved of their chronic suffering by early recognition and treatment of depressive conditions. The constellation of losses suffered by older persons makes them particularly vulnerable to depression; the constant loss of love objects, changes in body image, and other losses add to their loss complex. Many problems of older persons relate to the problem of loss.

Nurses have the responsibility of becoming cognizant of the mental state of their patients and of conveying their observations and clinical inferences to the attending physicians. Suggestions for psychiatric referral of patients are often welcomed by physicians who are frustrated and puzzled by the persistence of symptoms in the presence of negative diagnostic tests. The patient, too, is helped by the nurse in accepting psychiatric treatment because of the nurse's role as a sympathetic and knowledgeable person whose only interest is in his recovery.

The importance of listening has previously been discussed; listening carefully to the words that your patient speaks, the inflection, pitch of voice, and expression. For example, when the patient says, "Yeah, I'm really finished" with a sort of finality when you ask if he has finished his bath, he may be saying something extremely significant about himself. He may, for instance, be telling you that he did not pass his Ph.D. orals, that he is a failure as a father and husband, or that he has used up his life span. Tone of voice, inflection, and emphasis on certain words communicate feelings. Pick up verbal cues from your patient and analyze them. You may be saving his life.

Preoccupation with body functions, neglect of personal appearance, masked facies, and refusal to see loved ones may all be indications of depression. A spurt of angry words from a previously calm patient may furnish a clue as to how he has been feeling all along. Actions directed against self are also important, such as refusing to take medications or prescribed treatment, and refusing to eat. Tears or the traces of tears and sniffling as you enter the room or home may evidence depressed feelings. A patient who has lost his sense of humor is definitely depressed. A depressed person may injure himself; accidents should therefore be fully investigated.

The depressed patient may feel a chronic fatigue and discouragement because simple tasks become Sisyphus-like in nature. He may feel overburdened by his work load and be unable to take on any new responsibilities which demand a change in interaction. Depressive affects can easily be overlooked by physician and nurse, especially when they appear in a patient some time after treatment has begun. Nurses prepared to anticipate symptoms and to look regularly at the inner lives of their patients can perform primary preventive service in the interest of the mental health of patients and families.

Beginning students may look for just one etiological event to explain the onset of depression. In developing multifactoral concepts of human behavior, however, one must consider the totality of the patient's experiences in assessing his response to change. How the individual adapts to conditions at any developmental stage in his life is largely predicated on his total life pattern, his hopes, desires, and fears, and the successes and failures of past performances.

Therapeutic tasks

For the infant who has lost his mother, provision of a mother substitute serves as the balm. In the depressed patient, self-esteem must be regained; feelings that have turned inward must be turned outward. The first task of the nurse is to get acquainted and to learn the facts of a case. The next step has three aspects: getting the patient to talk, exploring the sources of pain, and encouraging catharsis. It may sometimes be necessary to use nonverbal communication as a starting point. Helping the patient to express his internalized anger is a central part of nursing action. With verbalization, the patient brings his feelings to the surface where he and the nurse can examine them, discuss them, and mitigate them through interaction.

Interest and concern alone are sometimes all that is needed. Emotional support is necessary, the support given through understanding, patience, and love. Love is the main thing—being with the patient and communicating to him that you are on his side; staying with him on a gradually diminishing basis, each day expecting more and more of him; calling on the telephone between visits if the patient is at home. You can do a lot in a five- to ten-minute phone call to help lift his spirits.

To be aware from the first of the individual's needs and his likes and dislikes is essential. The depressed person is physically immobilized; therefore, his needs have to be anticipated. Patients often lie or sit and wait to see if others are interested enough to make the overture to ascertain their needs. Keenly aware of the interactions of others, they easily feel slighted. They are crying for attention without knowing how to ask for it.

Relief from the punitive superego must be achieved when the severely depressed person accepts his fate and requests that you hasten his death. Provision for atonement needs to be made. Some patients feel that hospitalization is atonement enough; others feel that electric shock treatment is appropriate punishment and that they will rapidly come out of their depression after its administration. It is important for the nurse to make sharp assessment of each patient in regard to work assignment. For the depressed individual whose self-concept may be so poor that he thinks he is good for nothing, fulfillment of a daily responsibility may renew his sense of purposefulness. The provision for atonement will be different for various individuals. Menial chores may help some patients wash away theoretical sins symbolically. Such jobs could include scrubbing toilets and floors, washing windows and walls or dishes and clothes, cleaning cupboards and drawers. For some men, polishing and waxing cars, painting walls, and cleaning sidewalks are suitable menial chores. Polishing shoes is also a good menial task for men who can do this in a hospital or a home setting. Other kinds of jobs that regularly have to be done such as desk work may be suitable for other patients.

Depressed patients are accident-prone and should not drive a car or any other motorized vehicle. They can get along for quite a while without eating, but they must have fluids. The depressed person may have lost a lot of weight; therefore, a high caloric diet may be prescribed by the physician. Between-meal feedings may also help the patient's nutritional state. If he is at home, the nurse may need to teach the family member responsible for meal preparation to help the depressed patient meet his nutritional needs. The amounts of fluid intake and output require close attention; the temperature should be taken regularly, and all staff should be alert for infections or other manifest body changes.

The depressed person should be observed closely for sleep. Without sleep, exhaustion may occur and the mental state of the individual may become more severe. Personal hygiene may require assistance from the nurse—bathing, shaving, grooming, applying makeup, keeping clothes in order, and changing clothes. Setting a schedule for bathing, feeding, and other personal hygiene can help get the depressed person mobilized. *The nurse's presence also helps allay anxiety.* Depressed patients should be weighed weekly; an increase in weight will, in most cases, reflect the lifting of the depression.

Close observation of the patient and his environment is required for his safety. The dangerous time for the depressed person as far as suicide is concerned is when he is going into or coming out of a depression. It is important, however, to place responsibility on the patient for his own actions. Nurses have been known to go to pieces after a patient has killed himself, even though there was nothing they could have done to prevent it.

Depressed patients may prefer to eat by themselves rather than in the dining room at the regular dining hour. Sometimes they have to be spoon fed. To avoid constipation, they should be offered food that aids elimination, fluids between meals, and regular exercise. The release of internalized aggression in a socially acceptable manner through exercise and sports is therapeutic to the depressed person. Nurse and patient walking together and throwing a medicine ball back and forth may lead to longer walks and group sports such as volley ball.

Patients who are depressed should not be pushed into making decisions. At first all decisions may have to be made for them, with the nurse assessing and timing them each day until the patient can *very soon* assume responsibility. As the depression lifts, the nurse should watch for the turning point at which the patient can make decisions about his own care. Signs of this turning point may be the first good night's sleep in a long while, a relaxed, mobile facies, assisting another patient, or performing for himself some aspect of personal hygiene. Regaining appetite and gaining weight may be cues for the lifting of the depressive mood and the patient's ability to make more decisions for himself.

As early as possible, the depressed person should participate in group activity. Singing simple familiar songs is a beginning. Often the nurse will have to take the patient by the hand and sing with him the first time he is part of a group. Being with others in group singing or even just sitting evokes the herd instinct—described by one person as the "warm body" theory. It can be very comforting to the depressed person.

Individuals who are depressed frequently have no hobbies and have not participated in recreational activities since they were in grade school or high school. The nurse is the person who can best assess the appropriate time and activity for the patient in this area. At the beginning making simple things, easily finished in one session (the familiar pot holder, for example), is recommended. There is nothing quite so therapeutic as the sense of accomplishment, of creation, no matter how elementary the project.

Depressed patients receiving medication must be observed closely for therapeutic effects and other changes. They should be questioned about their symptoms and possible side effects, since they may not volunteer the information. Medication may be given to induce sleep, but with extra caution to guard against hoarding, since attempted suicide is a possibility. It is also necessary for the nurse to keep the menses record of the depressed female patient and to make sure she uses napkins or tampons during menstruation. Handing such items to the patient may be the beginning of her caring for herself.

If the patient is spoon fed, he should be offered the cup and the fork at each feeding to encourage self-help. Verbalizing to the patient that you know it is a difficult time for him acknowledges his pain and his depressed state, but it also connotes that the difficulty is time-bound and will not last forever.

There are no universals in the care of the depressed patient. You have to feel with each patient what he is like, what is most painful to him, and what can be done about his condition.

In summary, the level of depression is best measured by the ability of the person to function in his usual setting. The mildly depressed person is quiet, inhibited, and has an unhappy expression. His thoughts may be pessimistic and self-derogatory. Self-depreciating remarks are truly meant for the lost love object. He feels inadequate, discouraged, and hopeless, is unable to make decisions, and has difficulty with his usual intellectual activities. He is too concerned with personal problems and may complain a great deal.

The moderately depressed person has a feeling of unpleasantness, is tense, and feels pain. He is absorbed in a few topics of a very melancholy nature such as death and pseudoanhedonia.

The person who becomes more deeply depressed is dejected, feels rejected and unloved, and is anxious and perplexed. He is preoccupied; concentration, attention, and memory are impaired; he may have feelings of unreality and be unable to think. It is at this stage that the vegetative systems become affected, resulting in anorexia, constipation, loss of weight, and other symptoms. Delusions are likely to be self-accusatory or expressive of guilt and unworthiness. Suicidal thoughts tend to be present. He may be mono-syllabic, have psychomotor retardation, and show a neglected appearance and a dejected facies. The severely depressed person should be informed repeatedly that if he follows instructions he will gradually improve (Ayd, 1961). Reiteration of support, reassurance, and dissuasion from taking on anything difficult are also recommended. All instructions should be explicit and repeated frequently; rest and relaxation should be provided. If a patient cannot perform his job, his self-concept will receive a blow if he attempts to continue working. Taking a temporary leave of absence or reducing the work load may be advisable.

Depression may be reactive; that is, it may occur in proximity to a known event such as bereavement in which grief work is incomplete, business failure, broken love affairs, and other adversities. When not associated with a known event, depression may be the result of conflict between instinctual wishes and drives in which guilt, ambivalence (particularly love and hate feelings), and hostile impulses toward others are turned inward toward the self. The person who is wounded, hurt, and feels unwanted, neglected, and disappointed is prevented by a punitive superego from expressing his feelings outwardly. He is therefore compelled to direct his hostility to his own ego. Some features of melancholia, according to Freud (1917), are borrowed from grief; others have resulted from the process of regression from narcissistic object-choice to narcissism.

Involutional melancholia

Depression may be a symptom of many kinds of problems. It may be a component of mental disorders (e.g., schizophrenia, depressed schizo-affective type) or of the primary disorder itself. Depression appears in persons with major affective disorders when there is no discernible relationship to life experience.

Involutional melancholia is a depressive disorder occurring during the climacteric. Because of divided opinion as to whether this psychosis is a distinct entity, diagnosticians advise against use of this nomenclature until all other affective disorders are ruled out. "Involutional" refers to the return to a former nonsexual, physiological state in which the woman's uterus shrinks and the ovaries atrophy and the man's gonads are insufficient and the genitals atrophy. In men, this condition appears much later than in women and is called the andropause, analogous with female menopause. Involutional melancholia occurs more frequently in women and at a much earlier age, usually in the mid- or late forties.

It is thought that the compulsive personality is most susceptible to involutional melancholia. This is in accord with the psychoanalytic concepts of psychosexual development in which the early phases of development have an effect on all succeeding phases. Another related factor may be the "empty nest" phase of development, which coincides with the beginning of the menopause. This critical time of life may involve drastic role changes, both physiological and mental, especially in women.

> Mrs. Diaz, married at 16 and the mother of five children at the age of 22, was admitted to the hospital after two interrupted suicide attempts. While the children were growing up, she had devoted all her waking hours to them and to her husband, to the neglect of her own needs. By the time she reached her early forties, all her children had left home and she was denied her usual outlets of energy and her need to be needed. Her husband lost interest in her. Now in the hospital for a few weeks, Mrs. Diaz had no regard for her appearance, constantly derogated herself, and referred continuously to what she should have done when she was a child. Part of her preoccupation was also with all her well-intended acts that were not appreciated by either her husband or her children. She had insomnia, anorexia, and agitation. With her children gone and a husband who did not care about her, Mrs. Diaz had lost her vocation. She no longer had the opportunity to accomplish anything and to feel the gratification from being purposeful, so necessary to her well-being. The psychic wounds were already too deep at the time of admission for remedy. All attempts to help her regain her self-esteem failed.

PREVENTION

Much preventive work can be done with women in our society to avoid involutional melancholia. Since women in the middle-age group are a population at risk, efforts in homes and community agencies can be of benefit in reducing the number of cases of mental disorder. An understanding husband and family help, although they do not necessarily serve a preventive purpose. The woman who puts a great deal of energy and devotion into her activities in one phase of life may suffer a deficit of resources in other phases which provide no proper outlet for the same energy and devotion. Interests must be developed in all phases of life which can be carried over or renewed in the later periods when a woman needs to attain role functions other than those of wife and mother. In these times, there is a great deal of work that a middle-aged woman can do to retain her sense of usefulness after her children have left home. Unless she has prepared herself for this phase of life, she will not be able to assume a new and satisfying role. The old remedies of a change in environment by means of an ocean cruise or a trip around the world are ineffective.

Nursing students can be very helpful to women with whom they come in contact, at the same time preparing themselves for their own entrance into this life phase. Accurate information on the physiological changes during menopause can be reassuring to the uninformed person who has only heard old wives' tales about this being the period when women lose their minds. The physician's treatment may take the form of estrogen replacement therapy either orally or by injection. A thorough physical examination should be secured every year.

As in other depressed states, the person with involutional melancholia may omit some somatic complaints, so that health information must be elicited by specific questioning. Psychic energizers are often prescribed by the physician, sometimes together with tranquilizers if the patient is agitated. Severe cases require hospitalization, during which time the ancillary treatments afforded by the social, occupational, and recreational therapies are employed as fully as possible. Following is an example of nursing intervention with a man who was in the involutional phase of his life.

> Mr. Hirschbaum, a distinguished professor of law, was suffering from involutional melancholia and was just coming out of his depression. He was a tall, well-dressed, and serious man who had absolutely no hobbies. It was felt by the psychiatric team that it would be most therapeutic for him to acquire a hobby while in the hospital that he could pursue when he returned home. His reluctance and protestations against this prescription were ignored on his first visit to occupational therapy. Getting Mr. Hirschbaum to walk into the O.T. room was another matter. His nurse finally decided that he would not take "No" for an answer. When the time came to take him to the O.T. room, he simply took him by the hand and said, "Come on, Mr. Hirschbaum, I have the leather all laid out for you to learn how to make a key case, and I will stay with you and help." With one nurse pulling and another pushing, he was led into the room. His delight was evident as he began to work on the key case. A design had to be selected, the leather had to be cut, marked, pounded, and laced—all socially acceptable outlets for anger.

Nurse-patient relationship therapy for the patient with involutional melancholia is similar to that used with patients who are otherwise depressed. In the Forties, Fifties, and early Sixties, electroshock was used as primary treatment to alleviate the depressive affect. Psychotherapy, both individual and group, is now frequently used in combination with pharmacotherapy.

Manic-depressive illnesses

Other patients with major affective disorders have either the manic-depressive types of problems—in which there are severe mood swings of the patient toward elation or depression—or the circular type, in which there is both elation and depression. Patients may have recurrent manic or depressed states and remissions. Some psychiatrists doubt that a so-called manic-depressive disorder is that at all, but is actually schizophrenia. It is interesting to note that incidence of the disorder seems to be decreasing. It is thought to be more prevalent among the higher income groups, women, people from the Mediterranean area, and the Irish.

The new *Manual of the International Statistical Classification of Diseases, Injuries, and Causes of Death* (1967) now provides a classification for epidemiological studies which enables comparison of the prevalence of this disorder among countries throughout the world.

There are many theories with regard to the development of manic-depressive disorders. Their occurrence in the same family suggests an hereditary factor. Studies of monozygotic and dizygotic twins support the genetic point of view (Kallman, 1953). Other biological correlates have been described, such as, the pyknic[6] body build and the mesomorphic[7] somatotype.

Recently is has been hypothesized that elation is accompanied by an increase in brain catecholamines.

From the psychoanalytical side, mania is a flight into reality in which some regression occurs in both the ego and the superego. Mania is considered a defense against depression. An understanding of the psychodynamics of the depressive affect is therefore fundamental to comprehension of the elated joy of the manic patient.

---

[6] "One with broad head, thick shoulders, large chest, short neck, and stocky body" (Taber, 1965).
[7] The predominance of the structures of the body developed from the mesodermal layer of the embryo (Hinsie *et al.*, 1960; Patten, 1953).

Behavior

Manic patients are breezy, capricious, and extroverted. They may accomplish a great deal and may be well liked by their associates. They stand out in a crowd, seem to have limitless energy, and may be the life of the party. This stage is referred to as hypomania, and during this phase behavior is purposeful, much work is accomplished, and others wonder just how the person manages to be so vigorous.

In his spiraling *mood of elation*, the patient becomes expansive. He may consider himself increasingly powerful and wealthy, and will spend money wildly on luxuries at the merest whim. Bold schemes are devised which may easily fall apart. Irritability occurs, and hasty separations may ensue within families. Very little introspection seems possible for the elated patient; insight also varies with the degree of the mania.

The manic patient's witty comments have an infectious quality, and there is a saying in the profession that "everybody loves a manic." Immediately thwarting demands of the manic patient may, however, incur swift, uninhibited action from the patient. Professionals and others may become the focus of verbal attacks peppered with obscene expressions. The manic patient is very suggestible and distractible, flitting from subject to subject and from activity to activity. His attention span is short. The hypomanic patient writes copiously. Reams of letters may be forthcoming, which may create some turbulence. He can be absorbed with creating, even with a collection of rags which he may tear into bits and use as decorations for himself. His handwriting is large and bold, with words printed and underlined, and he often writes standing up. Constructing rhymes may occupy his attention, or making some elaborate drawing for a new invention. Clifford Beers wrote on wrapping paper (Deutsch, 1937).

All scraps of paper are, of course, precious to the patient and should be carefully saved for him. One patient in a manic state came to the hospital with rough drawings of a self-watering planter. He had great ideas of setting up an industrial plant near the hospital so that all the patients could be employed in it and make the planters for international distribution. He had planned that all proceeds would go to the hospital. Another patient designed a wheeled vehicle with a sail to travel over the Western prairies. Clifford Beers, hospitalized after a suicide attempt in 1900, while passing from a state of profound depression to one of extreme exaltation and approaching recovery, shaped in his mind a world-wide movement for the protection of mental patients. Later, *A Mind That Found Itself* (1908) resulted from the notes he made on wrapping paper while he was hospitalized. It is still widely read. Beers founded the National Committee on Mental Hygiene in 1909 (Deutsch, 1937).

Manic episodes are recurrent; thus someone within the family constellation and the patient himself may quickly perceive the hypomanic affect and seek treatment. The use of tranquilizers may eliminate the necessity for hospitalization. One patient I know gets so angry in her beginning manic phase that she tears up the linoleum at home. This is the signal to the family for taking her to the hospital and "farming out" the children to relatives.

As the hypomanic patient goes into an acute state of mania, if he is not furiously writing he will be talking continuously. He will have a constant and speeded up stream of speech in which he makes puns and rhymes; speech and laughter will be very loud. His ideas come so fast that, even though he is highly loquacious, he simply does not have time to express them in complete sentences. This results in a flight of ideas. The ideas will most likely be connected (one idea leading to another) although the first idea is only partially expressed. Ideas may be expressed which border on delusions of grandeur. Clang associations may occur in acute states in which the patient expresses himself with words that have similar sounds but different meanings. The nurse who is a careful listener will be able to capture some of this material, which is somewhat like free association. If she is able to understand it, she will better understand the patient and be better able to assist the physician in his treatment.

The psychomotor activity is accelerated in speech, and the muscular activity of the patient is also greatly increased. The manic patient is constantly on the go and in the hospital will soon learn a great deal about the other patients and the staff. He does not appear to feel fatigue. According to Morozov and Romasenko (Moscow, no date), this lack of fatigue is due to the increase of sugar in the blood and the utilization of more sugar. The level of lactic acid is low because it is rapidly eliminated from the blood. This explains why patients do not tire easily in the manic state if their carbohydrate intake is sufficient. Manic patients may decorate themselves with cosmetics until they have a garish appearance and wear brightly colored clothes in rather unusual arrangements. Numerous tinkling, jangling objects may be part of their costume. Some patients may remove their clothing and make erotic overtures to those around them.

Therapeutic tasks

If the manic patient is first observed by the nurse in the home setting, she may make an early referral and therefore possibly avoid a need for hospitalization. Environmental manipulation may be of therapeutic value to the hypomanic patient who is chronically unable to express his anger at being taken advantage of by family members. Treatment by the psychiatrist is most likely to be a combination of ataraxics and psychotherapy. Hospitalization may be required in acute states. Psychotherapy will not be of the uncovering type because discussion of conflict material may increase the overactivity. In these instances, psychotherapy will be rather direct reassurance. Lithium carbonate has been recently reported as highly effective in the treatment of recurrent and chronic mania (Kolb, 1968). In the past, electroshock, narcosis therapy, hydrotherapy, and other types of treatment were used for manic patients. These methods are still used by some psychiatrists here and in other countries. Hydrotherapy, called balneology in the Soviet Union, is a major part of treatment there.

Therapy advised by the physician or psychiatrist may be reinforced by the nurse in the home or in other settings. Nurses are usually nonthreatening and can often help a family member take responsibility for seeing that the hypomanic patient takes his medications and gets needed rest. In the nursing care of manic patients in the acute phase, the principal aim is to prevent exhaustion. Directing the patient, distracting him, and administering his medications to achieve ataraxia are three main points in nursing care. The patient therefore must be protected from himself. His sensorium is clear except in very severe mania, his memory is good, and his judgment is somewhat impaired.

The nurse must also assess the potentials of the patient and enlist his aid in his care. Examination of his body for neglected cuts and bruises or other traumata is important, as are observation and communication to him of the signs of his physical and mental state in a concerned and noncritical manner. For example, "You are really keyed up around all these people. Here is your coat. We are going for a walk."

Manic patients can be hypercritical of others, and the nurse should be prepared for criticism of makeup, coiffure, and perfume. If something about your appearance does not suit the patient, he will let you know about it. If the nurses are men, other criticisms may be made. Few are exempt. Amorous overtures to particular psychiatrists and/or nurses may be made by the manic patient. When they are absent, he may compose long amorous letters and poems to these individuals and fill up their mail boxes.

ENVIRONMENT

The protected *environment* of the hospital itself aids the patient, who is relieved of the demands of job or housewifely duties and family and surrounded by helping persons. The acutely manic patient is easily stimulated by bright colors, loud sounds, and other people. The nurse may use soothing, restful music as an aid. Maintaining the same nurses and providing a private room without bright lights and colors can help. Acutely excited patients may require the constant attention of at least one nurse because they tend to be impulsive and easily distracted. Visitors are inadvisable. After the acute phase is over, they may then be eased into group activities.

NUTRITION AND ELIMINATION

The manic patient is overactive and therefore too busy to eat. A high vitamin, high caloric diet will help prevent exhaustion and weight loss. In acute manic states, patients should be weighed daily. Frequent small meals will be taken by the overactive patient who is too busy to sit down and eat. He should be given finger food such as sandwiches, apples, celery, carrot sticks, and raisins or other dried fruit that can be taken and eaten *en passant*. Offering milk shakes and other fluids and holding the glass to prevent the patient from trying to throw it is one way to get him to take nutrients. Constipation is a problem which can be prevented by attention to intake of nutrients and fluids.

PERSONAL HYGIENE

The manic patient needs assistance with personal hygiene. Clothing should be durable and easily put on and removed. The excited patient has no time for tedious fasteners and otherwise complex arrangements, although he may festoon himself with available baubles. It is important to help the patient to control the use of cosmetics and jewelry. A male patient may take a quick shave upon suggestion. Since he is likely to hit only the high spots, someone else may have to complete the job. Bathing may present a problem with the busy, overactive patient. Assist him to gather needed articles for bathing; otherwise he may come from the bathroom *au naturel* looking for something like the soap! Attention should be given to the coiffure, nails, and oral hygiene of the manic patient, as well as to the maintenance of his wardrobe. The nurse should be alert to the fact that foreign objects may be stuffed into body orifices. During the bath a nurse can ascertain whether the patient has received any injuries during the day that might have gone unobserved.

Items from other patients may have been purloined. This may come to light only when the patient is getting his clothes ready for the laundry and emptying his pockets. Discreet return of such items to their rightful owners may avoid numerous headaches. Preventive measures such as asking other patients to keep their belongings inside cupboards and drawers can be instituted.

SOMATIC COMPLAINTS

Because these patients are so keyed up, they only inadvertently inform you about something that should receive attention such as chest pain or bleeding from some body orifice. If the patient has flight of ideas, he will include any symptoms in his flight of ideas. The alert nurse will *regard every complaint* with seriousness, explore it, record it, and bring it to the attention of the physician. Although the patient's primary diagnosis may be of psychogenic origin, he may develop other problems during the course of his disorder. Be careful to avoid the trap of considering only people's psychological needs when you are in a psychiatric setting.

MEDICATIONS

Administration of medications may pose a nursing problem. A refusal at one moment may be acceptance at the next. Make use of the suggestibility and distractibility of the manic patient, diverting his attention when required, and directing it to the task at hand. You might talk about something else, have the medications in one hand and a paper cup of water in the other, and say firmly and directly, "Mr. Zim, here are your medications, open your mouth," as you hold the medicine cup to his lips. Medications may have to be given by parenteral routes if the patient will not take them orally. All efforts should be made to administer medications with the least amount of exertion on the part of the patient. Usually at least one nurse on duty will be able to give the patient his medications orally. I have seen patients who would take medications only from other patients but would take them faithfully in this manner. A manic patient may hoard tranquilizers for patients who are "worse off than I am" or for "more difficult times." Some patients with recurrent episodes may persuade a new psychiatrist to give them larger doses than they really need for the purpose of hoarding.

SLEEP AND REST

Although most people need their daily rest, manic patients may not feel the need for sleep. Removing exciting stimuli from the patient's environment in the early evening will help prepare him for sleep. Playing a quiet game of cards or chess, or quiet conversation, a hot bath, warm milk, and a back massage will encourage sleep. These patients may go off to bed at their regular hour and awaken 2 hours later fully refreshed; adequate doses of medication may be required to ensure a full night's sleep. It is up to the patient and his nurse to make these judgments and request needed medication from the attending psychiatrist. Often orders for medication for excited patients are written *pro re nata*. As the mania subsides, patients sleep without so much medication; they also begin to gain weight. It is the nurse's responsibility to be aware of the amount of sleep of manic patients and to suggest tapering off the sleeping medication as soon as this is feasible. Enforcing daily rest periods can also help prevent exhaustion.

DIRECTING ACTIVITY

The excess energy of the manic patient should be directed into constructive channels. Exercise requiring the large muscle groups is appropriate if it is done in moderation. The excited patient cannot concentrate on precision work. In the hospital unit, making beds, vacuuming the floors, and mopping are all suitable. If the patient can safely perform his part of the chores in the milieu of the hospital unit, it will help his group relationships, which may have suffered as a result of his impulsive behavior. These chores may some-times be done after most of the other patients have gone out, in order to avoid overstimulation. Running, gymnastics, splashing in the swimming pool, walking, and building something are all appropriate activities.

Patients with manic-depressive disorders will most likely have recurrences. If there are alternating manic and depressive episodes, the condition is referred to as cyclothymic. Preventive techniques can be used to avoid extreme mania. An example is discussing with the patient how he feels when he is approaching a manic state and advising him how to get help. One patient I know regularly signs herself into the hospital when she becomes aware of symptoms; previously she was taken to the hospital by the police.

Patients may now be treated by their family physicians before they spiral into the dangerous delirious manic state. The overactive patient may also fall into the schizo-affective diagnostic category. The aim of nursing care with this group will also be toward prevention of exhaustion in addition to employ-ing the techniques necessary for working with schizophrenic patients (see Chapter 10). Patients with delirious mania may have developed it gradually, going through the two previously described stages of hypomania and acute mania. However, in some instances, a full-blown delirious mania may develop suddenly. The patient is incoherent, and his sensorium is clouded in all three spheres. He is highly overactive to no seeming purpose. Hallucinations and delusions are likely to be present. Exhaustion may be quickly reached, and signs of dehydration appear (e.g., dry mouth and lips, flushed face, fast pulse, and fever) unless preventive measures are initiated quickly.

From a psychotherapeutic standpoint, the goal of the psychiatrist is to aid the patient to progress to where he can consciously regard loneliness and separation without overactivity.

Care of the overactive patient is demanding for the nurse, who must be keenly aware of the "contagiousness" of his overactivity. As patients recover and spend weekends and other times at home before discharge, the nurse also aids them in dealing with lonely feelings by being an available and interested listener and reflecting feelings.

Following is a description of a manic patient:

> Mrs. Young is in the hospital for her third manic episode. There is history of a maternal aunt having a similar problem. Mrs. Young's first attack occurred 3 months after her first child was born, at which time she was hospitalized, receiving hydrotherapy, a series of electro-shock treatments, and continuous nursing care. She was discharged after 2 months. Eight years later she suffered her second attack and was again hospitalized, this time for 6 weeks, during which she was treated with phenothiazines. She came in for weekly psychothera-peutic interviews with her psychiatrist in the outpatient psychiatric department for 6 months. She has four children—21, 18, 16, and 10—and her husband is overseas. Her husband is in the regular navy. She is now 45 years old.

The present episode began with the return of her oldest son from Vietnam. He had volunteered for the service.

> Mrs. Young dyed her hair a fiery red, said she was "gloriously high" and "having a ball" and consequently went out dancing every night until the wee hours of the morning. She operates a specialty gift shop near her home and recently has been giving away her merchandise. She told the children to make their own breakfasts, ate none herself, and did not take time to prepare dinner, having so much to do. She left her gift shop several afternoons to go shopping and bought 25 different sets of beads and earrings. Her oldest child said that she had not slept for at least a week.

> Her makeup is excessive and carelessly applied. She is wearing a bright red dress, red coat, and very high-heeled red shoes and is carry-ing a red handbag. Nothing matches but the color. Her eyes are very bright, and she is in constant movement. During admission she sings and dances and hugs and kisses the admitting psychiatrist with a loud smack. She is unable to sit still. Her son says she must have lost 20 pounds during the past week. Her face is flushed, her pulse is 100, and her blood pressure is 150/100.

When more was known about the patient, it was ascertained that she became moderately depressed at least 4 to 6 days preceding the manic phase. With this information about Mrs. Young and her family, what nursing measures would you institute, and why? Stop now and think through the situation. Discuss your ideas with someone else.

The process of grief and mourning

Grief is a sequence of subjective states that follow loss and accompany mourning. Mourning indicates a broad range of reactions to loss and also refers to symbols of loss such as widow's veils and black arm bands. It is not a morbid condition; on the contrary, for the bereaved absence of mourning is abnormal. Mourning comprises the set of psychological processes aroused by the loss of a love object. In a broad range of reactions to loss, these processes are linked together and result in healthy or unhealthy adaptation to reality. Loss is a crisis to which the helping person can aid the sufferer achieve a healthy adaptation. Mourning is analogous to inflammation in physiology; several signs and symptoms may be included.

In grief, the loss of a loved person makes the world seem poor and empty. Other serious deprivations, such as loss of freedom in institutionalization, loss of country, and loss of neighborhood, will also produce grief. In the grieving person who suffers from object loss there is no significant fall in self-esteem, but there is some self-accusation. In contrast with melancholia in which the object loss may be trivial and the causative factors largely internal, the emotional loss in grief is attributed to an object which had been strongly desired, wanted, or loved and which had become part of the person's ego by a process of assimilation, incorporation, or introjection. A feeling of loss originates within the ego of the person; his hurt and disappointment generate hostile, angry feelings. The superego turns these feelings against the incorporated object and the ego, and the patient experiences the pain of depression.

Phases of grief and mourning

Bowlby (1968) describes four phases of grief and mourning. The first is the phase of numbing, the initial shock phase; the second phase has outbursts of anger or other distress signs; the third is yearning for the lost figure, a searching in the mind for the lost figure; and the fourth is healing and reorganization. Others have identified slightly different variations of the phases — for example, the following five stages: (1) denial and isolation, (2) anger, (3) bargaining, (4) depression, and (5) acceptance (Kübler-Ross, 1969). The bargaining stage is characterized by attempts to negotiate with the helping persons for more time to live or for a few days without pain. It has three qualities: postponement of death, a reward for the patient who does the best that he can, and a self-determined deadline. Mr. Lowenstein, who had Hodgkin's disease "bargained" with the hospital staff to "go home once more for my son's birthday." Pulling himself together for this event, he did go and returned to the hospital only to die a few days later.

Consider the experiences of loss that you observe in patients under your care: those who lose body parts (organ or limb); those whose body images change for other reasons; those who lose their homes because of a disaster, moving, or relocation (as in urban renewal); those who are dying; those who are bereaved; and those who lose pet animals. For a picture of the loss complex, add to these loss of money, job status, hearing, vision, sexual drive, and the ability to move about. The wish to remain whole and intact is fundamental to the human being. Since the first parts of the ego to develop are the body image, changes in it arouse the most emotional resistance (Rochlin, 1965). What Spitz (1946) called anaclitic depression is now included in the loss complex (Levin, 1965, p. 209). Everyone at some time experiences grief and mourning. Persons rebuffed or rejected, as in divorce and broken love affairs, may also experience the process.

There is a basic over-all pattern of grief and mourning in adults, amounting to a definite syndrome in acute grief. Intense emotional pain is felt—a feeling of loneliness accompanied by tightness in the throat, choking, sighing, crying, and an empty feeling in the abdomen. Others may vomit, lack muscular power, or feel another intense subjective distress described as tension or anguish. A feeling of emptiness prevails, and the mourner tends to avoid people, preferring to be left alone. Images of association with the deceased constantly occupy the individual's waking life. The mourner reviews all aspects of his life with the deceased; the fact that the love object no longer exists requires that the life energy be withdrawn from the lost love object (Freud, 1917). There is a struggle between reality and what used to be, with reality gaining ascendancy as the natural outcome.

The amount of time required for accomplishing grief work is an individual matter, but time is an important factor in giving needed help. The helping person must be at the patient's side right from the start. Waiting until the mourning period is over is useless, because by this time resolution will have been achieved, possibly in an unhealthy manner. For a healthy resolution, preventive techniques must be initiated early. In one community, quiet visitors from the mental health center keep the mourner company, wash the dishes, and help with other chores. In other communities such concern is shown by neighbors and church members.

During the time of grief and mourning, the bereaved is overwhelmed by a sense of helplessness and a concern that perhaps he could have done something to prevent the death. Tears and sobbing come without warning when memories of the deceased occur, when friends visit, and when sympathy is offered. The mourner lacks energy and feels as if he bears the burdens of the world. In the first phase of numbness, a definite sense of unreality prevails, as if all the happenings of the death were a bad dream. The voice of the deceased may be heard, as one hears voices or has mental images just before sleep, yet the mourner recognizes that it is unreal.

The mourner may evidence a loss of concern and warmth for others and show irritability and anger. He may wonder, "Why did this have to happen to me?" or, when reminded of the happy decades he spent with his love object, retort, "Well, I could have had a lot more!" The individual is overwhelmed with yearning for the lost object, and much of his mental life may be occupied with fantasies of its return.

The dream life of the mourner may be filled with nightmares, especially when there has been an accidental death of a loved one. Dreams of earlier relationships with the deceased may be frequent.

When the grief work is done, there is emancipation from bondage to the deceased; readjustments are made to the environment, and new relationships are formed. The lost object takes a different place in the individual's memory, and behavior is reorganized toward a new object.

In some cultures, such as the Anglo-American, thoughts and feelings with regard to loss are suppressed and de-emphasized. In others, loss may be dramatized. Patients should be viewed within the context of their cultures. The bereaved plead for sympathy and support, express anger, and seek understanding. In our culture these aspects of grief are not easily expressed. If grief work is unaccomplished, the thoughts and behavior of the mourner are still directed toward the lost object, hostility may be displayed, unreasonable appeals for help can be made, and the presence of the deceased will be felt in the home. The household may be maintained as before, with clothes and other belongings of the deceased kept in their places. Insomnia may become a problem, accompanied by preoccupation with body functions. Persons close to the deceased may feel that they are getting the disease or condition which caused the death of their loved one. When this happens, family members finally agree or are self-impelled to seek out their physician. For each family member it is a time of reassessment of family roles and rearrangement of family tasks. Hostility may be directed to others, especially the physician, and some recrimination may be expressed for his ineffectiveness in preventing the death of the loved one.

Adults have difficulty with grieving in a family in which attachment behavior[8] is regarded without sympathy—for example, where crying is

---

[8] Attachment behavior refers to instinctive behavior in animals. The function of attachment behavior is protection from predators.

discouraged because it is "babyish" and "bad." When a person who has grown up in such a family suffers loss, he may be inclined to stifle his grief; members of his family are the least likely to be able to help. A person whose family advocated courage and civilized behavior at all times, especially in the face of adversity, lost her mother at the age of 12 years. She did not shed a tear. Six months later, when her horse died, she wept uncontrollably.

During national tragedies (as, for example, when John F. Kennedy, Martin Luther King, and Robert Kennedy were assassinated), oceans of tears are shed by people who bottled up their feelings when disaster struck closer to home. For the first time in history, mass world-wide grief and mourning have become possible. The therapeutic effect on many people throughout the world of simultaneous mourning for a lost leader has been neither noted nor measured, but the possibility merits consideration.

Death, dying, and bereavement

One of the ways to learn about death is to recall your first experience with it. Attitudes toward death are strongly conditioned by the strength of the ties which integrate the individual within the social organization. The problem for each of us is how not to die alone. The first contact with death has important implications for life-long attitudes toward it. Stop now and think of the first death you recall. Share your thoughts with another person. My first memory is of my grandmother wrapped in a shroud and lying on a red couch. For years I carried this image until I checked it out with someone who attended her funeral. In actuality, my grandmother had been lying in a white casket, not on a red couch. What I had done in converting the image was associate the color of blood (red) with death.

In nursing and medicine, there is now an intellectual and social awakening to the needs of dying patients. This movement was spearheaded by Glaser and Strauss (1965) and Jeanne C. Quint (1967), who worked together at the University of California at San Francisco in a 6-year research project which gathered data from five schools of nursing in the Bay Area.

People prepare for their own deaths through experiencing those of pets, friends, classmates, and acquaintances as well as the deaths of family members and other loved ones. In our culture, only the aged are likely to refer to death in open conversation. Children and other young people may never have seen anyone die (except via the mass media) or been in the presence of a dying person. Death is denied in many ways, and various avoidance techniques are common in our culture, as shown by the many euphemisms relating to death.

In the hospital, reference to the dying person as the "terminally ill" or "the patient with a negative prognosis" and, in some cases, the furtive removal of the body to the morgue testify to these avoidance techniques. Funeral directors advertise the installment buying of funerals as "sunrise plans" and advise buyers of their services to purchase the watertight vault. In the funeral home, the corpse (man or woman) is often made up to look "lifelike," even if the person never wore makeup. The euphemisms describing death and the attempts of morticians to preserve bodies act as defenses for our helplessness in the face of death. The corpse is viewed in a "slumber room," and the deceased is referred to as the "dear departed."

At one time in America, the corpse was washed by close friends, wrapped in a shroud, and buried in a pine box.

Cultural beliefs about the dying ritual

The belief in an afterlife is pancultural. For the Buddhist, it is Nirvana; for the Scandinavians, Valhalla; for the pre-Christian Greeks, Elysium; for the Persians, the Abode of Song; and for the Western world, Heaven. Nirvana may be achieved at death, but it may also be achieved in life, when the spiritual struggle over Karma has brought to an end the series of deaths and rebirths and the long-sought state of extinguishedness ends the need for another rebirth.

A primitive view regarding death was that provision for the physical needs of the deceased helped him to a longer life after death. Archeologists have been able to describe previous cultures after studying their grave sites. The glorious treasures of the burial chambers of Tutankhamen show us, more than 3000 years after his death, the power of the belief in an afterlife. Fear of touching a corpse derives from the idea of death as something that comes and gets you.

Among the Romans, the attitude toward a corpse was mystical and supernatural; contact with one was alarming. However, the Romans did not manifest so much a fearful attitude toward spirits as they did an interest and desire through ritual to effect communion of the upper and lower worlds. The *dies parentales* held in February were holidays for performance of appeasement rites to the dead. The *lemuria* in May allowed the Romans to rid themselves of anxiety by spitting out black beans and saying, "With these I redeem me and mine," thereby banishing the spirits (Bendann, 1930). Holbein's series of engravings show Death as a dancing skeleton with clinging pieces of putrefied flesh, gathering people to him as he sees fit. The artist Rowlandson's "Dance of Death" deals with a similar theme.

The motif of the death dance is found in French literature and folk songs from the thirteenth century through the high point of its popularity, the middle of the sixteenth century. In the "theme of the three dead and three living men" (Huizinga, 1924; de Caumont, 1886), three young noblemen meet three hideous dead men who tell them of their past grandeur and warn the nobles of their imminent end. One can see this theme in the frescoes of the Campo Santo at Pisa, the oldest pictorial form of the death dance. The Church of the Innocents at Paris, which has been destroyed, had carvings on the same theme. A "dance of the dead" was actually performed in fifteenth-century France.

Since the thirteenth century, the mendicant orders had admonished the populace about death to such an extent that there were public outcries against the practice. By the fifteenth century the engraver and the carver made the dance of death graphic as well. The theme was widely dispersed throughout central and western Europe, possibly due to the revival of trade and commerce and the renewal and growth of city life. In addition to poetry, folksongs, sculptures, and woodcuts, manuscripts, performances, miniatures, and tapestries portrayed the dance of death. It represented or reflected the feeling of the populace toward the warnings made by the church, but it also showed that death was the great equalizer in that it took away pope, cardinal, bishop, friar, and priest. Wars and plagues made death a common acquaintance.

Burial customs

The burial customs of the Middle Ages were a constant reminder of death. Cemeteries were the preferred places of burial, and rich and poor were buried without distinction. Because of the belief that the human body decomposed in 9 days, bodies were quickly disinterred to make room for others; skulls and bones were heaped up along the cloisters and left for all to see. During the plagues, corpses were collected in the streets and piled in the charnel houses for mass burials. The rulers and potentates were put to rest in the cathedrals, frequently in coffins carrying life-sized representations of the decedents on their lids. The urge to be buried in home soil led to English soldiers abroad cutting up dead warriors (as was done with Henry V), boiling the remains, and returning them to the homeland.

In the daily life of medieval man, death was preached to him from the pulpit, bones of skeletons were stacked for him to see, and the power of death was felt all around him. He probably built his concept of things on a system which itself reflected his emotional state, opinions, interests, and necessities of life. On his way home from wars or from tilling the soil he probably thought of heaven, and of angels, devils, and death. Appearances of the latter were familiar to him from cathedral sculptures, chapel frescoes, descriptions by his priests, and the visible skeletons. He was daily reminded that death could strike at any time. The dance of death glorified death; the realism of death helped popularize the idea; without warning and without acceptance of bribes, Death dragged human beings of all stations and age into the dance and rejoiced.

Present customs

The contrast afforded by today's customs is marked, for the starkness of death is hidden away discreetly in hospitals, funeral homes, and distant cemeteries. People are usually taken to a hospital to die, and their care is turned over to the hospital personnel. When death does come, the body is removed immediately—impersonally, and even furtively. At one sanitarium situated high on a hill, corpses were sent to the bottom of the hill on a trolley running through a specially constructed tunnel, like soiled laundry down the chute. Although this measure was conceived to protect the patients from the sight of the corpse, all of them knew exactly when the trolley began its descent.

National mourning for great men has become familiar to all of us—flags are at half mast, schools close, work stops, and the funeral is televised for all to watch in the privacy of their own homes.

Following deaths in America black and purple wreaths are sometimes placed on the front doors of houses; men occasionally wear black armbands, and women dress in black and sometimes wear mourning veils. The hearse is black and, in military funerals, the caisson and horses are black.[9]

A cross-cultural study made of 127 elderly San Franciscans showed that death was the most frequently reported stress (Anderson, 1964). The loss of a spouse represented death's most serious threat to native Americans. Some Europeans, however, gave the loss of mother as the greatest of life's stresses. Persons with religious affiliations reported the death of loved ones as stressful more often than did persons without expressed religious affiliations. Women mentioned death more often than men, but men elaborated more upon the circumstances of death—the process of dying and the ordeal of death itself.

---

[9] It is a current fad among some young people to buy a hearse and ride around and sleep in it, as if in defiance of death.

Men also showed greater empathy in that they expressed suffering for the afflicted, while the women in their death recalls did not give empathy as the primary feeling. They were more likely to speak of the effect of the consequences of loss upon themselves, e.g., the misery of managing alone. In this study it was determined that loss of spouse was most stressful to the poor.

Therapeutic tasks

Ambivalence is common in mourning and is perhaps the cause of the intense pain of bereavement. Freud said in *Mourning and Melancholia* (1917) that no one gives up a love object, that there is a fixation of the memory of the lost object.

The work of mourning, the grief work, can be centered around a pool of shared images. Talking about the deceased with a friend or therapist will help create these. Some widows form groups that meet regularly for years and share remembrances of happier times and experiences with their spouses. The therapeutic potential of interpersonal relationships is mobilized and put to use in widow-to-widow programs being organized in community mental health programs. One such program noted that lending a friendly ear and a shoulder to cry on and helping other family members to be considerate were all of benefit to the bereaved widow (Silverman, 1969). People participating in these programs will remind a newly bereaved widow that the deceased husband would have liked her to do things in a certain way that will restore her equilibrium. The pain of bereavement is gradually neutralized by discussing the deceased in great detail. When the work of mourning is done, an unpainful picture of the loved one emerges, to be stored in the memory and recalled without suffering. The following is an example of unfinished grief work completed years later.

> The patient, a young boy now 16 years old, son of a prostitute, was placed in an institution by his mother at the age of 2 years. Later on he lived in foster homes. He was followed up by his psychiatrist several times a year in an effort to maintain continuity of the relationship (Bowlby, 1968). The boy made a plan to find his mother and then go to America to find his father, who he thought was an American serviceman. He discussed the plan with the psychiatrist, who listened but did not criticize it, although he thought it was quite impracticable. Eventually, the boy told the therapist that he believed the plan was difficult to accomplish and that, even if he succeeded in it, he might not be welcomed by his parents.

The boy finally came to accept his own reality—if he found his lost parents, they would be strangers. Maybe they would not be so glad to see him. He had a picture in which the lost person was present and one in which the person was gone. Someone's listening to him and showing care and sympathy helped him work through his conflicting images.

Immortality may be discussed and ideas about it reviewed. It is a very personal subject and may be expressed in terms of belief in an afterlife. Identification with the deceased may occur, not in the sense of one's becoming more like the dead person, but by retaining the image of the loved one painlessly through accepting certain thoughts and feelings.

CATHARSIS
One of the principal therapeutic tasks should be aimed toward securing catharsis, which can be defined as an effective discharge of feelings with resultant relief. It is the healthful release of thoughts and feelings through "talking it out" and experiencing the appropriate emotional reactions. If anger is expressed openly, the person gets over it. One newly bereaved widow beat up the physician; other people might get angry at the nurses. The climate can be set by the nurse for expression of angry feelings. Take the initiative to become acquainted with the family.

Nurses can take family members aside and help them to express their feelings about the dying patient. If the family knows that anger toward the physician and others may occur, it may help to advise them to engage in physical exercise for release of aggressive feelings. A long walk can be immensely helpful. Older family members who have experienced loss before and who understand the feelings may be enlisted to aid the younger ones during the crisis. An example of how a nursing student helped one family follows:

A student, during a visit to Mr. and Mrs. Johnson, learned that a grandson's divorced mother and father had just died within a few weeks of each other. Besides helping Mr. and Mrs. Johnson with their own grief and mourning about the loss of their son and former daughter-in-law, the student felt that they needed assistance in helping their grandson in this crisis. Since the new stepmother seemed unable to help Tommy, the student talked with Mrs. Johnson (the stronger one of the retired couple) about helping Tommy to express his feelings, informing his teachers about the loss of his parents, and getting the school counselor to talk with Tommy, all of which were carried out.

The manner in which grief is expressed is determined by the previous relationship with one's mother or mother substitute. If the person feels self-reproach or guilt, he needs someone who will listen to him. Thoughts that appear real to him may seem unreal to the therapist. The nurse can help the bereaved review their relationship with the deceased. A mourner who feels self-reproach or guilt needs to perceive the positive aspects of his relationship to the deceased and may require reassurance from the nurse that he did all he could to help the deceased get well or die without pain.

The unresolved grief of Doctor Zhivago resulted in his thinking that he saw his loved one on the street after the Revolution. Pursuing this image, he met his death (Pasternak, 1958). The therapist's work is to determine the feeling that is to be expressed and to help the mourner express it. If the person tries to turn back time he may become involved in a painful struggle with the past. If he is encouraged, however, to return to the time of bereavement and to review it in detail with a friend, relative, or therapist, he has a much better chance of relieving his sorrow. To give words to sorrow is important. The mourner's helper or therapist serves as a companion who gives emotional support and who has time to discuss his hopes, desires, plans for the future, regrets, reproaches, and disappointments.

We help our patients decide their own reality, as in the following example:

> Mrs. Potemkin, a patient who developed metastatic cancer, was greatly worried about her aged mother, who lived across the country. The old woman lived alone and held firmly to independence without accepting needed aid from physicians and acquaintances. The patient, preparing for her own death, was greatly relieved when she received news of her mother's death.

If the patient has not had time to grieve and mourn, as during a disaster or war, time and place should be set aside to complete the grief work. The treatment during World War II of grief-stricken Royal Air Force officers by T. F. Main (1968) is an example. The officers were removed from active duty with a diagnosis of combat fatigue. They sat and stared, neither eating nor moving. They had lost all their buddies. Dr. Main hypothesized that they needed time and a place for grieving. Each was then given a dark room for a few days with no interruptions, except for meals, in order to accomplish his grief work. Often this treatment was sufficient.

People need privacy to give vent to their feelings in our culture; many cannot cry in the presence of others. The nurse can ask others to leave while she is with the bereaved, or might ask the grieving patient to go to a secluded place. The climate is thereby set for the expression of sorrow, and the patient is encouraged to assume his role obligation of discussing feelings of loss, guilt, rage, and hostility if they are present.

Nurses should also help the patient who has lost a roommate or neighbor by death to express his feelings about the event. In a psychiatric unit, death is quite rare, but when it happens, it should be handled in a matter-of-fact manner and announced to the patients. Enough staff should be present at that time to help the patients express their thoughts and feelings within a group. Time must be found to accomplish this task.

The following excerpt is a beautiful example of some of the needs of the dying:[10]

> *Apart from this lying, or in consequence of it, the most wretched thing of all for Ivan Ilyich was that nobody pitied him as he yearned to be pitied. At certain moments, after a prolonged bout of suffering, he craved more than anything—ashamed as he would have been to own it—for someone to feel sorry for him just as if he were a sick child. He longed to be petted, kissed, and wept over, as children are petted and comforted. He knew that he was an important functionary, that he had a beard turning grey, and that therefore what he longed for was impossible; but nevertheless he longed for it. And in Gerassim's attitude toward him there was something akin to what he yearned for, and so Gerassim was a comfort to him. Ivan Ilyich feels like weeping and having someone to pet him and cry over him, but in comes his colleague Shebek and instead of weeping and being petted Ivan Ilyich puts on a grave, stern, profound air, and by force of habit expresses his opinion on a decision of the Court of Appeal, and obstinately insists on it. The falsity around him and within him did more than anything else to poison Ivan Ilyich's last days.*

The process of dying can only be experienced by the dying person himself. However, it is thought that the dying person goes through a process of grief and mourning for his own death. The last phase of life brings with it what was previously thought to be detachment from objects, but which now is viewed as an introspective involvement in holding one's self together. An extreme fear of death may be due to primitive fears of abandonment stemming from childhood.

Ask the family of the dying patient how the patient has reacted to a previous loss and about his philosophy of life. Relatives welcome the opportunity to talk about their loved ones. If there are no relatives or significant others, the nurse can get this information from the patient himself. Talking about what men live by is one approach. Another is to discuss the best and the most difficult things in life. Information about how previous losses have been met may be of help or they may not. New crises call for new adaptive mechanisms.

---

[10] Leo Tolstoy: *The Death of Ivan Ilyich* (1886). Baltimore: Penguin Books, 1960, pp. 143–44.

It is no longer claimed that the same defenses hold forth throughout the life span.

To determine how much the patient knows about his condition, ask the physician what information he has given the patient, his chances of survival, and how much time he has left. Awareness of oblique ways in which some patients may express their feelings must be uppermost in your thoughts as you care for the patient. Probing for feelings is not the answer.

Students often wish to hasten the process of verbalization of feelings with regard to death and fail to understand (in their own hastened learning process) that defense mechanisms actually function to protect the ego. A patient's fear of breaking down completely in front of the nurse or his family must be respected.

Inasmuch as dying patients will discuss their own deaths with their nurses, if with anybody, it is essential that nurses examine their own thoughts and feelings about death as they attend such patients. Fear of death is probably common to everyone.

HELPING CHILDREN VIEW DEATH

The age and level of development of the individual determine his manner of expression of grief. We need to know more about how children and adolescents express their feelings about death. One of the best films about how children view death is *Forbidden Games.* Some family members may consider it strange that children and adolescents do not cry but instead continue playing baseball or their other usual activities. If the young people cannot verbalize, these exercises may be their catharsis; in fact, the young mourner may display fierce competition. Retiring into seclusion to listen to music or a particular achievement at school may be other forms of catharsis. The child's behavior at a time of death is a dramatic example of the need to look beyond manifest behavior for understanding people and being able to help them. "Manifest behavior without analysis of its corresponding conflicts is a notoriously unreliable index to an understanding of psychology on a level that is beyond behaviorism."[11]

Parents who are experiencing loss, as of a spouse, need assistance in expressing their thoughts and feelings. They can be helped not to deny their feelings while in the presence of their children, but to express them. On the other hand, they can be advised to avoid becoming hysterical around the children. One child whose mother had died and whose father explained that she was dead and would be buried in the ground the next day asked him, "How will she breathe and who will feed her?" (Barnes, 1964). Children may feel

[11] Gregory Rochlin: *Griefs and Discontents: The Forces of Change.* Boston: Little, Brown & Co., 1965, p. 59.

that the death of a mother is contagious and avoid a friend whose mother has just died. If children see death only as sleep, which is one of the more common ways that parents explain death to a very young child, they may fear sleep themselves, and be unable to take naps and go to sleep at night. Clearly stating to a child that a dead person does not breathe, eat, or sleep may help him to better understand death.

A bereaved child may blame the surviving parent for his loss. Many children cannot cry at the death of parents because they are angry at being left alone. The surviving parent may be so absorbed in his own grief that he forgets about the child. The life style of the family will certainly affect their capacity for tension management and emotional support at the loss of one of its members. If you recall the death of Senator Robert Kennedy, and the help given to the children at the time of their loss, you have an example of children's involvement in the reality of the situation of death. It is of importance to note that the life style of the Kennedy family includes much support for its children. On the night that Robert Kennedy was shot, family friends checked the bedrooms of the children; 13-year-old David was found to have watched the tragedy of his father's death on television. The family friend held David in his own arms, giving him body contact comfort, and stayed in the room to share his grief (Caplan, 1968). The older children with the stronger egos were brought to their father's hospital room. The involvement of the children in the funeral— for example, standing guard at the casket; one was a pallbearer—kept them within the family circle during this tragedy.

The child can easily and immediately transfer affectional ties to a mother substitute. (The adult analog would be the widow who quickly remarries following the death of her husband.) The mourning period gives the adult mourner time for detaching emotional energy from the lost object. Only after a longer period of time does the adult mourner make the transfer. Denial is very strong in children. One child said, "If my mother were dead, then I would be all alone" (Wolfenstein, 1966). Here the child's concept of death is one of abandonment. He cannot conceive of his mother leaving him; therefore he cannot conceive of her death.

With children, there may also be magical thinking for the mother to return; it serves to bring back the lost parent. Children in a group may avoid talking of death if one of their members has lost a parent. Regression is common, often characterized by a return to thumbsucking and clinging to dolls. Games of playing dead enable children to act out their feelings about death. Displacement onto animals may also occur; their concern about the animals may actually represent concern for the dead parent. An active child may suddenly become quite passive or a naughty child unusually well behaved.

There is a difference of opinion about the age at which mourning occurs. Bowlby says it may occur at 6 months of age. Anna Wolf (1958) wrote that between the ages of 5 and 9 children may grasp the finality of death but not until 10 or 11 can they have something approaching adult comprehension of death. On the other hand, a child may intellectually understand death but the emotional impact will be too much for him. According to Furman (1964), mourning is dependent upon the ability to have a concept of death. The age that this ability occurs may certainly vary in different children.

ADOLESCENCE AND MOURNING

Adolescence can be considered the initiation into mourning; it must be experienced before the individual can perform grief work in reaction to future losses. Some view adolescence as a trial mourning itself—the breaking off of childhood ties and the detachment from parental figures. Adolescence then may be thought of as a necessary prerequisite for the mourning process. It is important not to confuse normal adolescent behavior and conflicts with the work of mourning. The renunciation of childhood may be accompanied by much pain unrelated to death.

In the adolescent mourner, particularly boys, crying may be considered a sign of weakness and will not be evident. The glorified and idealized parent of childhood is returned to in fantasy life. Mourning at a distance may occur, as in the previously cited example of the 12-year-old whose mother died and who remained stoical but cried profusely when her horse died. Mastery may be returned to as in childhood, where a very detailed verbal account of the death is given to another.

DYING, BUT NOT ALONE

In hospitals where there is staff transiency and turnover, it is imperative that information be passed on to nurses on different shifts so that each nurse who enters a dying patient's room does not expect catharsis. Usually, in a hospital with many staff members, patients will feel closer to one or two nurses. Know about and consider these nurse-patient ties in making patient assignments. Similarly, if the human relationship has become important to the patient, the nurse will not break it off but will remain with the patient throughout his last days. Nurses may have guilt feelings about their dying patients, especially those on clinical assignments where death is frequent. Discuss these feelings with others as they occur.

Everybody needs a confidante. Find out if the patient has anyone who shows care and concern about what is happening to him and make it possible for that person to stay with the patient during his last hours. People grieve and mourn for themselves in the process of preparing for death; be in tune with what your patient is experiencing. Students tend to look for formulas of behavior for themselves in relation to their dying patients. They sometimes blame the physician for not telling the patient what is happening to him. In discussing this matter in class one day, one student reported a change in her attitude when a young physician told her about a patient of his who committed suicide after he told her she was going to die.

PERCEPTION OF DEATH

Patients come to their own realization of death at their own pace. They can see expectation of it in our eyes, our manner, and our faces. Dying patients pick up clues from their relatives with regard to their deaths. When dying is prolonged, the patient can feel changes within his own body and come to his own conclusions. The patient perceives a decline in energy level. He is aware of losing or gaining weight and, often, of increasing infirmity. He knows he must depend on others to assist him because he can no longer get up to the bathroom and bathe himself, for example. He feels other changes in his body, e.g., increased or decreased pulse and respiration. Answering a simple question such as "how sick are you?" may help your patient to tell you what he knows about his condition. A dying patient may greet you with the announcement, "Nurse, I'm gonna die," or "Nurse, I'm dying," or "Nurse, I won't be here much longer." A calm acceptance of death by the nurse and a simple statement such as "I'll miss you," or "I am sorry that we all have to die" may be comforting to the patient. Those who cannot speak or hear may silently shed tears. The nurse can use touch—stroking the patient's hair, holding his hand, and drying his tears.

DETERMINATION OF DEATH

The determination of when a person is dead is changing from the traditional concept that death occurs when the heart stops beating to that of brain death determined by the EEG. At least one surgeon divides cadavers into two types, heart beating and nonheart beating. The impact upon the physician, nurses, and the family, of hearing that a patient is dead, even though he still has a beating heart, is difficult to assess. Determination of death has traditionally been made by a physician. Nurses now have to sometimes face requests from physicians to "pull the plug" that stops the heartbeat of the dead, though heart-beating cadaver. Legally, the heart-beating cadaver is dead because physicians determine death. The recent, widely televised flight of a heart-beating cadaver from out-of-state for transplant in Texas has set a precedent in the minds of the viewers for acceptance of death as brain death.

THE NURSE'S ACCEPTANCE OF DEATH

Since death is a concern of all nurses, you must recognize your own feelings about death before you can be of much assistance to dying patients and their families. Reviewing your earliest memories of death can aid in understanding feelings; sharing them with other students is also helpful. Many young people may never have experienced the death of a person, but almost everyone can recall the death and burial of a pet. Review what you did and what you felt the first time you had experience of death. Share your experiences with your peers. Although I had experienced death in my life several times before I went to nursing school, I still remember the first two dying patients I had, both of whom suffered from bacterial endocarditis. One was a 12-year-old boy, the same age as one of my brothers. He was the youngest patient on the unit, a large men's medical unit in a teaching hospital. The concern of the other patients in the 60-bed unit was touching. I was the only night nurse, and I was assisted by one orderly. This dying boy's needs were anticipated by the other patients, who were very sick themselves.

In the uninitiated, feelings of despair and frustration may be evoked by the dying patient. Guilt may also be felt because of one's failure to help the dying person. To overcome these feelings, nurses and other helping persons often feel impelled to make frantic efforts to save patients—suggesting, for example, surgery, parenteral feedings, or oxygen. Nurses who witness multiple deaths in a short space of time, as in an intensive care unit, or who otherwise take care of terminal patients need a defined place and time to discuss their feelings about dying and death. Such an arrangement is practiced by the head nurse of a cancer research unit in a large medical center, who invites the hospital chaplain to the weekly staff conferences (Stock, 1969). After the nurses ventilate their feelings about death, they proceed with the usual discussion of nursing problems.

STYLE OF DEATH

Everyone has a right to a dignified death. Nurses have a responsibility to the individual to assist him to die in the style which he chooses. Keep the patient as comfortable as possible. Instruct the family and all the staff that the sense of hearing is the last to leave the body. Admonish them to take care with what is said within the patient's presence even though he may appear totally insensitive to the world around him.

One of man's greatest fears is that of dying alone. If no friend or relative is attending the patient in his last hours, stay with him yourself. Patients who are being treated in large medical centers often come from long distances and may therefore not have the comfort of their families when they are dying. Old people may not have surviving friends or relatives to be with them. Reassure your patients that you will be with them to the end.

Family members who are visiting the dying patient may feel quite lonely, and they too will need the nurse's assurance and assistance. They may feel they are not doing enough, or they may wish unconsciously to hasten the death. Guilt may also be present because of old, unresolved conflicts with the dying.

A patient, Mrs. Quesada, has been in the hospital for 2 weeks and is now dying. She had been living with a daughter in San Francisco for many years and had had little contact with a younger daughter who lived across the continent. When the latter arrived, she made many complaints to the physician and the nursing staff about the care of her mother and insisted that none of the students touch her. It was felt that she was overcompensating for her guilt feelings for not having done anything for her mother in the past 20 years. A quiet reassignment was made of nursing staff, and the remaining complaints were handled matter-of-factly with care taken not to increase the daughter's guilt feelings by being oversolicitous.

PHYSICAL COMFORT
There are many books that deal with the physical needs of the dying patient. Following are suggestions of some things nurses can do to make the last days more pleasant for those who are dying. All things that we do for ourselves should be anticipated by the nurse and carried out without the patient's having to ask for them: oral hygiene for mouth breathing, care of the skin, repositioning, care of the hair and nails, helping the patient's intake by getting suitable foods and observing the output. Assisting the patient with the body arts, such as shaving, shampooing, and applying makeup, will help the family by minimizing to some extent the ravages wrought by the disease in the patient's appearance. Personal care of this nature is invaluable to the patient, who is made to feel that someone cares for him and who gets the basic comfort of being touched. *It is important that these procedures be carried out until the end; they convey to the patient that someone still cares about him.*

ATTITUDES TOWARD DEATH
The nurse has a responsibility to help her patients use their last moments to the fullest. The following is an excellent example of a caring staff:

Mr. Campbell had leukemia. He was in his late twenties and had a wife and a 3-year-old son. He was told by his physician that he had probably 3 months to a year to live and that he would be helped during his illness. The nursing staff and the physician helped him to plan his time so that he could be with his family as much as possible. He spent much of his time at home, returning to the hospital when he had an infection. Eight months later he went into terminal coma while in the hospital.

It should be noted that many people approach death with a minimum of fear. The following is an example of the serenity of an older person approaching 90 years of age. Her husband had predeceased her and three of her six children had died, one only two weeks earlier. She lived alone in the old house where she had spent most of her life. She told her visiting nursing student:

> I don't really have a great fear of dying. In fact, sometimes when I get lonely, I almost pray that God will take me. I guess He just isn't quite ready for me yet.

The fear of dying can be present in any patient. The following situation is an example of a patient who verbalized his fear of death.

> The patient is an Italian man, Mr. Bottesini, in his older years, who raised vegetables on the outskirts of the city when he was younger and now lives in the same house, surrounded by subdivisions. He has a deeply lined face, a thin body, and an unsmiling demeanor. Now in his second week postsurgery in which he had a prostatectomy, he complains bitterly to all who will listen that his bed has been wet all night, that no one came to check him but the little Chinese girl, and that he is afraid that he is ready for Colma.[12]

> It was difficult to get across to the night staff that Mr. Bottesini was very shy and could not bring himself to allow a young girl to change his dressings and his bed. As a result, he did not ask for help and no one took the initiative to check his bed. Mr. Bottesini became more and more anxious and began to complain about the meals, the small bathroom, and being ready for Colma. The nursing staff became more and more irritated, held a conference, and decided to set limits on his behavior. They felt very pleased with themselves when Mr. Bottesini stopped complaining. At this point they learned that he had developed a fistula and would require a colostomy as an interim measure. Then guilt arose in some of the nurses and they became very solicitous of the patient.

What are the nursing problems involved in the case described above? What actions would you have taken and why? Discuss them with others.

SPIRITUAL NEEDS

Nurses who are sensitive to the needs of the dying will give priority to these needs. Reading part of the patient's Bible to him may be a help; comfort may also be received from the presence of a minister or priest. Some dying patients who have broken their ties with the church may not think of asking for religious consolation until the nurse suggests that the chaplain come in and talk with them. The following situation is an example of how a nursing student helped a patient to establish contact with the minister of his church:

---

[12] The location of the burial grounds for citizens of San Francisco.

Mr. Adams was diagnosed as having lung cancer and was told by his physician that he has perhaps two to three months to live. He is in a ward with three other men who have minor surgical problems. The student learned that the patient lives alone. He is divorced and his children live across the continent and do not write to him. The student, thinking of spiritual needs, asked the patient if he would like to see his minister. When the patient refused, the student pursued the matter until he told her that he had not gone to church for 20 or 30 years, that his old church was far across the country, and that he did not know any ministers. The student dropped the subject and went on to something else. Later, she found out the days the Episcopal minister regularly visited the hospital and arranged a meeting at which she told him about her patient, mentioning that he had a fatal disease, that he had not been to church for a long time, had no family in the area, and needed a friend. The minister agreed to visit the patient who, when he was subsequently informed of the fact, seemed pleased and relieved.

At the time of death even unbelievers may become believers or agnostics.

MEDICATIONS
Nurses sometimes require assistance in making decisions about whether to give p.r.n. (at their own discretion) medications to the dying person; they may feel that the patient himself should be consulted and his wishes honored during his final days. Judgment about pain medication requires a thorough knowledge of many factors: the patient's pain tolerance, severity of pain, and whether or not the patient himself wishes to remain aware of what is happening to him. A frank discussion with the patient may elicit his own thoughts and feelings about his style of dying. Some people wish to be fully conscious even when they are suffering. Incorporate the wishes of such patients and their families into your nursing care plan and team conferences. Others prefer to be "knocked out" or "unaware." Time is also a factor in this type of decision. Many things need to be done—letters written, a will drawn up, farewells made to family and friends. These matters should not be delayed too long, because dying patients are no longer interested in what they are leaving behind and may not be capable of handling their affairs.

The silence of death

Two months before my father died I went with him to his physician for treatment of the sarcoma that had suddenly enveloped his body. In spite of his increasing fatigue, he went about his work as usual. Finally becoming bed-ridden, he read his Bible, made his peace with God, and one morning called all of us individually to his bedside to say goodby. "Be a good girl and don't forget me," were his last words for me. He went quietly into coma that afternoon and died 2 hours later. Because his face was disfigured, his body was prepared by the mortician and placed in a pine box in the same room where he died. Friends and neighbors called and sat with the coffin until it was time for the funeral, which was held in the local church. Burial was in the adjacent graveyard among the wild flowers of the earth that he loved.

I have given this example as a contrast to the more common style of dying, most likely to occur in hospitals with nurses in attendance.

After all of the pertinent knowledge of medical science has been exhausted in treating the dying person, the family and nurses wait. Family members may be torn between the wish to prolong the contact and the desire to get it over with. Help the family members to decide among themselves that at least one person will take the responsibility for staying with the dying relative. Sitting, caring, touching, and showing concern become all that is left for the nurse to do. The nurse who sits at the side of a dying person and holds his hand until the last breath feels a oneness with the experiences and suffering of mankind and realizes the evanescence of life. When life finally leaves the body, the stillness and silence of death can leave the living with the feeling of hope that someone will do the same things for them when their times come.

Summary

In this chapter, some aspects of the problem of loss have been discussed. Depression, as a frequent outcome of feelings of loss, is differentiated from normal states. The prevalence of depression is described and ways for the nurse to recognize depressive affects outlined. The mental disorder of involutional melancholia is discussed, with emphasis on preventive measures by the nurse. Nursing care of patients with manic-depressive illnesses is considered. In a section on grief and mourning, the central aim of the nurse to help the bereaved complete their grief work is stressed. Some aspects of the social and intellectual movements in nursing designed to enable better understanding of the dying patient and the bereaved family are discussed, with a focus on the nurse's therapeutic tasks.

References

American Psychiatric Association: *A Psychiatric Glossary*. Washington, D.C., 1969.

———— *Diagnostic and Statistical Manual of Mental Disorder*, II. Washington, D.C.: 1968.

Anderson, Barbara Gallatin: "Death as a Subject of Cross-Cultural Inquiry." Presented at the International Congress of Social Psychiatry, London, 1964.

Ayd, Frank: *Recognizing the Depressed Patient*. New York: Grune and Stratton, 1961, pp. 118–25.

Barnes, Marion J.: "Reactions to the Death of a Mother," *The Psychoanalytic Study of the Child*, Vol. 19. New York: International Universities Press, 1964, pp. 334–57.

Beck, Aaron T.: *Depression*. New York: Harper and Row, 1967.

Beers, Clifford Whittingham: *A Mind that Found Itself* (1908). Garden City, N.Y.: Doubleday, Doran and Co., Inc., 1921.

Bendann, E.: *Death Customs, An Analytical Study of Burial Rites*. New York: Knopf, 1930.

Berezin, Martin A., and Cath, Stanley H., eds.: *Geriatric Psychiatry: Grief, Loss and Emotional Disorders in the Aging Process*. New York: International Universities Press, Inc., 1965.

Bowlby, John: Notes from Symposium on "Separation and Loss." San Francisco Psychoanalytic Institute, San Francisco, 1968.

Caplan, Gerald: "Lessons in Bravery," *McCall's*, pp. 85ff, September, 1968.

Caumont, M. A. de: *Abecedaire en Rudiment d'Archéologie*. Caen: F. Le Blanc-Hardel, 1886.

Deutsch, Albert: *The Mentally Ill in America*. Garden City, N.Y.: Doubleday, Doran and Co., Inc., 1937.

Forbidden Games (*Jeux Interdits*), Film, Robert Dorfman, 1952.

Freeman, Lucy: *The Cry for Love*. New York: The Macmillan Co., 1969.

Freud, Sigmund: "Mourning and Melancholia" (1917), in *The Collected Papers*, Vol. IV. London: The Hogarth Press, 1949, pp. 152–70.

Furman, Robert A.: "Death and the Young Child," *The Psychoanalytic Study of the Child*, Vol. 19. New York: International Universities Press, 1964, pp. 321–33.

Glaser, Barney, and Strauss, Anselm: *Awareness of Dying*. Chicago: Aldine Publishing Co., 1965.

Goodman, Louis S., and Gilman, Alfred: *The Pharmacological Basis of Therapeutics*, 3rd ed. New York: The Macmillan Co., 1965.

Hinsie, Leland E., and Campbell, Robert Jean: *Psychiatric Dictionary*. New York: Oxford University Press, 1960.

Holbein, H.: *The Dance of Death*. London: Hamilton, Adams and Co., 1887.

Huizinga, Johan: *The Waning of the Middle Ages*. New York: Anchor Books, 1954. (First published in 1924.)

Kalkman, Marion E.: "Recognizing Emotional Problems," *American Journal of Nursing*, **68**:536–39, March, 1968.

Kallman, F. J.: *Heredity in Health and Mental Disorders*. New York: W. W. Norton, 1953.

Kolb, Lawrence C.: *Noyes' Modern Clinical Psychiatry*. Philadelphia: W. B. Saunders Co., 1968.

Kübler-Ross, Elizabeth: *On Death and Dying*. New York: The Macmillan Co., 1969.

Levin, Sidney: "Depression in the Aged," in Berezin, Martin A., and Cath, Stanley H., eds.: *Geriatric Psychiatry: Grief, Loss and Emotional Disorders in the Aging Process*. New York: International Universities Press, Inc., 1965.

Lieberman, Morton A.: "Observations on Death and Dying," *The Gerontologist*, **6**:2:70–73, June, 1966.

——— "Depressive Affect and Vulnerability to Environmental Change in the Aged." *Proceedings of Seminars, 1961–1965, Duke University Council on Gerontology*, April, 1965, pp. 328–35.

——— Prock, V. N., and Tobin, S. S.: "The Psychological Effects of Institutionalization," *Journal of Gerontology*, **23**:3:343–53, July, 1968.

Lindemann, Erich: "Symptomatology and Management of Acute Grief," *American Journal of Psychiatry*, **101**:141–48, 1944.

Main, T. F.: "The Hospital as a Therapeutic Institution," in Barnes, Elizabeth, ed.: *Psychological Nursing*. London: Tavistock Publications, Inc. (Barnes and Noble, Inc., in U.S.A.), 1968.

Maoz, Benjamin: "Female Attitudes to Menopause," *Social Psychiatry*, **5**:1:35–40, January, 1970.

Menninger, Karl: *Man Against Himself*. New York: Harcourt, Brace and Co., 1938.

Morozov, G., and Romasenko, V.: *Neuropathology and Psychiatry*. Moscow: Moscow Peace Publishers (no date).

Motto, Jerome: Notes taken from lecture at symposium on "Psychiatric Problems of Aging," Mendocino, 1968.

Pasternak, Boris Leonidovich: *Doctor Zhivago*. New York: Pantheon, 1958.

Patten, Bradley M.: *Human Embryology*. New York: Blakiston Co., Inc., 1953.

Pirenne, Henri: *Economic and Social History of Medieval Europe*. New York: Harcourt, Brace and Co., 1936.

Quint, Jeanne C.: *The Nurse and the Dying Patient*. New York: The Macmillan Co., 1967.

Reik, Theodor: *Listening with the Third Ear*. New York: Grove Press, 1956.

Rochlin, Gregory: *Griefs and Discontents: The Forces of Change*. Boston: Little, Brown and Co., 1965.

Schwab, John H., Brown, Judith M., Holzer, Charles E., and Sokolof, Marilyn: "Current Concepts of Depression: The Sociocultural," *The International Journal of Social Psychiatry*, **14**:3:226–34, 1968.

Silverman, Phyllis Rolfe: "The Widow-to-Widow Program," *Mental Hygiene*, **53**:3:333–37, July, 1969.

Spitz, René, and Wolf, Katherine M.: "Anaclitic Depression," *The Psychoanalytic Study of the Child*, **2**:313–43, 1946.

Stock, Irene (Head Nurse, Cancer Research Unit, University of California Medical Center, San Francisco): Personal communication, 1969.

Taber, Clarence Wilbur: *Taber's Cyclopedic Medical Dictionary*, 10th ed. Philadelphia: F. A. Davis, 1965.

Tolstoy, Leo: *The Death of Ivan Ilyich* (1886). Baltimore: Penguin Books, 1960.

Webster's Seventh New Collegiate Dictionary. Springfield, Mass.: G. and C. Merriam Co., Publishers, 1965.

Wolf, Anna: "Helping Your Child to Understand Death," *Child Study*, **35**:36ff., Winter, 1957–58.

Wolfenstein, Martha: "How Is Mourning Possible?" *The Psychoanalytic Study of the Child*, Vol. 21. New York: International Universities Press, 1966, pp. 93–123.

——— "Loss, Rage and Repetition," *The Psychoanalytic Study of the Child*, Vol. 24. New York: International Universities Press, 1969, pp. 432–60.

World Health Organization: *International Classification of Diseases*, Vol. I. Geneva: 1967.

Suggested readings

Alpert, Augusta: "A Brief Communication on Children's Reactions to the Assassination of the President," *The Psychoanalytic Study of the Child*, Vol. 19. New York: International Universities Press, 1964, pp. 313–24.

Barckley, Virginia: "Grief, a Part of Living," *Ohio's Health*, **20**:34–38, April-May, 1968.

Burnside, Irene Mortenson: "Grief Work in the Aged Patient," *Nursing Forum*, **8**:4:416–27, 1969.

Eissler, K. R.: *The Psychiatrist and the Dying Patient*. New York: International Universities Press, 1955.

Freedman, Alfred M., Kaplan, Harold I., and Kaplan, Helen S., eds.: *Comprehensive Textbook of Psychiatry*. Baltimore: The Williams and Wilkins Co., 1967.

Gerber, Irwin: "Bereavement and the Acceptance of Professional Service," *Community Mental Health Journal*, **5**:6:487–95, December, 1969.

Grollman, Earl A.: *Explaining Death to Children*. Boston: Beacon Press, 1967.

Hamovich, Maurice B.: *The Parent and the Fatally Ill Child*. Duarte, Calif.: City of Hope Medical Center, 1964.

Hinton, John: *Dying*. Baltimore: Penguin Books, 1967.

Kastenbaum, Robert: "Multiple Perspectives on a Geriatric 'Death Valley'," *Community Mental Health Journal*, **3**:1:21–29, Spring, 1967.

Laufer, Moses: "Object Loss and Mourning During Adolescence," *The Psychoanalytic Study of the Child*, Vol. 21. New York: International Universities Press, 1966, pp. 269–93.

Levin, Sidney: "Depression in the Aged," *Geriatrics*, **18**:302–307, 1963.

————— and Kahana, Ralph J., eds.: *Psychodynamic Studies on Aging: Creativity, Reminiscing and Dying*. New York: International Universities Press, 1968.

McDonald, Marjorie: "A Study of the Reactions of Nursery School Children to the Death of a Child's Mother," *The Psychoanalytic Study of the Child*, Vol. 19. New York: International Universities Press, 1964, pp. 358–76.

Mitford, Jessica: *The American Way of Death*. Greenwich, Conn.: Fawcett Publications, Inc., 1963.

Moriarty, David M., ed.: *The Loss of Loved Ones: The Effects of a Death in the Family on Personality Development*. Springfield, Ill.: Charles C Thomas, 1967.

Quint, Jeanne C., and Strauss, Anselm L.: "Nursing Students, Assignments and Dying Patients," *Nursing Outlook*, **12**:24–27, January, 1964.

————— "The Threat of Death: Some Consequences for Patients and Nurses," *Nursing Forum*, **8**:3:286–300, 1969.

Rheingold, Joseph C.: *The Mother, Anxiety and Death*. Boston: Little, Brown and Co., 1967.

Rochlin, Gregory: "Loss and Restitution," *The Psychoanalytic Study of the Child*, Vol. 8. New York: International Universities Press, 1953, pp. 288–309.

————— "The Dread of Abandonment," *The Psychoanalytic Study of the Child*, Vol. 16. New York: International Universities Press, 1961, pp. 451–70.

Silverman, Charlotte: *The Epidemiology of Depression*. Baltimore: Johns Hopkins Press, 1968.

Solzhenitsyn, Alexander: *Cancer Ward*. New York: Farrar, Strauss and Giroux, Inc., 1969.

Sudnow, David: *Passing On*. Englewood Cliffs, N.J.: Prentice-Hall, Inc., 1967.

Toynbee, Arnold: *Man's Concern with Death.* London: Hodder and Stoughton, 1968.

Travelbee, Joyce: "What Do We Mean by Rapport?" *American Journal of Nursing,* **63**:70, 1963.

Ujhely, Gertrud: "Preventive and Therapeutic Nursing Care," *Nursing Forum,* **5**:2:23–35, 1966.

———— "What Is Realistic Emotional Support?" *American Journal of Nursing,* **68**:758, 1968.

Velda, Jacoba van: *The Big Ward.* New York: Simon & Schuster, 1960.

Verwoerdt, Adriaan: "Communication with the Fatally Ill," *Southern Medical Journal,* **57**:787–93, 1964.

———— *Communication with the Fatally Ill.* Springfield, Ill.: Charles C Thomas, 1966.

———— "Communications with Fatally Ill Patients—Tacit or Explicit?" *American Journal of Nursing,* **67**:2307–2309, November, 1967.

Wagner, B. M.: "Teaching Students to Work with the Dying," *American Journal of Nursing,* **64**:128–31, November, 1964.

Wallace, Elspeth, and Townes, Brenda D.: "The Dual Role of Comforter and Bereaved," *Mental Hygiene,* **53**:3:327–32, July, 1969.

Waugh, Evelyn: *The Loved One.* New York: Random House, 1948.

Weisman, Avery D., and Hackett, Thomas P.: "Predilection to Death: Death and Dying as a Psychiatric Problem," *Psychosomatic Medicine,* **23**:232–56, 1961.

8   Aggression

Patriotism is not enough;
I must hold no hatred in my heart for any man.
   Edith Cavell

Freud (1930) postulated that aggression derives from and is part of one of the two major instincts of man—the instinct for death (Thanatos).[1] (The other is Eros, the instinct for life.) The frustration-aggression hypothesis of Dollard (1939) purports that frustration increases with rank and territory of man. Berkowitz (1962) views aggression as not automatically accompanying frustration or threat. Instead, he sees it as relative to the degree and amount of frustration, the power of the individual to react against the aggressive act, and one's values against aggression. In past centuries aggressive acts might lead, for example, to a duel—a type of confrontation unlikely today. Duelling served as a sanctioned outlet for individuals or groups in conflict. After the duel, amicable relations were expected to be resumed.

In modern times, in the highly ritualized sport of fencing one may symbolically "pick off" one's adversary by winning a bout; afterward both parties remove their protective masks, approach each other, smile, shake hands, and thank each other. Competitive sports are ritualized forms of aggressive behavior.

While some groups are more aggressive than others, all cultures experience aggression to some degree. The evocation of aggressive behavior depends on a number of antecedent conditions, e.g., the arbitrariness of the frustration, the power to retaliate against the aggression, and the presence of values against aggression.

Aggression has been described by an ethologist as the fighting instinct[2] in beast and man directed against members of the same species (Lorenz, 1963). Aggression in the psychiatric sense can be either appropriate or inappropriate, directed outward, or directed toward the self.[3]

----

[1] In Greek mythology Thanatos was the personification of Death, the son of Nyx (night) and brother of Hypnos (sleep).

[2] "*Instinct* is generally understood to be a specific response pattern—invariant in its development, maturation, and expression—that occurs to some quite specific cluster of stimuli from the environment" (Holloway, 1967, p. 40). (Copyright, 1967, The American Museum of Natural History.)

[3] "*Aggression* is a forceful, physical, verbal, or symbolic attack. It may be appropriate and self-protective, including healthful self-assertiveness, or inappropriate. It also may be directed outward toward the environment, as in explosive personality, or inward toward the self as in depression." (From *A Psychiatric Glossary*, copyright 1969, American Psychiatric Association.)

Aggression is usually easily perceived, and the concept of constructive aggression is well known. The child who uses magical thinking to release aggression may also experience guilt when, for example, he wishes that his father would die and the parent does die. A guilt reaction to unexpressed aggression is probably normal for the adolescent. In the 10- to 15-year-old, depression is linked to unexpressed aggression. Sadism and murder are extreme forms of outward aggression; masochism and suicide are examples of extreme inward aggression. A study by Silver (1969) covering three generations of families of abused children supports the view that violence breeds violence and that a child who experiences violence has the potential of becoming a violent member of society as he grows older.

Displacement

Aggression may be aroused by frustration, threats, or annoyances. Displaced aggression directs hostile feelings toward a person or an object other than the one which causes the frustration. The man who has a hard day at the office and comes home and yells at his wife or kicks the dog is one example of displacement.

The need for expression of aggression arising from intrapsychic tensions, and the need for resolving an external conflict are dissimilar. Intrapsychic tensions may be released toward one of several different people, whereas external conflicts between persons or groups may be resolved by arbitration or negotiation.

Need for release of aggression

Release of aggression as in play, hunting, work, and other physical activities may be greatly altered when patients are hospitalized, at times of other stresses, and when the usual outlets for aggression are not available. For example, a blind person may verbally attack an agency, reject it, or make excessive demands on it. His family may also join in the attack. Nursing students are familiar with the many biting remarks that some patients make about the institutions serving them, and about the professionals caring for them. The intimacy, sustained close contact, and heightened interaction that nurses experience with patients provide fertile ground for arousal of hostility and tension as well as the more positive affects of rapport (Coser, 1956). The rivalry—e.g., the traditional dislike of the French for the Germans and vice versa—between nations also serves as a channel for release of aggressive feelings. The competitiveness between nations symbolized in the Olympic Games can now be vicariously experienced throughout the world through the medium of television.

Inappropriate aggression: suspicion and hostility

Suspicion is the imagination of the existence of some fault, defect, guilt, or falsity when there may be slight evidence for its existence or none. It precedes hostility. The suspicious person tends to question motives of others over minute matters, mull over the consequences, and later confront individuals with long and involved analyses of their motives. Hostility refers to an unfriendly, antagonistic manner, to resentment, grudges, and resentful acts. All humans experience hostility. It is common for everyone to feel aggressive when frustration is encountered and handle it by adjusting, adapting, changing one's perceptions, or leaving. In a nonhuman primate society, there is no alternative to bluffing; if the bluff is called, fighting occurs. Humans, however, have language—they can explain, reason, and negotiate (Washburn, 1969). Hostility usually emerges after much rumination over an imagined slight. Buss (1961) makes the point that a hostile remark such as "I hate you" voiced by a person who is alone is not aggressive until there is someone to hear it. Hostility is one way that patients who are threatened react to the threat. If the threat can be removed, the hostility is not needed.

The following terms describe behavior of hostile persons: picky, resentful, argumentative, antagonistic, uncooperative, aggressive, irritable, caustic, sarcastic, rude, critical, resistant, begrudging, ignoring, demanding, complaining, scapegoating, gossiping, blocking, derogating, threatening, and rejecting (verbally and nonverbally). Inflicting physical injury, making barbed remarks, and joking at someone else's expense are all examples of hostility.

Nursing intervention

Aggressiveness in patients may stir up anxiety in the nurse. The patient who is sarcastic, irritable, and resentful and who constantly complains about the hospital, the physician, and the other staff may put you in a defensive position without your actually knowing whether his complaints are justifiable. Try to discover if there is indeed a basis in fact for the sarcasm. If there is none, perhaps your patient is releasing aggression because his normal manner of handling it is unavailable. The nurse can help by listening, offering alternative solutions to problems, and helping the patient to be secure enough so that aggressive behavior is no longer necessary. One nurse's approach to a patient whom most of the nurses described as "demanding" was to simply explain to the patient what she was going to do and how she would do it before she started anything. The patient responded in a receptive way, and the student was satisfied with her discovery. Taking the initiative, after explanation to the patient—what Ruesch (1961) calls "unaggressive directness"—indicating that the patient is expected to carry through his therapeutic regime, may really communicate to him. One student reports a situation as follows:

> The patient was called "demanding" by the other nurses, but I could tell that she was frightened and insecure the moment I met her. Throughout the evening she continuously asked for things. When I encouraged her to get out of bed and walk, she said that she didn't want to. I explained the reason why I was getting her up and that I would be with her all the time. I didn't ask her again. I just prepared to ambulate her. After she had walked down the hall and back to bed, she said to me, "It's all to your credit that I got up tonight. You were good enough to spend time with me."

The student had noted the insecurity and apprehension of the patient when she had asked what other patients she would be taking care of that evening. The student made herself available and used her professional authority for leverage only after assessing the individual needs of this "demanding" patient.

Patients with more severe problems, as in the psychoneuroses, who cannot express anger and hostility may be aided by the psychiatrist to do so. The patient immediately past his psychotherapeutic hour often is upset and may require a release of aggressive feelings.

The nurse can help by providing support to the patient who is learning to express anger and by not denying one's own anger. Make clear to the patient that destructive aggression is not acceptable. The use of suggestion can direct the patient to socially acceptable outlets such as pounding. Fear of losing self-control may accompany release of pent-up hostility; the patient may request you to help him not to lose complete control. Breaking all the windows in a day care center may temporarily release tension, but the destruction remains as a reminder of the guilt involved. The nurse sets limits here in that property and people are not to be physically attacked and helps the patient verbalize hostility or work it out in other ways. Talking through events that lead to expressions of hostility can help the patient learn new ways of handling aggression. Assist the patient immediately when he is able to talk about it, not tomorrow or next week.

Signs of mounting tension can be noted by the nurse, who can prevent the patient from hurting others, destroying objects, and injuring himself. Increased motor activity, angry facial expressions, stereotyped movements, and tremulousness may be some of the cues. Doing some habitual thing in a different manner than usual may be another sign of mounting tension. Remove the patient from the group to his room or similar privacy, remain with him, touch him, hold him, and talk with him. If possible, the same person assigned to help him meet his needs should be available to him through periods of aggression.

ACTIVITIES FOR THE RELEASE OF AGGRESSION

Activities that involve pounding, running, hitting, and cutting release aggression. For immobilized patients, a set of exercises requiring muscles that are not immobilized can be run through regularly. Vicariously "participating" in a much-loved television game may afford an effective outlet. Watching boxing and wrestling matches where someone else does the "clobbering" perhaps enables the vicarious releases of aggression. Being able to discuss a favorite competitive game and how effective one is in it can also release aggression. The identification with a particular ball team, horse, or driver of a racing car, and watching, hearing about, or discussing their competitive actions help release aggression. For example, one older patient in his nineties now almost blind, home bound, living alone, with all relatives dead, loved horse racing. The nursing student enlisted the aid of her *beau* to learn something about racing so she could discuss it with him. The animation on his face was the reward for her. For some, a punching bag, ping pong, hammering, tennis, or a fast fencing bout provides for release of aggression.

In a hospital setting, pounding metal as in copper work or metal sculpture and the pounding and kneading necessary to prepare clay for the potter's wheel are outlets. The classic example given for the sublimation of aggression is the surgeon who instead of expressing his aggression just by cutting people up does it by performing a precise operation. Typing and piano playing and various tasks carried on each day in a hospital setting can be made available to the patient. The nurse can help by learning the patient's needs and meeting them.

Running away from the hospital is sometimes attempted by patients, and efforts by staff to thwart such attempts will probably be met by aggression. The nurse should be aware of the usual habits of patients. A sudden decision to join a group of patients for an outing which has previously been consistently refused or a frantic accumulation of possessions when visitors are about to leave are nonverbal cues to what the patient may have on his mind.

The hostile patient expects the nurse to be hostile in return. If the nurse rises to the challenge, the positive feedback is likely to increase the patient's tension and result in a fight. Other ways of responding may disarm the hostile patient. Turning a verbal attack into something that can be laughed about can drain off tension (Ruesch, 1961, p. 150). Humor is one of the popular coping mechanisms; having a good laugh makes almost anything seem less formidable.

> A patient, Miss Lee, a beautiful model in her early twenties who was very caustic and belittling, especially of men, was diagnosed as being passive-aggressive. She kept after me to read the *Diagnostic and Statistical Manual of Mental Disorders* so that she could find her diagnosis. One day I handed it to her, and she studied it very closely for several hours. Later she approached me and demanded to know whether or not her selection of diagnosis was correct. She had chosen *involutional melancholia*. When I explained that this disorder was of the menopause, she had a big laugh and was quite relieved. Her sarcasm was temporarily discharged.

Hostility from patients is probably one of the most difficult things to deal with in nursing. Some people are more sensitive to hostility than others. When hostility is encountered for the first time in a patient, you may have a tendency to flee the situation or to make a counterattack, both of which are quite natural but neither one of which benefits the patient. Help him identify what is threatening, frightening, or annoying to him, and accept the patient as he is. Accepting him as he is implies that you will not pass moral judgment on him. It does not mean abandoning the patient in his psychological state but implies that you perceive the strengths within the individual and can therefore help him to move on to greater potentials. Setting limits on behavior and disapproval of behavior communicate to the patient that you care about him but not particularly about some of his behavior. *Avoid reacting to hostility as if it were personally directed toward you*. It is important to accept the feelings of the hostile patient and to give him the opportunity to clarify them with you. The following is an example of what one nurse did with *action language* and *the herd instinct*.

> A teen-age patient, Valerie, became belligerent, rude, and abusive to a nurse who took it personally and retaliated by becoming abusive to the patient. The nurse thereby lost control of the situation and the patient's abusiveness spiraled. Another nurse, observing the event, went over quietly to Valerie, took her by the hand, walked to a corner with her, sat with her until she calmed down, and then interested her in something else.

The action of the nurse let the patient know that she was accepted for herself. The nurse's presence and calm manner acted as comfort and negative feedback to the patient. Since anxiety itself communicates rapidly to others, the nurse, to be helpful to the patient, learns to control her own anxiety. The serene, authoritative manner of the nurse communicates to the hostile patient whose whole personality is *not* hostilely oriented. Retaliation or the use of the talionic principle is discarded in therapeutic work. A word of caution is included here: students should not mistakenly use these therapeutic techniques in life situations where their own self-preservation may be at stake.

The therapeutic task of the nurse is to help the hostile patient regain and perceive self-esteem. Removing his working defenses is opening a psychic wound and should be avoided. Belittling others (derogation) is a defense; as the patient belittles others, they become less threatening to him. Hostile individuals, beneath their thorny and bristly exteriors, are really insecure; their aggression may be a facade covering up their insecurity. Belittling the nurse may result when the nurse has not gained the patient's trust and supported his ego.

TRUST

Suspicious and hostile patients watch every move you make, every nuance and inflection of your voice, and mull them over. Take the initiative and make the overture to your patient, even if you anticipate a hostile encounter. This bolsters self-esteem of the patient. Trust is not likely to be established right away, but persistent interest communicates to the patient.

If you are on a home visit, the way you react to other members of the family—or, if in hospital, to other patients—communicates to the suspicious, hostile patient. An impersonal hasty manner of one staff member may also communicate to the hostile patient that he may expect the same treatment from all the members of your profession and therefore further eliminate possibilities for the development of trust. Empathize with the patient and assess his particular situation so that you can be more aware of his expectations of you. Patients who are suspicious and hostile are keenly aware of actions of staff and patients that are different from the particular culture of that psychiatric unit—e.g., staff members who give their attention to each other instead of the patients. If the whole ward is going on a picnic, the suspicious patient will wait to see if the nurse has remembered his special needs, for example, his medications, and ponder possible motivations if these have been overlooked. A promise for the smallest item is not forgotten.

THE NURSE'S HOSTILE FEELINGS

Any feeling of hostility in the nurse toward a patient must receive careful attention and self-examination through introspection and discussion with others. The continuous giving to others may drain the nurse emotionally, and hostile behavior may ensue. In at least one large medical center where many organ transplants are done, the nurses who care for these patients have psychiatric nursing consultation available to them and also regular group sessions with a psychiatrist.

The paranoid personality

The paranoid person has excessive suspicion, hostility, and rigidity. Reality testing is impaired. Possibly throughout their lives they have been unable to trust anyone. The paranoid person may not be able to get along with anyone and therefore lives alone, or at odds with those with whom he does live. He has a basic insecurity, is full of pride, and has been unable to develop satisfactory social skills. He is rigid and self-centered in his personality organization. He is sensitive to situations that make him feel inferior and most likely had a childhood in which his parents made demands of him that he could not meet. As a child he was sensitive and narcissistic. He uses overcompensation for feelings of inferiority, and his compensatory mechanisms involve status and prestige. He tends to deal with problems by brooding and introspection. There may be delusions, ideas of reference and influence, and extramarital affairs.

Since counteraggression reinforces the patient's delusions, in the nurse-patient relationship a lack of counteraggression is necessary; intellectual challenges may be encountered with the patient, and relationships explored matter-of-factly. Truthfulness and promises are rigidly adhered to by the nurse. A promise made, however small, is remembered by these patients, and if unfulfilled, is taken as rejection and becomes further food for insecurity. The nurse does not agree with the patient's delusions, but instead helps him use other defenses in adaptation. The account by the therapist who entered into the delusion of his patient is dramatically presented in the "Jet-Propelled Couch" (Lindner, 1955).

Summary

This chapter presents aggression from the social, ethological, and psychiatric points of view. The need for release of aggression is discussed as being common to everyone. Suspicious, hostile, and paranoid behavior are described and implications for nursing presented.

References

American Psychiatric Association: *A Psychiatric Glossary*. Washington, D.C., 1969.

Ardrey, Robert: *The Territorial Imperative*. New York: Atheneum, 1966.

Berkowitz, Leonard: *Aggression: A Social Psychological Analysis*. New York: McGraw-Hill Book Co., 1962.

Brooks, Beatrice R.: "Aggression," *American Journal of Nursing*, **67**:12: 2519–22, December, 1967.

Buss, Arnold H.: *The Psychology of Aggression*. New York: John Wiley and Sons, Inc., 1961.

Clack, Janice: "Nursing Intervention into the Aggressive Behavior of Patients," in Burd, Shirley F., and Marshall, Margaret A., eds.: *Some Clinical Approaches to Psychiatric Nursing*. New York: The Macmillan Co., 1963.

Coser, Lewis A.: *The Functions of Social Conflict*. New York: The Free Press of Glencoe, 1956, p. 62.

Dentan, Robert Knox: *The Semai; A Non-Violent People of Malaya*. New York: Holt, Rinehart and Winston, 1968, p. 58.

Dollard, J., Dobb, L. W., Miller, N. E., Mowrer, O. H., and Sears, R. R.: *Frustration and Aggression*. New Haven: Yale University Press, 1939.

Freud, Sigmund: *Civilization and Its Discontents*. London: Hogarth Press, 1953. (First published 1930.)

Holloway, R. L.: "Human Aggression: The Need for a Species-Specific Framework," *Natural History*, **76**:10:40–43, December, 1967.

Jourard, Sidney: "How Well Do You Know Your Patients?" *American Journal of Nursing*, **59**:1568–71, November, 1959.

Lindner, Robert M.: *The Fifty Minute Hour*. New York: Rinehart, 1955.

Lorenz, Konrad: *On Aggression*. New York: Harcourt, Brace and World, Inc., 1963.

P. O. Reprints: "Understanding Hostility," *American Journal of Nursing*, **67**:10:2131–50, October, 1967.

Ruesch, Jurgen: *Therapeutic Communication*. New York: W. W. Norton and Co., Inc., 1961.

Silver, Larry B., Dublin, Christina C., and Laurie, Reginald: "Does Violence Breed Violence? Contributions from a Study of Child Abuse Syndrome," *American Journal of Psychiatry*, **126**:3:404–407, September, 1969.

Stringer, Marge: "Therapeutic Nursing Intervention Following Derogation of the Nurse by the Patient," *Perspectives in Psychiatric Care*, **3**:4:36–38, 1965.

Washburn, Sherwood L.: "The Origins of Aggressive Behavior," *Mental Health Program Reports-3*. Washington, D.C.: U.S. Department of Health, Education, and Welfare, 1969, pp. 255–72.

Suggested readings

Berkowitz, Leonard, ed.: *Roots of Aggression*. New York: The Atherton Press, 1969.

Grier, William H., and Cobbs, Price M.: *Black Rage*. New York: Basic Books, Inc., 1968.

Jahoda, Marie: *Race Relations and Mental Health*. Place de Fontenoy, Paris: United Nations Educational, Scientific and Cultural Organization, 1960.

Kiening, Sister Mary Martha: "Hostility," in Carlson, Carolyn E., ed.: *Behavioral Concepts and Nursing Intervention*. Philadelphia: J. B. Lippincott Co., 1970, pp. 187–205.

Kneisl, Carol R., and Kelly, Holly S.: "Introduction to the Conference on Hostility in the Nurse-Patient Interaction," *Perspectives in Psychiatric Care*, **7**:4:153–58, July-August, 1969.

LeBon, Gustave: *The Crowd*. London: Ernest Benn Limited, 1952.

Stastny, Joy P.: "Helping a Patient Learn to Trust," *Perspectives in Psychiatric Care*, **3**:7:16–28, 1965.

9 The suicidal crisis

There is but one truly serious philosophical problem,
and that is suicide.
    Albert Camus, "An Absurd Reasoning,"
from *The Myth of Sisyphus*

Operatic suicides are very dramatic and the affects are diverse. They range from the fear of *Peter Grimes* to the jealousy of *Wozzeck* and the despair of *Tosca*. The theme of romantic love and the unwillingness of one to live without the other is exemplified in the tragedy of *Romeo and Juliet*. Suicide prevention in antiquity probably began with Plutarch, A.D. 46–119 (Choron, 1968).

In England the Salvation Army established an antisuicide department as early as 1906 (Stengel, 1964, p. 118). The Samaritans, founded in 1953, comprise a group of ministers and lay people with physician consultants. Similar organizations exist in many towns and in other countries. The Samaritans help others by offering friendship, care, concern, and love and have become international (Varah, 1965).

The incorporation of suicide prevention centers within public health services at both federal and local levels gives a new emphasis to this problem of humanity. More research into suicide has therefore been made possible. The National Institute of Mental Health Center for Studies of Suicide Prevention was established in October, 1966. Founded in 1967, the American Association of Suicidology is the first nationwide organization to be dedicated to the scientific study of suicide prevention. The Association stimulates research, education, and training in suicidology,[1] disseminates knowledge through programs and publications, and encourages the application of research to the understanding and reduction of self-destruction in man. The first Annual National Conference on Suicidology was held in Chicago in 1968. Subsequently the International Association for the Prevention of Suicide has been formed and is involved in much-needed investigations. The fifth International Conference for Suicide Prevention was held in London in 1969.

A new school of suicidology open on an interdisciplinary level gives impetus to better understanding that may lead to more effective preventive techniques. *The Bulletin of Suicidology*, first published in 1967, aids in communication of findings, knowledge of organizational structures, and so forth.

The study of suicidology is aimed at reducing the self-destruction of man. The purpose of the National Institute of Mental Health Center for Studies of

---

[1] Suicidology is the study of suicide and suicide prevention as well as related phenomena of self-destruction.

Suicide Prevention is to assist, encourage, support, and catalyze research, in addition to training, supporting, and demonstration activities related to suicide theory and suicide prevention throughout the country. It is designed to further basic knowledge of the problem of suicide and to develop techniques for aiding the suicidal individual.

In the study of suicide, the psychological autopsy has given further understanding that may lead to more effective preventive efforts. The psychological autopsy focuses on the intention of the deceased in relation to his own death. It represents an attempt by a team of professionals to clarify cases in which the motivation for suicide is unclear. Information is secured from a number of persons and a reconstruction is made of the life style of the deceased and the last few days of his life. After the information is discussed by the team, a confidential written report is given to the medical examiner (Curphey, 1968). Family members and others involved have remarked on the benefits of talking with the team performing the psychological autopsy. The team therefore performs a double function—research into the conditions surrounding the suicide and the therapeutic function of aiding the bereaved.

A new profession of suicidology thereby emerges, with fellowships available to qualified members of the mental health disciplines, including psychiatry, psychology, social work, psychiatric nursing, anthropology, sociology, and public health education.

The new community mental health centers made possible under the Mental Retardation and Community Mental Health Centers Act of 1963 (Public Law 88–164) are now being realized. One of the important services receiving federal funds is 24-hour psychiatric emergency service. Such a service will be available for people who are in suicidal crises, at any time of the day or night. The success of suicide prevention depends upon the action of local communities and on other factors yet to be determined. On the other hand, Dr. Henry W. Turkel (1967), coroner for many years in San Francisco, declares that efforts of his city's Suicide Prevention Center have not affected the statistics in his office. Basic nursing students in a local state college in a small northern California community were catalysts in the formation of a suicide prevention center. They recognized the need for one and went about learning the organization of their community to attempt to meet some of the needs of its suicidal residents. They had learned something about populations at risk and took direct action through community organization to do something about the problem.

Epidemiology

There are more than 20,000 reported suicides annually in the United States. It is generally believed that a more accurate figure would be two to three times greater. Stigma is attached to suicide, and attempts to cover it up are made by physicians and families.

Suicide is the second leading cause of death on college campuses, with the rate for men twice as high as for women (Ross, 1969). There is also a high rate in the aged population. Suicide ranks among the ten leading causes of death in the nation at large. There are 10 suicides for every 100,000 people in this country (1969). In the 15–19 age group, suicide is the third leading cause of death, exceeded only by accidents and cancer. Since this is a vulnerable age group, all schools and college campuses should have access to suicide prevention centers. A report on former students from two universities made by Paffenbarger (1969) showed that paternal deprivation through early loss or death of the father was dominant among the distinguishing familial characteristics. Disrupted affectional relationships figure prominently in the suicides of persons who suffer from alcoholism. Loss of this relationship within 6 weeks to 1 year of the suicide has significant effects (Murphy, 1967).

Most observations on the incidence of suicide show that it is relatively rare among children. There is also evidence that it is more prevalent in those who have incurable diseases and those in war, although the incidence of suicide in the population at large decreases during wartime. Suicide through self-neglect may be more widespread than documented, especially among those experiencing the crises of aging, poverty, loneliness, and desolation. Suicide is linked with alcoholism and homicide. Suicide in accidents, especially automobile accidents, may go unrecorded as suicide. Studies of the psychodynamics of death have resulted in changes in the concept of the modes of death, e.g., the NASH classification—natural, accident, suicide, and homicide (Shneidman, 1969).

Suicide is higher among the single, widowed, separated, and divorced; males outnumber females. In the United States, it is more prevalent among whites than nonwhites. However, there is a high incidence of suicide among the Chinese in San Francisco and among the Cheyenne Indians (Dizmang, 1968). Migrants to a district, foreign-born, the aged, and those living alone have distinctly higher suicide rates. In most areas of the world, physical and mental illness, social isolation, death of a loved one, and loss of status

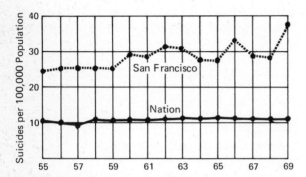

Figure 8 Comparison of suicide rates of San Francisco with the over-all rates of the United States. (Sources: U.S. Department of Commerce: *Statistical Abstract of the United States*, 1962, 1965, 1967, and 1969; San Francisco Department of Public Health; and the Metropolitan Life Insurance Co.: *Statistical Bulletin*, **51** : 10, May 1970.)

(particularly upon retirement), together with the sudden lowering of income, are associated with suicide in the aging (World Health Organization, 1968). In San Francisco, which has been called the suicide capital, a study by Seiden (1967) shows that only 5 percent of suicides are from the Golden Gate Bridge. Suicide is shown to be a local problem; internal migration does not affect the death rate from suicide. The fact that San Francisco leads the nation also in alcoholism influences its suicide rate. From autopsies conducted by San Francisco's coroner, Dr. Turkel, it has been shown that ingestion of poison leads all suicide methods in San Francisco. San Francisco is a relatively small city, but there is a large area in the central city where suicide rates are high. San Francisco's median age is 8 years higher and the single population 35 percent greater than in the country as a whole. All these factors contribute to the high suicide rate.

Etiology

The motivation for suicide was considered by Freud to be directed against the introjected love object, a kind of murder of the self. It has been a generally accepted view that suicide is internalized aggression. Durkheim (1951) categorized suicide into three types: *egoistic*, where man no longer finds life palatable and therefore kills himself; *altruistic*, that is, required by society; and *anomic,* in which society is lacking in its supports to the individual. Added as a footnote to these three types of suicide was another, which has received little attention: *fatalistic* suicide.

> the suicide deriving from excessive regulation, that of persons with futures pitilessly blocked and passions violently choked by oppressive disciplines . . . the suicide of very young husbands, of the married woman who is childless. . . . But it has so little contemporary importance and examples are so hard to find. . . . Do not the suicide of slaves . . . belong to this type, or all the suicides attributed to excessive physical or moral despotism? To bring out the ineluctible and inflexible nature of a rule against which there is no appeal, and in contrast with the expression "anomy" which has just been used, we might call it fatalistic suicide.[2]

No more than half a century has elapsed since the time of Durkheim; therefore such cases of fatalistic suicide are now perhaps more evident. The all-too-familiar example of the person who kills himself when his fraudulent activities are discovered or who is jailed for minor violations of authority may fall into this category. In a study of 42 black men who killed themselves in New Orleans the critical factor of fear and impotence in dealing with the police and other authorities was seen as relevant to suicide (Breed, 1969).

Menninger (1938) described three components of every suicide: the wish to kill, the wish to be killed, and the wish to die. He also pointed out that self-mutilation is a "compromise form of suicide" constituting a victory of the life instinct over the death instinct (Menninger, 1938, p. 285). Meerloo (1962, p. 25) notes that "there is also the secret belief in mystical rescue and revival; an urge to make a magic offering to the gods; and many other motivations contributing to the act."

Because children are so dependent on love objects for gratification and since identification and other levels of growth have not been completed, destruction of introjected love objects is too painful. Therefore, children rarely commit suicide (Schechter, 1957, p. 131). However, in the suicidal child, the hostility toward the parent is turned inward and desperate attempts are made to regain contact with the parent. Feelings of rage, helplessness, and worthlessness are developed. Although there are many motivations for suicide in children, the primary one is real or threatened loss of a love object (Schechter, 1957, p. 141). The treatment of the suicidal child is to re-establish gratifying object relationships.

---

[2] Emile Durkheim: *Suicide.* New York: The Free Press, 1951, p. 276.

If the target of aggression is another person rather than oneself the homicide rate increases—as in the legitimized act of war (Henry, 1954, p. 102). Aggression, instead of being directed against the self as in suicide, is directed outwardly in war.

Disruptions of social relations have also been postulated as etiological factors in suicide. For example, broken homes and parental loss in childhood predispose to depression and suicide in later life (Dorpat et al., 1968). Since children are the age group likely to have the most status integration on a wide scale, this may account for their low suicide rate (Gibbs, 1964).

Cultural determinants of suicide must be studied in every case. The influence of society in the determination of the particular kind of human being under consideration requires emphasis. In the black culture, abandonment by husband or boy friend, guilt about pregnancies, and rejection of their children are factors in the suicide of women (Hendin, 1969). Also, a history of childhood rejection in black men and women may add to the higher urban suicide rate among young black adults than that of their white counterparts (Hendin, 1969, p. 106). A connection between conscious overt violence, including homicide, and self-destructive behavior, including suicide, is made by Hendin, who describes the experience of being black in our culture as generating violence. The black man is thus faced with the problem of controlling it (p. 48).

In adolescence, the reawakening of the Oedipal conflicts, the emergence of heightened emotional stresses, and sexual urges that may be strongly tabooed are etiological factors. The Icarus complex has been noted as a factor in suicide, especially in Japan and the Soviet Union, where failure in exams denotes loss of status and wounded ambition (Meerloo, 1962).

Suicidal equivalents are alternate expressions of self-destruction. Accidental injuries, antisocial acts, engagement in dangerous activities, and cigarette smoking are familiar examples.

The patient feels love and hate together; ambivalence is marked. He also feels the urge for life and the urge for death. The instinct for life (Eros) and the instinct for death (Thanatos) present in everyone are in conflict (Freud, 1922). The suicidal person slashes his wrist and cries for help at the same time. The first person who survived the suicidal leap from the Golden Gate Bridge decided between the time she jumped off and before she hit the water that she wanted to live and, despite broken bones, swam to safety.

On the other hand, there is more to suicide than hostility (Shneidman, 1966). Shneidman refers to dependency as a factor with critical affects of helplessness and hopelessness. "I can't survive in this world" and "I'm too far gone for anyone to help me" are expressions of these affects.

Patients who are depressed may be particularly suicidal, although not all suicidal patients are depressed. The most vulnerable times for the depressed patient are when he is going into or coming out of a depression.

The following facts and fables about suicides are pertinent to the practice of all helping persons.

Facts and fables about suicide

1. **Fable** *People who talk about suicide don't commit suicide.*
   Fact *Of any ten people who kill themselves, eight have given definite warnings of their suicidal intentions. Suicide threats and attempts* must *be taken seriously.*

2. **Fable** *Suicide happens without warning.*
   Fact *Studies reveal that the suicidal person gives many clues and warnings regarding his suicidal intentions. Alertness to these cries for help may prevent suicidal behavior.*

3. **Fable** *Suicidal people are fully intent on dying.*
   Fact *Most suicidal people are undecided about living or dying, and they "gamble with death," leaving it to others to save them. Almost no one commits suicide without letting others know how he is feeling. Often this "cry for help" is given in "code." These distress signals can be used to save lives.*

4. **Fable** *Once a person is suicidal, he is suicidal forever.*
   Fact *Happily, individuals who wish to kill themselves are "suicidal" only for a limited period of time. If they are saved from self-destruction, they can go on to lead useful lives.*

5. **Fable** *Improvement following a suicidal crisis means that the suicidal risk is over.*
   Fact *Most suicides occur within about three months following the beginning of "improvement," when the individual has the energy to put his morbid thoughts and feelings into effect. Relatives and physicians should be especially vigilant during this period.*

6. **Fable** *Suicide strikes much more often among the rich or, conversely, it occurs more frequently among the poor.*
   Fact *Suicide is neither the rich man's disease nor the poor man's curse. Suicide is very "democratic" and is represented proportionately among all levels of society.*

7. **Fable** *Suicide is inherited or "runs in the family."*
   Fact *Suicide does not run in families. It is an individual matter and can be prevented.*

8. **Fable** *All suicidal individuals are mentally ill, and suicide always is the act of a psychotic person.*
   Fact *Studies of hundreds of genuine suicide notes indicate that although the suicidal person is extremely unhappy, he is*

> *not necessarily mentally ill. His overpowering unhappiness*
> *may result from a temporary emotional upset, a long and*
> *painful illness, or a complete loss of hope. It is circular*
> *reasoning to say that "suicide is an insane act," and there-*
> *fore all suicidal people are psychotic.*[3]

Ritual suicides

In Japan, *hara-kiri* may be carried out when there is a change of status of the individual. The *kamikaze* pilots of World War II achieved a form of *hara-kiri* which accorded them great honor. The rite of *suttee* in which the Hindu wife throws herself on her husband's funeral pyre and is cremated with his body is still illegally practiced in India (Carstairs, 1958, p. 74). Recent public immolations by persons protesting events in their individual countries signify the intensity of feelings involved for the act itself and the martyristic nature of the suicides. These immolations perhaps exemplify asceticism and martyrdom in their most dramatic form.

Alienation

There is a resurgence of loneliness in our society; it is not physical loneliness, but the loneliness of the crowd or loneliness of self. Loneliness refers to being without company, destitute of friendly companionship. Being lonely refers to self. That there is more loneliness today is symbolic of the fact that institutions do not offer a sense of belonging. Being human is inseparable from being social; yet loneliness can be experienced in relation to others and to oneself. It can therefore occur when one is physically close to others. Alienation in modern society is real. The power and attraction of groups such as Esalen, Encounter, NTL (National Training Laboratory Institute for Applied Behavioral Sciences) and others which invite the individual to examine his mirror-image self and the mirror of his social image through the group experience is a possible indication of the alienation in contemporary society.

---

[3] Shneidman, Edwin S., and Farberow, Norman L.: "Some Facts About Suicide." Washington, D.C.: Superintendent of Documents, Public Health Service Publication No. 852, pp. 3–5, 1965.

Even families involve themselves in these group experiences for better understanding of individual members and the unit as a whole. The technological modern society seems to have discarded the church social, the annual family reunion, and other kinds of small gatherings where people could observe the yearly differences, take in new members by birth and marriage, note the members missing either by death or other reasons and thereby feel an identity of self and with the group. Can our institutions in the mass society provide a sense of belonging?

In our society, although we may sympathize with others, it is culturally forbidden to feel sorry for ourselves. It is important to distinguish between social isolation and loneliness. The former is an objective condition such as the situation of a hermit. It refers to having few contacts with family, neighbors, or significant others. Loneliness is subjective; it is a feeling and may be unrelated to social isolation (Townsend, 1963).

We as a people are dissatisfied with self and are generally striving for some kind of improvement of self. It is not uncommon to see students in their sixties. At one local college recently a talk by a noted author was interrupted by an activist student who in subsequent conversations was referred to as "kid"; he was actually 37 years old! People with higher degrees attend evening classes and take trips to foreign countries to "sit in on classes there." Students with perfectly respectable grades of "C" and "B" often say disappointedly, "I *could* have gotten an A." People in our society are not taught to be alone—there is push for conformity, to be with others, to be beset with decibels and other stimulants. Children are not taught the value of solitude or how to deal with it and derive benefit from it. For the most part, the solitary experiences of mountaintop, prairie, desert, taking an ocean voyage, or being snowbound have disappeared; ways of finding solitude are seldom sought in the crowded city. Perhaps the alienation results from the daily physical closeness and encounters with hundreds of people in an urban environment. Alienation may be a defense since interacting to any personal degree with all the individuals one meets in an urban environment would quickly deplete one's energy sources.

Fromm (1962) points out that in our society, a society of consumers, we are surrounded by innumerable *things* in whose creation we have not participated directly—we know only how to use or to consume them—and that this alienates us from ourselves.

The love of solitude and time for contemplation as a method of self-renewal has been virtually lost in our society where a man who is not at work feels he must be constantly entertained. Stimulus flooding may leave us with a psychological numbness (Keniston, 1967). Toynbee (1968) states that one of the features of human nature that makes us human is the faculty of spiritual contemplation.

The dynamic interaction of self-worth, degree of ego strength, and number and availability of alternatives offered by our culture determines the amount of alienation for each one of us.

The era of transitory relationships may require alienation as a method of survival. On the other hand, however, nursing students are asked to overcome alienation. In nursing, there is an intimacy between the nurse and the patient that calls for involvement. The student's wish to be needed is met by the helpless, dependent, horizontal patient who depends on one for his sustenance and comfort. When one is needed, one is not likely to be lonely. Understanding oneself and one's relation to the society in which he lives is a prerequisite to being an effective nurse. It is not all learned at once and in fact all throughout life there are continuous glimmers of further understanding, if one seeks it. It in part prepares the nurse to better help patients who are lonely, fear death, are helpless, have financial problems, are paralyzed unexpectedly, and who can never resume the level of wellness formerly experienced.

It is quite significant to recall one graduating student's remark that all his class wanted in the university was "to embrace each other." The popularity of sensitivity groups on various campuses underlines his remark.

The intensive study of suicide during the Sixties reveals it as a method of communication. Causes for suicide are likely to be multiple and one traumatic event may be the precipitating factor after a series of preceding ones. To save a life, all professionals need to learn to be sensitive to the nuances of those individuals under their care. The profound loneliness of the suicidal patient with the subsequent cry for help is now receiving more attention in this country.

Nursing intervention

With the suicidal patient the only significant intervention is prevention. The principal preventive technique is for a concerned person to show to the suicidal person that he really cares for him in a very deep way—that he is truly a friend and that he will not desert him. Nurses are with patients and families throughout many stresses and can readily encourage this attachment behavior. Attention to their needs during these emotional crises may prevent suicide. Over 75 suicide prevention centers have now been established in the nation for receiving telephone calls from the distressed potential suicidal person; others send out teams for home visits. With Public Law 88–164 now enabling the establishment of community mental health centers in all states, suicide prevention services will most likely become an integral part of these centers or will develop a relational system with them, since one of their requirements is to provide 24-hour emergency psychiatric care.

Suicide is now viewed as communication: when, how, and where it takes place; to whom it is directed; and what is the content of the message. Nursing has previously been mostly concerned with patients who were hospitalized; now in the era of community mental health, nursing is concerned with preventive efforts in an anticipatory way. When the suicidal attempt comes, it may be too late. The challenge is to find populations at risk and to assist these individuals and families to meet their basic needs and crisis situations.

Recognition of the suicidal crisis

Aggression directed inward toward the self may result in suicide or the contemplation of suicide. Most suicidal patients give a warning. It is up to you to hear it and to respond. Cues may be verbal or nonverbal. The stresses of life and the process of passage through the usual developmental phases of life are all danger points. Changing jobs, leaving home for school, loss of job, marriage, inability to keep up grade point averages, divorce, death, and rejection are phases of the life arc in which anticipatory work is needed for prevention. A child who requests a blue casket and a blanket of flowers if he dies is telling you something serious. There are two dynamics found in lethal attempts: hostility and anxiety; therefore, these two facets of human behavior are critical phases and it is up to the helping person to note behavior and to do something about the suicidal person.

Asking how to leave one's body to a medical school is a hint of suicide, and saying "I'm going to shoot myself" is a direct announcement. A fellow student who says that he cannot concentrate or who declares, "I'm all washed up," or who keeps saying over and over, "I'm no good," "It's my fault— I'm responsible," is asking for help. A sudden change in a person from being happy-go-lucky and cheerful to irritability, solemnity, and anger may be indications of suicidal thoughts. Giving things away, making a will, and checking on insurance are indirect cues. In over one half of suicidal deaths, the person who kills himself indicates that he will do so to others. There seems to be a 3-month interval following the suicidal crisis in which the patient is dangerous to himself (Shneidman, 1959). School problems, family problems, and drug abuse are some of the precursors of suicide. Early secondary prevention at this stage can be effective.

Preventive efforts include observation and assessment of developmental tasks, and helping patients to attain those tasks they have not accomplished.

Suicidal children are often those who do not take part in school activities and who do not have any close friends. In the adolescent, if the drive toward independence from parents is interfered with by cultural problems and a low opinion of his self, there is increased alienation which may make him more vulnerable to suicide.

With a distressed person, emergency evaluation is required to assess his self-destructive potentiality. Psychiatric first aid may be administered via the telephone interview where a relationship must be established and maintained, and trust secured if one is to provide the needed help. Taking a history from the distressed individual reminds him of his identity; it also provides information about the strengths of the patient. Emergency evaluation may also involve a home visit or a visit to another institution such as a school or hospital. For a potentially suicidal person, the emergency evaluation requires that the therapist get information, assess the lethality, and decide on action very quickly. The suicidal crisis calls for help on the spot.

For patients who telephone or who come into the Suicide Prevention Center in Los Angeles, at least five steps are designated in the treatment process: "(1) Establishment of a relationship—maintain contact and obtain information; (2) identification of and focus on the central problem; (3) evaluation of suicidal potential; (4) assessment of resources and mobilization of outside resources; and (5) formulation and initiation of therapeutic plans."[4] At least ten criteria to evaluate suicidal potential have been developed: (1) Age and sex; (2) suicide plan; (3) precipitating stress and the patient's reaction to the stress; (4) symptoms; (5) resources; (6) characteristic functioning; (7) communication; (8) reactions of significant other; (9) medical status; and (10) prior suicidal behavior (Farberow, *ibid.*, pp. 389–92).

Hendin (1964) evaluated suicidal patients on a scale of one to three with regard to their suicidal intent: the patient with (1) minimal intent; (2) moderate intent; and (3) maximal intent. Patients with maximal intent to die may accidentally survive and will continue in the maximal intent group unless atonement has been reached by the intended act. Those with minimal intent may also accidentally die, as in the rejected lover's simulating taking poison which actually *is* poison. The patients in the moderate intent group are indecisive. They may be the ones who jump from bridges and decide during the fall and before they hit the water to swim to safety.

If the patient is not hospitalized, the nurse first encountering the suicidal patient has the responsibility to assist the patient and his family or friends to get help. Knowledge of the particular community facilities is therefore *very*

[4] Farberow, Norman L.: "Crisis, Disaster and Suicide: Theory and Therapy," in Shneidman, Edwin S., ed.: *Essays in Self-Destruction*. New York: Science House, Inc., 1967, p. 388.

necessary, in addition to the ability to assess the situation and to give psychiatric first aid. The book *Doctor Zhivago* portrays all too well the hushing up of the suicidal attempt in former times which is still all too prevalent in the twentieth century (Pasternak, 1958). The frantic pleas to the physician, the anguish, the pain, and the hushed-up episode, all speak eloquently of society's attitude toward the person who tries to kill himself. It is time now since we are approaching the twenty-first century to abolish the hidden suicide attempt and to do all that we can to assist those who cry for help. They may be our dearest firends, family members, professors, roommates, colleagues, or complete strangers. The message is the same.

Patients in the hospital

Nurses in hospital settings encounter patients of all three degrees of intent. The following is an example of how one patient felt and what the nurse did:

> Mrs. Jorgensen, a patient in a special precautions unit, usually spoke of subjects other than herself. The nurse, however, recognized her need to express her feelings and encouraged her to do so. Mrs. Jorgensen stated that she just wanted to rot and didn't want anyone to take special precautions with her or even give her any kind of care. "I just want to get out of my misery."

It was important in this situation that Mrs. Sanderson was able to ventilate her feelings about having an infection without fear of being rejected. Ventilation to a concerned, sympathetic listener who cared about her greatly unburdened the patient. The nurse conveyed to the patient that she cared for her and helped her to perceive that she was healing rapidly and that the isolation period would not last much longer. Patients who state to you "I don't want to be a burden" and who appear hopeless and helpless may be suicidal. The silent patient who has had a drastic change in body image or other crises may be suicidal.

Depressed patients who find the early morning hours black and melancholy may rush into activity in efforts to ward off suicide. The tension of some depressed patients can be easily felt, i.e., a very tense, determined gait, vigorous scrubbing of the face, bathing and splashing water. A depressed patient who had killed her best friend was subsequently in psychiatric treatment. Some months after her release, she suggested a suicide pact for the entire family, while on a trip. Rehospitalized, she persuaded the intern on duty one Sunday afternoon to give her permission to go out with her family to visit friends where she jumped to her death from their high-rise apartment. Depression often lifts after a suicidal attempt as though atonement has been achieved. When patients confide in you their fantasies in which death is a means of gratification, suicide is a very great danger.

Prevention of suicide

Detention may propel the depressed person into a suicidal attempt. Careful attention must be given to the psychodynamics of each individual. The traditional nursing safeguards such as 24-hour observation and removal of harmful objects from the environment are not used in some areas such as Northern State Hospital, Washington, which is an open hospital; in the United Kingdom and in Colorado the same approach is used. The responsibility put upon the patient is considered to be of value in prevention of suicide. Where nursing staff use the traditional safeguards, it may further lower the ego of the depressed patient. Even with the most vigilant observation and removal of harmful objects from the environment, patients manage to attempt to kill or do kill themselves. Before entry to a hospital, one patient hid a razor blade in the innersole of her shoe and carefully reglued the innersole back into place. Another had hidden a large box of phenobarbital tablets in a facial tissue box which she brought with her to the hospital. Still another patient had 30 Nembutal capsules in the bottom half of a pack of cigarettes, having cut the cigarettes in half, put the capsules in the package, and replaced the halved cigarettes. Another patient in bed under the watchful eyes of nurses managed to turn over and slice his veins with a piece of glass which was previously hidden in the pocket of his pajamas. One patient who succeeded in his suicidal attempt had taken phenobarbital, iodine, slashed his throat from ear to ear as well as his wrists, and his antecubital veins. Due to his poor condition, physicians were unable to suture his throat, although they did succeed in lavaging his stomach with starch. The patient was conscious until death and wanted to live. I still remember the suffering in his eyes.

Suicide reflects hopelessness, helplessness, and fearfulness within individuals. It can be recognized and help can be given to prevent it. Suicide prevention centers and others have the working philosophy that one must convey to the suicidal person that someone cares deeply. However, if one's own philosophy and affect is one of hopelessness, this may itself push the potential suicide over the brink. People live up to expectations and how the nurse feels deeply affects the patient and his family. Hope must be sought by the nurse—all thoughts and actions (behavior) pyramid toward this point.

The following is an interaction between a nursing student and her suicidal patient, a teenage girl:

The patient Diane feigned illness, avoided group therapy, and finally, after being questioned, said that she wanted to get sick so she would not be sent home. She stated that she had already caused her parents too much sorrow.

> **Nurse** Why?
>
> **Patient** I've saved my medications since I've been here. I've intended to kill myself ever since I've been here. (She sat forward in her chair with her head hanging down and looking at the floor.)
>
> **Nurse** Do you still feel like taking your own life?
>
> **Patient** I don't know.

The student and the patient proceeded to talk about love and friendship and the patient related how her best girl friend closed the door in her face when she went to visit her the last time she had been home on leave. The interaction ended with the student's saying forcefully and earnestly to the patient.

> **Nurse** Diane, I feel very strongly that you can get well and gain a desire to live. It's something each one of us has to discover. Life in some ways is very good and in other ways is very bad. Now, we can talk about this for a long time but ultimately the decision is yours. Let me help you. We can find some of the things that make life worthwhile.
>
> **Patient** O.K.

The student acknowledged the feelings of Diane, especially the feeling of rejection. She also immediately and openly asked her about suicidal thoughts. She expressed directly her belief in Diane as a person and quite pointedly put some responsibility on Diane's shoulders. After working with this patient $4\frac{1}{2}$ months the student terminated, as required by the curriculum. The student received the following note:

> Dear Miss H.
>
> I call you this because it really takes a lady to do what you did. I haven't even opened the gift yet, but I feel I should write and let you know how thrilled I am. I'm writing this in pencil because tears blot ink, and I do want you to be able to read this.
>
> I'm also writing this to thank you for all you have done for me. I would probably be doing all my foolish things if it hadn't been for you yet.

Believe me I am very grateful, and always will be. I was afraid the hospital wouldn't be able to help me, but now that I see they can and already have, I'm going to do my best to get well.

Thanks again for everything. With all my love, D.

P.S. Please write.

There were many other examples of emotional support given to this patient by the student and others in the mental hospital. The foregoing interaction represents part of an interaction at a time when Diane was quite suicidal.

Hospitalized patients may take the time of weekend leaves to commit suicide. Often it is the psychiatric nurse who knows the moods of the patient: as part of the psychiatric team playing a most vital role in the determination of the appropriate timing of weekend leaves in the course of the patient's mental disorder. The circumstances of leaves should be known and include what the family and patient plan to do, where they will be, what help can be secured if the suicidal feelings emerge.

Within the psychiatric unit itself, the change of shifts and meal time are times that patients use to commit suicide. Other times when staff and other patients are occupied may be sought. Weekends and holidays where the policy is to provide only a "skeletal" staff and where the patient may feel very keenly alone may be the times chosen.

Visiting hours when the depressed person receives no visitors is another crucial time. It is of significance that at least one senior center in San Francisco remains open on Sunday to aid aging individuals in overcoming loneliness. The importance of doing special things appropriate to the season for patients who stay in the hospital on weekends and holidays is of significance in prevention. Verbal acknowledgment that it is difficult to be in the hospital at these special times may be of benefit to the patient, who may express anger or other emotions related to his condition. The thoughtfulness of the dietary department in providing traditional foods, decorations made by the patients for the dining room, and initiating group discussion of former holidays and family traditions may be especially helpful. Celebration of birthdays provides recognition of the patient as a person.

Initiation of discussion of various traditions may be a catalyst, especially if the patients are of different cultural backgrounds. Here is where knowledge of anthropology is useful to the nurse, especially in the great melting pot of urban America. If she has not already learned something about the cultural background of her patient, then she will certainly be stimulated to read, inquire, and find out. Knowledge of the great religions of the world, their holidays, and religious practices is of considerable import in acknowledging individual identity; it also strengthens family identity, which may be important to the developing teen-ager or the elderly individual who may be facing death alone.

It is important to be aware of whether or not your suicidal patient is sleeping at night. With this person, who most likely suffers insomnia, the dark sleepless night may culminate in a particularly difficult time during the early morning hours. It may be at these times that the patient needs the nurse the most. Recognition should be given by the supervising staff to the particular nursing requirements of the patient population in a psychiatric unit.

Times within the psychiatric unit in which inexperienced nurses and others are in charge should be avoided, if possible. Patients may watch and wait for such a time to talk the inexperienced person into giving him permission to go out with relatives and, in turn, persuade the relatives to take them to places where suicide is possible, for example, to visit friends in high-rise apartment houses. Absences of helping persons involved with the suicidal person must be prepared for very carefully.[5]

It is important to be aware that the patient who suddenly becomes better or who suddenly begins making decisions or whose depression has lifted is at a vulnerable point and requires particular forcefulness of help and hope at this period. The person who is feeling better may have the psychic energy to do away with himself, whereas he did not have this energy when he was severely depressed.

If you find that your patient is suicidal, get someone to stay with him—an experienced nurse who does not leave the room unless relieved by another experienced nurse. For patients who take sleeping pills, slash their throats, and fill themselves with poisons, the general hospital is the most likely place they will be taken. The emergency room of a general hospital is usually equipped with antidote charts, drugs necessary in treatment, lavage equipment, and other aids to assist in overcoming suicidal attempts. Nurses who first encounter patients who have attempted suicide should be able to elicit from the patient exactly what he has done without adding to the guilt which is usually already present over the attempt of the person to take his own life. This very first encounter is her chance to instill hope in the patient. The nurse may also be able to assist families and friends who accompany the patient in this crisis. If hospitalization occurs, the patient and his family will be under the care of a physician and psychiatric consultation provided. Nurses have a responsibility to see that the patient gets the help he needs. Many patients have an idea of

---

[5] Some suicide prevention centers advise their staff to be available for some of their patients on a 24-hour basis, due to the rapport established between the two people.

how to help themselves, and the nurse can use the resources within the patient himself. There is nothing more important than follow-up. A person who has temporarily been without hope sees no hope for the future. Therefore, follow-up is crucial. Patients who have survived suicidal attempts also often have suggestions about how to help others.

Although some professionals advocate stripping the environment of the hospitalized suicidal patient of all suggestions and methods of suicide, I have found common sense to be of help here.

It is good judgment to have the patient in the general hospital on the ground floor, if possible, close to the nurse's station, and in a private room. The watchful eyes of the nurse on the suicidal patient can be likened to those of the nurse in a surgical recovery room who watches his patients recovering from the effects of anesthesia. This idea of caring, simultaneously with surveillance can have a therapeutic effect.

The nurse caring for patients who have suffered a debilitating disease or who have been diagnosed as having cancer should be especially aware of the effects upon the patient, who may choose to have his own style of death—that of suicide. One patient who had a stroke and after recovery participated in a class for students advised the students to never leave a razor around as a temptation to their patients who had just suffered a stroke. Patients with chronic disease may give up and subsequently die as a result. Patients admitted to homes for the aging may give up and die within 6 months of entrance, with a secret belief in rescue. As hospitalized patients recover, temptations that are obvious should not be sought out, for example, visits to places of great heights and easy access to self-destruction.

Effects of suicide upon the nurse

In caring for patients who have attempted suicide, the nurse's anxiety level may rise. Repressed self-destructive urges are aroused in others by the suicidal act. The suicides and suicidal attempts of others bring to our own consciousness aspects of death and consideration of our own death. The nurse has the responsibility for management of anxiety within self and avoiding communication of it to others. In addition, the nurse has the responsibility for helping other personnel on the psychiatric team handle their anxiety by role modeling to them.

Effect of suicide upon the survivors

The two-sidedness of death is a fundamental feature of death—not only of the premature death of the spirit, but of death at any age and in any form. There are always two parties to a death: the person who dies and the survivors who are bereaved.
  (Toynbee, 1968)

Suicide has a stigmatizing effect upon the survivors—the "psychological skeleton in the closet" with the resultant search for the motive for the death (Shneidman, 1969). All family members and/or significant others need help to come to terms with their feelings about the suicide. Provision of emotional support at these times is important to the mental health of the survivors in the bereavement crisis. Being available, being undemanding, and assisting in practical ways all help. Emotional support from the nurse may be the decisive factor between successful adaptation and maladaptation.

Summary

In this chapter, attention is given to recent national and local organizational structure to study and prevent suicide. Populations at risk are named and etiology of suicide is discussed. Responsibilities of the nurse in the recognition of the suicidal crisis are discussed and interventions outlined.

References

Breed, Warren, in Hendin, Herbert, ed.: *Black Suicide*. New York: Basic Books, Inc., 1969, p. 135.

Camus, Albert: *The Myth of Sisyphus*. New York: Vintage Books, 1960.

Carstairs, G. Morris: *The Twice-Born*. Bloomington: Indiana University Press, 1958, p. 74.

Choron, Jacques: "Notes on Suicide Prevention in Antiquity," *Bulletin of Suicidology*, pp. 46–48, July, 1968.

Curphey, Theodore J.: "The Psychological Autopsy," *Bulletin of Suicidology*, July, 1968, p. 41.

Dizmang, Larry H.: "Suicide Among the Cheyenne Indians," Center for Studies of Suicide Prevention, National Institute of Mental Health, 1968.

Dorpat, Theodore L., Jackson, Joan K., and Ripley, Herbert S.: "Broken Homes and Attempted and Completed Suicide," in Gibbs, Jack P., ed.: *Suicide*. New York: Harper and Row, 1968.

Durkheim, Emile: *Suicide*. New York: The Free Press, 1951 (first published 1897).

Farberow, Norman L.: "Crisis, Disaster and Suicide: Theory and Therapy," in Shneidman, Edwin S., ed.: *Essays in Self-Destruction*. New York: Science House, Inc., 1967.

———— and Shneidman, Edwin S., eds.: *The Cry for Help*. New York: McGraw-Hill Book Co., 1961.

———— "Suicide Prevention: A View from the Bridge," *Community Mental Health Journal*, **4**:6:469–74, December, 1968.

———— and Palmer, Ruby A.: "The Nurse's Role in the Prevention of Suicide," *Nursing Forum*, **3**:1:93–103, 1964.

Freud, Sigmund: *Collected Papers*, Vol. 5. London: The Hogarth Press, 1950, p. 135 (first published 1922).

———— *The Standard Edition*, Vol. 17. London: The Hogarth Press, 1955, pp. 7–64.

Friedman, Paul: *On Suicide*. Discussions of the Vienna Psychoanalytic Society—1910. New York: International Universities Press, Inc., 1967.

Fromm, Erich: "Alienation Under Capitalism," in Josephson, Eric and Josephson, Mary: *Man Alone: Alienation in Modern Society*. New York: Dell Publishing Co., 1962, pp. 56–73.

Gibbs, Jack P., and Martin, Walter T.: *Status Integration and Suicide*. Eugene, Oregon: University of Oregon, 1964.

———— ed.: *Suicide*. New York: Harper and Row, 1968.

Hendin, Herbert: *Suicide and Scandinavia*. New York: Grune and Stratton, 1964, p. 14.

———— *Black Suicide*. New York: Basic Books, Inc., 1969.

Henry, Andrew F., and Short, James F.: *Suicide and Homicide*. New York: The Free Press of Glencoe, 1954, p. 102.

Keniston, Kenneth: "Drug Use and Student Values," in Hollander, Charles: *Background Papers on Student Drug Involvement*. United States National Student Association, 1967, pp. 121–30.

Meerloo, Joost A. M.: *Suicide and Mass Suicide*. New York: Grune and Stratton, 1962, p. 25.

Menninger, Karl: *Man Against Himself*. New York: Harcourt, Brace and Co., 1938.

Metropolitan Life Insurance Co.: *Statistical Bulletin*, **51**:10, May, 1970.

Murphy, George E., and Robins, Eli: "Social Factors in Suicide," *Journal of the American Medical Association*, **199**:5:303–308, 1967.

Paffenbarger, R. S., King, Stanley H., and Wing, Alvin L.: "Chronic Disease in Former College Students," *American Journal of Public Health*, **59**:6: 900–909, June, 1969.

Pasternak, Boris Leonidovich: *Doctor Zhivago*. New York: Pantheon, 1958.

Ross, Mathew: "Suicide Among College Students," *American Journal of Psychiatry*, **126**:2:220–25, August, 1969.

San Francisco Department of Public Health, personal communication, 1970.

Schechter, Marshall D.: "The Recognition and Treatment of Suicide in Children," in Shneidman, Edwin S., and Farberow, Norman L., eds.: *Clues to Suicide*. New York: McGraw-Hill Book Co., 1957.

Seiden, Richard H.: "Suicide Capital? A Study of the San Francisco Suicide Rate," *Bulletin of Suicidology*, pp. 1–10, December, 1967.

Shneidman, Edwin S., and Farberow, N. L.: "Suicide and Death," in Feifel, Herman: *The Meaning of Death*. New York: McGraw-Hill Book Co., 1959.

———and Farberow, N. L.: *Some Facts About Suicide*. Washington, D.C.: Superintendent of Documents, Public Health Service Publication No. 852, 1965.

——— "Preventive Suicide," *American Journal of Nursing*, **65**:5:111–16, May, 1965.

——— Notes taken from lecture on "Depression," Napa State Hospital, Imola, Calif., 1966.

——— ed.: *Essays in Self-Destruction*. New York: Science House, Inc., 1967.

——— ed.: *On the Nature of Suicide*. San Francisco: Jossey-Bass, Inc., 1969.

Stengel, Erwin: *Suicide and Attempted Suicide*. Baltimore: Penguin Books, 1964.

Townsend, Peter: *The Family Life of Old People*. Baltimore: Penguin Books, 1963.

Toynbee, Arnold: *Man's Concern with Death*. London: Hodder and Stoughton, 1968.

Turkel, Henry W.: Notes taken from a symposium on "Suicide," San Francisco State College, San Francisco, 1967.

U.S. Department of Commerce: *Statistical Abstract of the United States*, 1962, 1965, 1967, and 1969.

Varah, Chad, ed.: *The Samaritans*. New York: The Macmillan Co., 1965.

World Health Organization: *Prevention of Suicide*. Public Health Papers No. 35, Geneva, 1968.

Suggested readings

Bakan, David: *Disease, Pain and Sacrifice*. Chicago: University of Chicago Press, 1968.

Batchelor, I. R. C.: "Suicide in Old Age," in Shneidman, Edwin, and Farberow, Norman L., eds.: *Clues to Suicide*. New York: McGraw-Hill Book Co., 1957, pp. 143–51.

Beall, Lynnette: "The Psychopathology of Suicide in Japan," *The International Journal of Social Psychiatry*, **14**:3:213–26, Summer, 1968.

Bell, Karen Kloes: "The Nurse's Role in Suicide Prevention," *Bulletin of Suicidology*, **6**:60–65, Spring, 1970.

Blaker, Karen: "Crisis Maintenance," *Nursing Forum*, **8**:1:42–49, 1969.

Choron, Jacques: "Concerning Suicide in Soviet Russia," *Bulletin of Suicidology*, December, 1968, pp. 31–36.

Douglas, Jack D.: *The Social Meanings of Suicide*. Princeton: Princeton University Press, 1967.

Dublin, Louis I., and Bunzel, Bessie: *To Be or Not To Be: A Study of Suicide*. New York: Harrison, Smith and Robert Haas, 1933.

——— *Suicide: A Sociological and Statistical Study*. New York: Ronald Press Co., 1963.

Farberow, Norman L.: *Bibliography on Suicide and Suicide Prevention*. Washington, D.C.: U.S. Government Printing Office, Public Health Service Publication No. 1970, 1969.

Goethe, Johann Wolfgang von: *The Sorrows of Werther* (1774). New York: F. Ungar Pub. Co., 1957.

Jacobs, Jerry, and Teicher, Joseph D.: "Broken Homes and Social Isolation in Attempted Suicides of Adolescents," *The International Journal of Social Psychiatry*, **13**:2:139–49, Spring, 1967.

Kloes, Karen B.: "The Suicidal Patient in the Community: A Challenge for Nurses," *ANA Clinical Sessions*. New York: Appleton-Century-Crofts, 1968.

Maris, Ronald: *Social Forces in Urban Suicide*. Homewood, Ill.: The Dorsey Press, 1969.

McLean, Lenora J.: "Action and Reaction in Suicidal Crisis," *Nursing Forum*, **8**:1:28–41, 1969.

Seiden, Richard H.: "Campus Tragedy: A Study of Student Suicide," *Journal of Abnormal Psychology*, **71**:6:389–99, 1966.

——— *Suicide Among Youth*. Prepared for the Joint Commission on Mental Health of Children, Task Force III. Washington, D.C.: U.S. Government Printing Office, December, 1969.

10　Relating to withdrawn and autistic patients

Patients in different age groups and with numerous diagnostic categories may evidence withdrawal and autistic behavior. The psychosis in which these behaviors is most dramatically presented is schizophrenia. In the *Diagnostic and Statistical Manual of Mental Disorders,* II (1968), there are now eleven diagnostic categories for schizophrenia.

Recognition of withdrawal

With the new focus on preventive intervention, nurses in all areas of practice aid in the early recognition of withdrawn and autistic behavior so that something can be done about it in its early stages. The withdrawn person will not ask for things for himself. He is often alone. He may be described by his teacher and family as being a "model child," "bright," and "never in any trouble." He may regard himself as unpopular and unliked; he avoids people, stays in his room at home, sleeps a lot, and more and more drops out from daily associations and activities. Withdrawal is not to be confused with solitude which is necessary to think things through, reflect upon previous actions, and plan new ways of doing things. The temporary bizarre habits and patterns of life occurring during adolescence are not to be mistaken for autism and withdrawal. There is a belief in some psychiatric circles that adolescence is a schizophrenic period itself. The withdrawn person's fantasy world more and more occupies his thoughts and he behaves according to the pleasure-pain principle instead of the reality principle. Withdrawal strikes at the ego, and the activities of daily living no longer seem important. The patient may stop bathing, shaving, eating, and spend his days and nights in bed. Bizarre gestures, mannerisms, activities, and use of body arts may be the first cues in the recognition of withdrawal and autistic behavior. Since the prodromal signs and symptoms may pass unnoticed by family members, the condition may be underway long before it comes to the attention of professionals. In our technological urban society, it will probably first come to the attention of people where the person works or goes to school. School and industrial nurses may be able to institute secondary preventive measures.

293

Acceptance of mental disorder

Negative attitudes toward persons with mental disorder need to be overcome in our society. Some people still regard any concern for mental health as having the stigma of being crazy. Your attitude toward people with mental problems is carefully observed by your patients and their families as well as others with whom you come into contact. As a nurse, you encounter a wide range of people. It is your responsibility as a *professional*, at all points of life to be cognizant of the fact that when you are speaking of your own attitudes about mental disorder, you are not only a citizen, you are a professional and others listen intently and carefully to what you have to say. Peculiarities and idiosyncrasies of family members may be ignored or even encouraged by others within the family. One teen-ager patient of mine had developed a language of neologisms—no one else understood this language but her mother.

Hospital admissions are often likely to occur when the patient no longer fulfills his family role. For example, the child who runs away or suddenly shoots someone without provocation, the young mother who neglects feeding and otherwise caring for the needs of her new baby, the housewife who doesn't cook meals, the husband who suddenly and without explanation quits work and remains at home.

Cultural determinants

Although there is as yet no anatomy of culture, the most primitive cultures recognize mental disorder. The cultural background of the patient may be part of the key to understanding his behavior. Some neighborhoods and communities may tolerate a psychotic person whereas in another he may be confined immediately. One of my patients, newly admitted to the mental hospital, said that when she still had money she was considered by her neighbors as being eccentric and when she had spent all her money, she was considered a mental patient. Due to her obesity she did not have money to buy clothes, so she entered the hospital wearing a sheet.

What the symptoms of the patient mean to the family and involved others may determine whether or not he remains at home or is hospitalized. The complexity and plurality of social roles required by members of the modern urban family may make psychic disturbances less tolerated by them than the more simple roles required in rural and other areas.

Still other factors may be the health status of the other family members, population density, frequency of occurrence of the deviant or abnormal behavior, traditions within the family, type of housing, and conditions at work. The social class of the person of deviant or abnormal behavior is still another factor. Middle-class patients have been more able to afford out-patient and home treatment than lower class patients.

With the enabling legislation of Public Law 88—164 and Public Law 89—105,[1] and the development of community mental health centers that are in the process of being established over the country, availability of services to all classes of people may change this statistic.

Persons with symptoms such as delusions and hallucinations which are generally indicative of psychosis in western society may in more primitive societies be assigned highly respected religious roles. It must also be remembered that not many generations ago, demoniacal possession was practically universally believed in; in this country persons who deviated from the norm were labeled witches and hanged.

The degree to which the family feels mental disorder is a stigma will influence their readiness to seek psychiatric care. One patient, in an acute psychotic break, who also had epileptic seizures, was prayed over by his family all night before admission to hospital. They belonged to one of the fundamentalist religious sects and were attempting to remove the devil from the possessed patient. The anxiety of the neighbors in this instance led to the admission of the patient to the mental hospital.

The observations by nurses of the prodromal signs and symptoms of psychoses can add to the understanding of mental disorder since the nomenclature only includes the full-blown pathology.

How the patient feels about himself

The withdrawn, autistic patient may imagine that he "smells funny" or "looks peculiar." He may feel that people look at him in a condescending manner and are out to get him. He may assume grotesque body positions. The patient may appear to be preoccupied with a dream world but he is acutely aware of

---

[1] Public Law 88—164 is the Mental Retardation and Community Mental Health Centers Act. Public Law 89—105 is the Act that provides for staffing of the centers; subsequent amendments affect these two.

everything said and done within his presence. His posture and stance may indicate a turning inward. He may not be able to look at anyone face to face because, as one patient expressed it, "everyone knows more than I do." Plans for the future are vague and unrealistic. The patient suffers from a feeling of rejection and lack of self-esteem. The way he protects himself is by withdrawal from emotional involvement with people. He does not trust or confide in anyone and others may view him as indifferent. He seldom shows emotion about his likes and dislikes and doesn't feel much enthusiasm for anything.

Depersonalization

Depersonalization refers to feelings of unreality or strangeness concerning either the environment, the self, or both. In the patient with autistic behavior, there is a loss of ego boundaries—the ego cannot differentiate between the real world and the inner world. Interest and affect, formerly directed toward conscious aspects of existence, become attached to the unconscious, and withdrawal results. The behavior of the patient seems mechanical. The patient feels himself changed—he seems unable to identify his own personality; it seems indistinct. In attempts to rationalize these feelings the patient may develop nihilistic ideas that parts of himself are strange and do not belong to him. He may develop further nihilistic ideas that he is dead. Feelings that one side of his body is different from the other, that fluids are backing up into the blood, that he is turning into the opposite sex, that he is being charged with electricity, that he has no stomach, that he is drowning or dying may preoccupy the patient.

The following is an example of a patient who verbalized her nihilistic ideas:

The setting is a psychiatric unit in a hospital and the nurse is sitting in a side room with a patient who is receiving intravenous therapy. Another patient enters and begins—

Patient   I'll carry my coat and skirt over my arm or tie mine up in a plastic bag and throw it over my shoulder on a stick. Nurse, I want to go home. When I swallow my food it doesn't go down—it stops right here (points to the upper chest). I don't have any stomach. Look at me—this is all I have (rubs abdomen which is covered with varicose veins).

Nurse   You will be able to eat and you will feel better.

Many autistic patients, however, will not verbalize their feelings and fantasies. Withdrawn patients are hypersensitive to nuances of feeling, ordinary communication is dropped, and attention is shifted to absorption with the self.

Protected environment

A protected environment may relieve the withdrawn and autistic patient of some of his fears: or it may bring on still others. One of my teen-ager patients, when hospitalized, thought that the round windows on the doors of the hospital rooms were portholes and that he was therefore in a ship—not only a ship but a sinking ship and that he was drowning. His facial expression and actions expressed terror at this time. However, he was also mute upon admission and it was only much later, as he recovered, that he related this fear to me. Unverbalized fear can be felt by the nurse who is sensitive to the needs of her patients. Being with the individual who is afraid, in a non-threatening manner, aids the patient to perceive your support. Stating and restating to the fearful patient the reality of time, place, and person will help.

A warning note must be made here about a protected environment for withdrawn patients. The open-door policy of hospitals may give the patient freedom to further withdraw. It becomes rather easy for the patient to spend his entire day on solitary walks, sleeping, or wound up in other activities by himself. In a large mental hospital setting, it is quite common to observe autistic patients sidling up to the hollows of trees so as to be inconspicuous or standing under covered areas talking and gesturing to themselves. On the hospital unit you may find an autistic patient in remote areas of rooms or sitting under a table with his jacket pulled over his head unraveling bits of cloth or tearing paper into little pieces.

Developing rapport

For the withdrawn and autistic patient, it may take a long time before he can display affect toward you. Attempts to pull away the veil of the dereistic world and bring in reality requires that you convey persistent interest in the patient, that you show consistency in amount and time of communication with him and that contacts with the patient allow enough time to do this.

The autistic patient fears closeness because of the hurt that he has received. Being close entails being able to feel and to express feelings with the other person. Autistic patients may not be able to do this. Feelings may be discussed but the autistic patient will often discuss them in terms of someone else's feelings, *not his own.* Since parents were perceived as being too cold or too threatening or too close and rejecting, he does not feel that anyone can love him for what he is and is ambivalent about what he should be like. In fantasy, he may have developed his own identity in a "community" such as the "Yeeries" of Deborah in *I Never Promised You a Rose Garden* (Green, 1964), and feel reluctant to give up this fantasied identity. His wishes for love and to be loved are confused with feelings about formerly painful relationships. The first task of the nurse is to assure the patient of his identity and worth as a person by conveying to him that you are interested and care about him.

Mothering care

In the establishing phase of the nurse-patient relationship, most of your time may be taken up with helping the autistic patient to meet his mothering needs, that is, bathing, feeding, personal hygiene, dressing, and grooming. Patients may perform some of these things for themselves; others will require assistance in most all of them. Still others will only partially attend to their needs. For example, it is quite common for the autistic patient not to tie his shoelaces. A simple act such as tying the patient's shoelaces for him may be the key to establishment of rapport. Your body language communicates clearly to the patient how you feel about him. No two people, for example, bathe a patient exactly alike. Gertrud Schwing (1954), assuming that autistic patients were primarily orally deprived, used physical ministrations including feeding and caressing to relate to her patients. Rosen (1953) forcefully confronted the patient with interpretations of unconscious motivation and a mystique of personality. With the aid of attendants he assumed total care of his patients, often adding them to his household. Sechehaye (1951) used what she called symbolic realization to contact withdrawn patients through a symbolic return to mother. Bettelheim's work (1955, 1968) with autistic children documents the influence of the human relationship. Fromm-Reichman's (1950) technique of intensive psychotherapy with autistic patients was shaped on the empathic response. Sullivan (1953) focused on the interaction between the therapist and the patient at the moment that it occurred. The "here and now" received emphasis in his approach. Bateson and Jackson (1956) using the "double-bind" theory treated the entire family. The social psychiatric approach used in treatment by Main (1946), Jones (1953, 1968), Wilmer (1958), Bierer (1948), and others added a new dimension to the intensive psychotherapeutic approach.

Awareness that mutual withdrawal can occur is a spur for the nurse to pursue the establishment of rapport. Verbalize to the patient how you think he feels and aks him whether or not you are correct. Indicate that you think he is capable of recovery and tell him that he has to make the decision to want to be helped. Restate your expectations so that the patient still knows that you have them. It is here with the autistic patient that your conversations and other efforts may be one-sided for a long time, before the patient develops trust and is otherwise responsive to you. The work of Ward (1969) with her silent patient records one verbal sound—a grunt—during her entire contact with him. One-sided relationships are at first difficult. You learn to be alert for small changes in your patient that indicate movement toward trust; for example, when your patient first looks at you, gets up when you present yourself, or takes your hand.

When nurse-patient relationships are one-sided and there is little movement toward progress, there may be a tendency to depreciate one's own efforts since no effects are discernible. Nurses may fall back on one facet of interpersonal relationships, i.e., "to accept people as they are," and steadfastly defend their position. Part of this position is to stoutly declare that they have no right to delve into the lives of their patients, that they furthermore do not have the skills to help mental patients or the time to spare to do it if they could. If you should find yourself approaching this position, try to look at the fact that if you understand something about human motivation and also accept people as they are, you are much better equipped to help those who cannot help themselves. If understanding the "why's" of behavior is necessary for the health of our patients, why not help search for it in order to help each person realize his greatest potential—whatever that may be for him?

Fantasy life

The autistic patient's fantasy life defends the ego. In his dereistic world, hallucinations, delusions, and illusions may act as defenses; they are accessory symptoms of autistic patients and may all occur in the same patient. When the nurse enters the world of the patient in such a manner that the patient no longer needs these defenses, he gives them up for more healthy ones.

Hallucinations

An hallucination is a false sensory perception. The visual hallucinations immediately preceding sleep and other somnolent states are known to almost
everyone. The hallucinations resulting from fatigue, dehydration, and exposure
are epitomized in the mirage of the desert traveler. As sleep loss progresses,
there is an increased unevenness of mental functioning (Williams *et al.*, 1962).
Sensory deprivation produces hallucinations, mostly visual, but some kinesthetic. Those individuals who have had anesthetics preceding surgery have
probably had the experience of both visual and auditory hallucinations.
Hallucinations induced by hallucinogenic drugs are now well known. The
environment of the patient in a general hospital in which he is isolated from
loved ones and rather powerless may contribute to altered mental states and
resultant hallucinations.

One autistic patient who was talking to herself, when asked to whom she
was speaking, stated that sometimes her thoughts became so intense that she
could hear her mother and father saying threatening things to her. She said she
knew that her father and mother were not present but that the thoughts
persisted and she answered them out loud. People who live alone or who may
be doing very concentrated work often talk to themselves in response to their
own thoughts. In these instances, the hold onto reality is kept, however.
Hallucinations may involve any of the senses: auditory hallucinations are
most prominent in patients with autistic behavior. Their presence, if not
verbalized, may be inferred from behavior. The listening posture and demeanor
of your patient may indicate that he hears voices. Impulsive and aggressive
actions on the part of the patient may be in response to inner voices as well as
the inactivity and dream world of withdrawal. Threatening, unfriendly, inner
voices may issue commands or caustic apprisals. They tend to occur during
periods of mounting anxiety and to represent voices of "significant others"
in the life of the patient: parents, spouses, children, and grandparents. The
voices may be helpful to the patient in that they accompany him through
various activities. One patient reported voices that were active in achievement
of orgasm (Modell, 1962).

Patients may also verbalize their hallucinations very directly.

Illusions

Illusions are mistaken sensory perceptions. An illusion can affect any of the senses. For example, a patient who heard airplanes flying over the hospital said that their sound was the voice of her estranged husband.

Delusions

A delusion is a false belief. It is to be differentiated from illusions and hallucinations in that it involves thought, not sensory perceptions. A patient in his home expressed the delusion that he was being hypnotized by a public address system for the purpose of being brought to believe in the Roman Catholic Church. Another patient expressed the delusion that the President had put a Bible into orbit and that it gave off mercury. She thought, however, that she was secure in an automobile and therefore only went outdoors if she could ride in one.

Nursing intervention

The principal aim of the therapist is to relieve the anxiety of the patient, the difficulty he has in communication, and the feeling he has of being unrelated to others. This can best be done by limiting the environment of the patient to a simple one with the same people in it who give attention to him. Showing him the physical layout if it is a hospital allays anxiety. Identifying the specific needs of the patient conveys the idea that you care for him. Since anxiety influences and interferes with communication, all communication should be simple and easily related to the real world. Patients should be in a milieu in which they can exert some control and in which simple social relationships are possible. Powerlessness, isolation, and purposelessness merely add to hallucinations. As a therapeutic relationship is established, the patient feels more secure and the need for hallucinations as defenses against anxiety disappears. On the other hand, the hallucinations met in long-term autistic patients are likely to be rather stereotyped.

Anxiety is hypothesized to be the antecedent of hallucinations, illusions, and delusions. These symptoms are reflections of hopes, wishes, and fears of the patient; they are defenses against anxiety. They are indicators of the unconscious life of the patient and require careful attention to be understood. The work of the nurse is focused toward helping the patient to relieve his anxiety where these defenses are no longer required.

There are periods in which patients seem free of hallucinations; it is important for the nurse to be cognizant of these times and to show interest and concern for the patient and to convey interest in him as a person and not just in his hallucinations.

If the patient's behavior indicates to you that he may be hearing voices, ask him about them. For example, "Tell me about the voices. . . , whose voices are they? Are they friendly to you? Are they unfriendly to you? When do you hear them? Have you heard them at similar times before?" If the voices or other hallucinations frighten the patient, the nurse should be ready to provide a safe environment for him. Stating to the frightened patient where he is and who you are and that it is a safe place may provide the needed comfort.

The work of the nurse is centered around helping the patient to establish what is real and what is unreal. The patient may, for example, believe that you are a spy. Establishing contact with the patient, gaining trust, and being with him in an ego-supportive role can help him to perceive the real world. Establishment of ego boundaries aids in anxiety reduction. If the hallucinations, delusions, and illusions are defenses against anxiety, they will not occur when the patient's fractured ego is once more whole. Man is a social animal; he is gregarious; for the most part, he is comfortable around others. Assisting the autistic patient to relate to other patients may help him to give up his world of unreality. The nurse and other members of the therapeutic team do not agree with the delusions, hallucinations, and illusions of patients. Neither do they argue about them. A simple forcefully put response such as "I don't hear any voices" or "you might be mistaken" helps the patient to distinguish between the real and the unreal world. Use of the concept of negative feedback in which the delusions, illusions, and hallucinations receive little attention from the nurse is one approach. Verbatim recording should be done which gives a lead to the inner life of the patient that may be of central importance in his care. There is a need for more research and knowledge about hallucinations as well as other behavior of autistic patients.

All these interventions cannot be done at once. It may take a long time for the autistic patient to trust you enough to confide in you what is on his mind.

Regression

Regression with symptoms of dependence occurs in almost every illness. It may be temporary or, as in patients with autistic behavior, prolonged. Regression implies a return to a former level of development. A healthy person can regress as in play, and then return to his developmental level quite readily. This has been called regression in service of the ego (Kris, 1952). Regression may also occur in crisis situations such as the birth of a new sibling, childbirth, hospitalization, or with the debilitating diseases and conditions in which there are disturbances of body image. It is a human tendency to regress under stress. The psychotic patient is only more severely regressed—the nursing approach is similar.

The nurse may be repulsed by the severely regressed patient. Anger is commonly felt and the thought may occur that the patient really could do something himself about his regressed state. On the other hand, the regressed patient may progress rapidly forward only to regress back to his former state. You may find yourself discouraged or lose interest in the patient who seems unable to recover. You may also feel that you have personally failed. The problem of withdrawal, autistic behavior, and regression may cause you to be perplexed and bewildered. It may be difficult to comprehend the meaning of such behavior, especially in adults. Some scientific people seem to be able to work more comfortably in situations where causes of phenomena are quickly and easily identified. Since there are no exact formulas to follow in interpersonal relationships, you will need to develop and to follow your own way in working with people. An assessment of ego strengths of the patient is one way to begin. Determine where the patient is and work from that point. This knowledge will help you to set more realistic goals. Severely regressed patients in great numbers are no longer seen on the back wards of some mental hospitals as they were 20 years ago where great efforts in "habit training"[2] were made by the nursing staff. But regression still occurs. The degree of regression can also be assessed and a picture put together of what the patient was like before the regression. Avoid attempting to get the regressed patient to achieve a level of wellness unknown to him or impossible for him to

---

[2] Habit training refers to the retraining of severely regressed patients to use the toilet themselves and to otherwise meet their own needs in personal hygiene and to feed themselves.

achieve. Knowing what kind of person you are dealing with—his assets and liabilities—will help you to make a more realistic nursing care plan and therefore better aid the patient to achieve the highest potential of which he is capable. In order to do this, you will need to know the following:

His patterns of coping
How the patient views himself
How the patient has adapted himself
How the patient has coped with the crises in his life cycle
The nature of his relationships with others

Pooling the information about the patient and his situation by the therapeutic team gives each person involved the opportunity to give and to take information and to formulate a better plan of care. If you get to know something about your patient's goals in life, his educational background, how his life has been spent, i.e., jobs held and jobs aspired to, his hobbies and his other interests, you will have the beginnings of assessment of his strengths.

When you develop a fundamental cognitive understanding of the patient's problem, you may feel discouraged because you have the problem of the patient in the forefront of your mind instead of the patient as a person. You may also feel angry because you are doing all the work in the relationship and the patient is making no effort whatsoever. Hope for recovery of your patient may then disappear. If you perceive that the patient himself appears not to want to get well, you may feel further hopelessness. It is well known from the studies of Stanton and Schwartz (1949), Caudill (1952), Greenblatt *et al.* (1957), Tudor (1952), and others that how the staff feels readily communicates to the patient. Adverse feelings influence behavior of the patient; therefore, the nurse's feelings of frustration, hopelessness, and discouragement have to be dealt with. Frustration may be high on your list because you have tried everything that you know how to use. You may feel worthless and inadequate and wonder whether or not you will ever be able to help the patient or anyone else. You may feel angry at the patient because of the way he has made you feel.

Students who have developed countertransference to their patients, for example, as a sibling, often become angry at the psychiatrist and psychologist who diagnose the patient as schizophrenic or some other classification and adamantly champion the patient's cause. Once a patient who had been a member of my social club and a student at the same university had a psychotic break while playing the role of Ophelia in her drama group on campus. She was admitted to the mental hospital, and I found her on the unit where I was assistant head nurse. Later on, she was presented at "Grand Rounds" as a possible candidate for prefrontal lobotomy. I persuaded and encouraged her as well as

I could to present the part of herself that I knew as a contrast with her state of mutism. I felt angry at her psychiatrist who had not been able to achieve rapport with her and was therefore recommending that the answer to her problem was a prefrontal lobotomy. I felt a kind of sibling loyalty to her and a strong urge to protect her from the neurosurgeons. As it turned out, at "Grand Rounds," she was quite open and responded readily to the questions of the interviewer, the chief of psychiatry. In spite of her accessibility at that event, the staff recommended that she have a lobotomy, which was refused by her mother.

There is no substitute for this kind of experience with regressed patients. Talk it over with someone with more contact with regressed patients than yourself. Try to understand the limitations of other professionals as well as your own. Remind yourself that the condition of the patient did not occur overnight and that predicting an end point to regression is a tricky endeavor for the most experienced professional. Hope for recovery of your patient can re-emerge as you develop self-insight and a better understanding of motivation underlying the regression.

As you get to know your patient better, you will be able to observe his healthy behavior and, in the development of your short-term and long-term goals in nursing care, get a better idea of what can be accomplished and the next steps to take in that direction. Looking for the strengths of your regressed patient and nurturing these like a delicate plant helps him to blossom into full flower and gives the impetus for recovery.

It is the consistency of daily goals and daily expectations that convey to the patient that you care about him. Weekly or monthly goals may also be set in collaboration with the therapeutic team. Patients may have periods of great forward spurts toward recovery and then go backward. The nurse can be ready for these reverses and starts and not get too excited about them but calmly set about expecting the patient to move forward again. In the case of acute physical illnesses in individuals, regression may be life saving and therefore encouraged. However, in mental disorder, regression is a fundamental issue. A psychiatric milieu which fosters powerlessness, regression, conformity, and provides no ways for patients to perform purposeful activity and to take responsibility will most likely not enable the regressed patient to make much progress.

During regression, magical thinking (see page 14) may particularly emerge. Try to be aware of what your patient is expecting by the process of magical thinking and point out social reality to him.

In psychoanalytic theory, ambivalence derives from the oral stage of development and subsequent phases. Your patient who has regressed to an earlier phase of development will show other characteristics of that period of development. If your patient is regressed to the oral stage of development, ambivalence[3] is therefore activated. There is an element of indecisiveness in the patient's behavior. The ambivalent patient may agree to play ping pong with you and stop right in the middle of the game. Another example is the patient who expresses love on one hand and hate on the other. For instance, the patient who hugs you delightedly and, at the same time, unconsciously wants to kill you. Another example is the patient who alternately reaches out toward people and subsequently withdraws from them. The nurse can support behaviors that move toward reality testing and assist the patient to be more cognizant of social reality, as below:

>**Patient** What would do if I pushed you off a five-story building? What would you do?
>
>**Nurse** I would probably be dead and you would lose a friend. Then how would you feel?

Another patient, in his twenties, who lives at home and tells you that he does not trust his mother—that he would like to be on his own but at the same time cannot accept different living arrangements as in a foster family— is expressing ambivalence. Extremes of ambivalence coupled with negativism accompanying regression may result in marked indecision. The nurse makes decisions for the patient where necessary and helps the patient move toward making his own decisions.

Terminating with autistic patients

The anger felt by the patient toward the nurse who is leaving him may help the patient to achieve independence. If he can feel anger, tolerate it, and express it in an adult manner, without feeling that he is disintegrating, a definite advance has been made. Anger may be expressed obliquely as, for example, the patient who does not keep his appointment with you. Or he may "forget" his appointment with you because he fears that he may be unable to control his anger. The nurse begins discussion of termination upon first contact with the patient and again long before the last contact with him. If you have talked about loss and expressed feelings about it during the nurse-patient relationship, termination will be better understood. Former losses are

---

[3] Ambivalence refers to the presence of opposite emotions, ideas, attitudes, or wishes toward a situation or an object.

reactivated and it is the work of the nurse to help the patient express his feelings about these losses. One patient, Mr. Cohen, now 47 years old, at termination spoke of the girl that he dated in high school. Others speak of death, perhaps not their own, but the death of other patients. Nearing termination, Mr. Cohen noted the hearse at the hospital morgue and commented "that someone must have died—sometimes two die within a day on the wards where the old people are. Most of these people do not have anyone to think about them." Although Mr. Cohen could not express directly his feelings about termination, through the death of someone else, he made an appeal to the student to be remembered and perhaps be mourned for when he died (Doane, 1963). (The reader is referred to the section on Grief and Mourning in Chapter 7 for review.) The patient mourns for the nurse with whom he has developed a meaningful relationship and with whom he has been able to be himself. Autistic patients need a great deal of help to express feelings. Saying directly that "It is all right to cry when you say goodbye," may be the cue. Another may be to simply state your own feelings as "I feel sad that we have to say goodbye," or "Leaving is like leaving high school." Emotional termination may occur before the last meeting. Help the patient to review the time that you have spent together by reviewing it before the last meeting and mentioning the date that you began and the events of the relationship. In the terminating phase, patients may suddenly open up with a rush of feelings. In the reluctance to terminate, they may express loneliness, self-depreciation, and guilt. An example of self-depreciation at termination occurred between an autistic patient and student on a downtown outing during part of the terminating session. The patient stopped in front of a photography shop:

> **Patient**   (observing the photographs) It's kind of sad that everyone is so much more beautiful than I am. I look at T.V. and each woman seems more beautiful than the last—it's discouraging.
>
> **Nurse**   You are pretty. You have very nice hair.

The student's reply is ego-supportive and also conveys directly to the patient what the student thinks of her appearance. The nurse can counteract the reluctance to terminate by discussion of the patient's growth and maturation and by encouragement (Fromm-Reichman, 1950). Although one student and patient had spent many hours together during the semester—the student had assisted the patient to fix her hair, fold her sleeve, etc.—it was only during the last 5 minutes of the relationship that the patient herself could "reach out." She did this by grabbing the student's hand, squeezing it, and exclaiming, "Oh, Margaret, please don't forget me. . . ." The student held her hand with both of hers and said, "I won't forget you."

Patients may tell you about their former physical ailments or newly developing ones as in an effort to keep you with them. They may also praise others on the team and say that these people helped them more than you did. In this, the patient is disdaining any transference which implies that you are important to him in any way. One patient at the time of termination got a job and informed the nurse, "I'm leaving you."

Nursing students often use a cultural ritual to assuage termination pangs of their patients and of their own by holding farewell teas, coffee hours, picnics, and other outings. Sometimes the patients themselves plan these events for the students. If such an event is planned, the other work of termination should have already been accomplished. Teen-age patients in particular often manage to get cake and coffee for their departing students.

The factor of time is very important—last appointments should be made so that you can be with your patient longer than usual if he requires it. Much work of the relationship is often accomplished during the last few nurse-patient contacts. If your interaction has centered around an activity such as a walk or card-playing, you may wish to continue this during the last visit. Sometimes another patient may join you—which can also be a catalyst for expression that this is the last time you and your patient are meeting and also may provide a basis for therapeutic patient-patient interaction after you leave. Other staff may also be of assistance at termination. One staff member said to the student who was with her patient, "It was good to have you here. How long have you been here?" The patient, usually taciturn, proceeded to answer, "Four months," and went on to tell of all the things he and the student had done together.

Students and their patients sometimes plan group outings and during the terminating phase these can be used to help the patient perceive that others are terminating at the same time and to talk about loss in a group. If the student and patient are also known to other staff and patients, when the nurse leaves, the patient has someone with whom he can communicate a pool of shared images. Helping your patient plan to fill up the appointment time that you have had with him is an important facet of termination. Other patients are often sensitive to this need and their help can be enlisted. If the patient is being reassigned to another nurse, inform the patient and inform the nurse of your work with the patient. A summary should be made and added to the patient's record.

SEPARATION OR "LITTLE TERMINATIONS"
Autistic patients seem to find separation difficult and may regress during the absence of the nurse unless careful attention is given to holidays, vacations, intersessions, and illnesses of the nurse. Nurses can prepare their patients for their absences by informing them of the time and occasion for them. If the

absence is lengthy, during the interim write a note to your patient reaffirming your next appointment date. The use of professional calling cards with dates for the next appointment can be something for the patient to refer to and consider. Reminding the patient that other staff are available in case of need and informing the other staff yourself that you will be gone can indicate to the patient that you are concerned about him. Concentration on the patient's feelings of loss during these separations can act as focal points for understanding his feelings of loss. Holidays alone can be periods of life in which loss is most acutely felt. The nurse can aid the patient to discuss those former holidays and his feelings about them. Nursing students often send their patients a commemorative card at these times. Some psychiatrists on vacation send cards to their patients to indicate that they are remembered.

NURSE'S NEEDS
Termination with autistic patients may be particularly anxiety provoking for the nurse. If there is no one to continue the nurse-patient relationship, the student may wish to continue on as before. The student needs guidance to consider the reality of the situation as well as support for one's feelings. The student may also feel pushed to get the patient "well" before leaving, not recognizing that the patient's recovery cannot be so easily tied to a schedule. If the nurse can perceive the efficacy of preventive techniques at the time of termination, the patient will derive more benefit from the nurse-patient relationship than a hurried push for recovery which is not in tune with the timetable of the patient. How the patient himself reacts to termination will clearly affect the nurse's needs. The nurse directs all possible attention to prevention in the terminating phase. *Figure 9* is a device for seeing how what you do in the terminating phase can add a meaningful chapter to the life of the patient. Therapeutic termination or prevention of desolation becomes your aim—not to get the patient 100 percent well the day that you leave.

RECORDING
Written nurse-patient interactions help the nurse to analyze and interpret communication with the patient. Evaluation, introspection, and reflection upon the events between you and your patient can lead to insights which are filled with affect and poignancy. In learning to work with patients, one of the major educational aims is to become conscious of one's own communicative behavior. In addition to introspection, written work aids objectivity and can be put aside after its initial use for future reference. Since almost all professionals who work in a similar intensive manner with patients have supervision and/or consultation by a more experienced professional or in the case of the experienced worker, a colleague, both written records and verbal accounts are helpful to both participants. As a student, your instructor is your preceptor

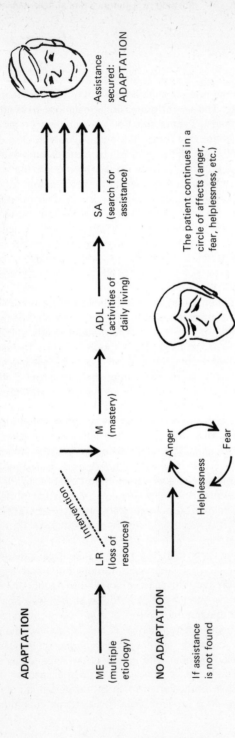

ADAPTATION

ME
(multiple
etiology)

LR
(loss of
resources)

Intervention

M
(mastery)

ADL
(activities of
daily living)

SA
(search for
assistance)

Assistance
secured:
ADAPTATION

NO ADAPTATION

If assistance
is not found

Anger

Fear

Helplessness

The patient continues in a
circle of affects (anger,
fear, helplessness, etc.)

Figure 9 Nursing intervention occurs at *LR* where loss of the person on whom the patient has learned to depend becomes an experience in which there is growth instead of a painful psychic wound. In the process of nurse-patient interaction, both the nurse and the patient grow, and after termination, each takes a place in the memory of the other.

and will usually require either written nurse-patient interactions, tape recordings, or video tapes for your perusal, analysis, and also as an initial basis for discussion in individual conferences with you.

Other therapies

In addition to the human relationship, various other therapeutic endeavors have been attempted and many are still being used in some parts of the world for these patients. Since the etiology of autism is unknown, various therapies are prescribed. Physicians and psychiatrists who are oriented to the biological school tend to use biological therapies. Those oriented to the psychological school tend to treat their patients with the human relationship or a combination of psychotherapy and the biological treatments. The effect of the human relationship pervades all the therapies, and some psychiatrists, learning of new therapies for autistic patients, advise less experienced colleagues to hurry up and try the new treatment "while it is still effective." Since there is considerable attention given to all patients who are receiving new therapies, the effect of a new treatment may be due to the human relationship instead of the particular treatment being administered.

Regardless of the ailment of the patient, the nature of human beings remains the same. When old problems are faced and conquered, new ones arise. As you contact and work with autistic patients you will develop your own theories about the etiology of their problem.

Insulin coma therapy was introduced by Manfred Sakel of Vienna in 1938. Electroshock therapy was first used by Dr. Lucio Bini and Dr. Ugo Cerletti in 1937 and introduced in this country about 1940 (American Psychiatric Association, 1944). During my practice as a psychiatric nurse I have seen the following therapies used for the autistic patient.

Metrazol shock
Electroshock
Insulin coma
Subcoma insulin therapy
Combined insulin and electroshock
Lobotomy
Hydrotherapy
Total push therapy
Industrial therapy
Narcosis therapy

Work therapy
Recreational therapy
Occupational therapy
Music therapy
Kinesics
Educational therapy
Individual psychotherapy
Group psychotherapy
Family therapy
Diet therapy
Remotivation groups
Social group work
Milieu therapy
Ataraxic drugs
Operant conditioning

The reader is referred to any of the standard textbooks of psychiatry for further knowledge of these therapies.

Work therapy

The importance of performing a purposeful activity such as a job cannot be overemphasized in our technological society where one's identity is closely connected with work. The film *Woman in the Dunes* is a graphic portrayal of the ordering of life around a daily task.

Patients in large public mental hospitals have too long been involved in institutional peonage, that is, long hours of work without pay. Some get the idea that if they work hard and long enough they are working their way out. Others, long accustomed to the hospital, perform 8-hour daily jobs and say that when they grow too old to work they will enjoy sitting in the sun on the grounds and talking with their friends. One patient who had worked on a food truck delivering food to the various wards felt that he was helping the other patients by doing this and was therefore living a useful life. He felt that his work paid for his room and board, which indeed it did. The employees helped keep him supplied with cigarettes. In the hospital for 16 years, and now at the age of forty-seven, this patient seemed content to stay exactly where he was. To him, his work on the food truck justified his staying in the hospital. Until the whole system is changed with regard to patients' performing the work within large institutions without pay, the patients who are there will most likely continue to do the work because it meets one of the basic needs— *to achieve and to do something purposeful.* The turn toward work and helping others is a significant event in the recovery of the autistic patient. It is of interest to note that all patients in mental hospitals in the Soviet Union are expected to work and I have seen the most regressed schizophrenic patients making beautiful flowers and other objects for the market. Work therapy is an integral part of the rehabilitation of the mental patient in Holland and in some parts of England. Praise for a job well done is ego-building for almost everyone. The knowledge that the nurse has of the patient and his particular situation can be of great aid to the psychiatric team in helping the patient obtain and hold a job. The nurse is likely to know the patient's stress points, some of his strengths and weaknesses, ways to bolster his ego and to help him deal with problems encountered at work. The motivation of patients with institutional recoveries is particularly challenging for the nurse, for it is often difficult for them to leave the security of the hospital for the outside world.

In some mental hospitals, patients assist in the care of animals and gardens. The trend in the United States is for the state mental hospitals to discontinue growing and providing their own food because it costs more than buying it. At the Colony of Gheel in Belgium, mental patients do agricultural work.

Discharged patients who cannot compete in the labor market may be able to work in a sheltered workshop where some guidance and supervision are provided, if your community has these workshops available.

Nursing care of two patients

The following summaries demonstrate the influence of milieu and some aspects of the nurse-patient relationship in the care of two autistic patients. For Annette, the extent of rehabilitation needed was great:

> Annette had been cared for at home by her mother and sister for 11 years, during which time she had not uttered a word or helped herself in any manner. She is now 22 years old. Following a sickness at age 11, which had been diagnosed at a local hospital as encephalitis, she had "lost her ability to speak and to move." During the ensuing years, she had been taken to several clinics by her mother. In the clinic at the university hospital an observant neurologist sent her to the local psychiatric hospital for observation and diagnosis. Although Annette had not spoken to anyone for 11 years, her sister and mother had read to her and left the radio on in her room. However, she gave few responses to them that indicated she was aware of her environment.

Since Annette had several contractures due to her long years in bed, the physical therapist came and spent 2 hours each day with her. Nursing care involved establishing a relationship with Annette. Since she was a bed patient, the first contacts were made with her through bathing, feeding, and grooming. All staff expected that Annette could speak and care for herself and each day verbalized this and offered her the chance to perform her own care. After 2 months she began to speak and with the work of the physical therapist was soon able to walk.

The next step in the nursing care plan was to help her to feed herself, carry out her own personal care (she had to learn how to apply lipstick, for example), and join the other patients in the dining room for meals. Annette relearned to socialize with others—she seemed completely out of tune in relating to peers—she was, however, most comfortable in the presence of older women who "mothered" her. Nursing care also involved sex instruction, helping her to know the value of money, to choose appropriate clothing for her age, to shop for herself, and to use the public transportation. Recreation was a problem for Annette who had some permanent curvature of her spine which limited activity. The nurse also helped her to learn to enjoy herself by going on a walk or to a film. Outings to Chinatown, museums, and the park helped Annette to explore the outer world of the city, to learn independence, and to handle approaches by strangers. Further rehabilitation involved education and vocational rehabilitation.

Although the nurse-patient relationship is telescoped below within this one paragraph, it is intended that the reader perceive some of the nursing care of this patient before the use of ataraxics and without the use of any of the therapies such as electroshock treatment. It is intended to portray the influence of a person on a person.

Another patient—Opal Sullivan—was mute, withdrawn, autistic, and restless. She did not stay in her room or sit alone but paced up and down the hospital unit a great deal. Most of the early contacts with Opal centered around mothering care such as feeding, grooming, elimination, cigarettes, and medications. In Opal's dereistic world, verbal messages were ignored. For example, suggestion that she take a shower and get ready for bed went unheeded. But getting her clean clothes and other personal effects ready, taking her by the hand and stating simply, "Opal, it's time for your shower, come on, your things are ready," and giving her a tug gave her the aid that was needed. At times, her negativism was so strong that she refused all approaches by pulling away. In these instances, compromises were made, such as agreeing that she did not have to shower today if she did not feel like it but to wash her face and hands, brush her teeth, and change her clothes, and take one the next day. At times Opal became very angry, shadow-boxed, and was assaultive to the nurses. Signs of mounting tension were clearly observable in her increased pacing, rapidity of smoking, angry facial expression, and tremulousness. Removing her from the group, sitting down with her, holding her, lighting her cigarette, and talking with her about how you thought she felt were calming actions. If her tension went unnoticed, it spiraled rapidly into attacking someone or some object in the environment. If the nurse assigned to Opal to help her meet her needs was available, it seemed that calming her down was accomplished somewhat more easily. Since Opal was mute, her needs were anticipated by nonverbal cues, her facial expression—especially her eyes—and her body language. Displeasure, pain, pleasure, ambivalence, and determination were evidenced by this type of communication and were very useful to the nurse in ascertaining her needs. It was also important to convey to her that she could tolerate anger and not be consumed by it. The firm touch and voice of the nurse through these aggressive periods were intended to convey to her that the "bad me" had not eliminated the caring person from her dereistic world.

In the case of Opal, ataraxic drugs were administered after $2\frac{1}{2}$ to 3 months of the condition described above. She was also seen in psychotherapy by her psychiatrist all during her hospitalization and was discharged when she became able to handle her own affairs under his continued care.

The patient's preference for one nurse may create jealousy among staff members. Discussion of all patients at nursing care conference helps to clarify that all patients and all nurses do not relate in the same way to each other. It is important, however, that all patients have at least one person on the nursing staff with whom they feel comfortable and in whom they feel free to confide. One of the advantages of the availability of a diverse staff in a psychiatric setting is that the chances are increased that the patient will be able to relate to at least one staff member. I have rarely observed patients in a treatment setting who did not have some member of the staff they related to quite positively.

Long-term illness

Patients who have long-term illness with conditions such as cerebrovascular accidents and subsequent loss of ability to speak and move parts of their bodies may react by withdrawal and regressive behavior, although the affect is different than that of autism. In emphasis on mothering care, the nursing care is quite similar. The nurse's feelings may also be similar when she is primed for the quick recovery of her patient and finds instead that progress is slow, recovery is long, and the little things that one does *every day* with long-term patients carry the ingredients of recovery, not some big dramatic one-day treatment. These daily acts include consistently caring for him as a person, provision of emotional support as he needs it, and doing this over and over.

Day treatment

The concept of day treatment is now made possible on a widescale basis within the neighborhood of the patient through community mental health centers. As these centers are established, the treatment and care of acute and long-term patients will be under their jurisdiction. In this type of setting, families can also be easily involved in the treatment process.

   The following schedule is from a day treatment center in one of the five catchment areas of the city of San Francisco:

Day treatment center schedule

Monday morning	Staff only	
	9:15–10:45	Day treatment staff meeting
	12:00–1:00	Lunch
Monday afternoon	1:00	Day members arrive
	1:00–2:30	Optional activities (e.g., current event group, art therapy, drama reading)
	2:30–3:30	Activity meeting
	3:30	Day ends
Tuesday	9:00	Staff meetings, teams A and B separately
	9:00	Day members arrive
	9:30	Small group meeting, A and B
	10:45–12:00	Psychodrama
	12:00–1:00	Lunch, bring lunch to eat here or can find nearby restaurants

	1:00	Meet at day center for after-noon activity
	3:30	Day ends
Wednesday	7:00–10:30	Doughnut sale at the general hospital to earn money for field trips, activities
	10:30–11:00	Day members arrive from home or doughnut sale
	11:00	Community meeting
	12:00–1:00	Lunch, bring lunch or find near-by restaurant
	1:00	Meet at day center for after-noon activity
	3:30	Day ends
	7:00–9:00	Family group therapy (for day members referred by their primary therapist)
Thursday	8:30–10:00	Staff meeting, all staff
	10:00–10:30	Day members arrive
	10:30	Small groups meet, A and B
	11:30–12:00	Get ready to leave on outing
	3:30	Day ends
Friday	9:00	Day members arrive
	9:00–9:30	Staff meets separately, teams A and B
	9:30–10:30	Separate group meetings, small groups A and B
	10:30–11:30	Team B, medication group
	12:00–1:00	Lunch, bring bag lunch or find nearby restaurant
	1:00–3:00	Activity possible—volleyball
	3:00–4:00	Head nurse meets with nursing staff

Aftercare

Although aftercare services affect all mental patients, they are discussed under this heading because autistic patients now make up a large portion of patients in mental hospitals who subsequently need prolonged aftercare services and who are high on the readmission rate. More than 200,000 individuals are now hospitalized with schizophrenia, and at least 2 percent of persons born in 1960 will have an episode of schizophrenia at some time during their lives (Mosher, 1969). In 1966 the Center for Studies of Schizophrenia was organized in the National Institute of Mental Health. A major goal of the Center is to coordinate the efforts of research, training, and service throughout the country. Attention will also be given to the treatment of patients in new types of facilities so as to provide for individualization of care and to avoid the chronicity of "warehousing" the patient.

An interesting development is the view of schizophrenia as a developmental crisis through which patients have to be helped to achieve higher levels of integration and functioning; this will result in study of nonbiological treatment (Mosher, 1969).

Although the ataraxic drugs have enabled many patients to be relieved of their symptoms, there are still many who have prolonged hospitalization and many of those who do leave the hospital continue with functional impairments (Mosher, 1969). Visits to the home of the mental patient during his hospitalization afford an opportunity to assess whether the patient is wanted at home and whether the home is conducive to his mental health. The family that has already adjusted to the absence of the patient, or excluded the disordered member before his hospital admission, will require different help than the family anxious to have the patient back (Merrill, 1969). The effect on the family of the presence of the patient can also be assessed and recommendations subsequently made to the therapeutic team. The positive potentials of the family system can also be determined and the help of relatives elicited and acknowledged. The experience of the nurse in the observation and assessment of the mental state of individuals is now extended to families. The work of Spiegel (1957), Ackerman (1958), Caplan (1964), and others contributes to the necessary theoretical knowledge (see Chapter 4). Caring for patients and families in a community setting provides a broader knowledge of family dynamics and concepts of role.

Upon leaving the hospital, autistic patients may require aftercare. Help may be given to them in the form of (1) finding a job and a place to live, (2) follow-up and psychological support, (3) assisting the patient and his family through crisis periods, (4) general health supervision, (5) supervision of medications, and (6) socialization. Silverstein (1968) made a study of 10,786 released patients who left 18 state mental hospitals in Pennsylvania. In his study, he found that three of the aftercare services (medication, counseling, and psychotherapy) constituted over 75 percent of the aftercare recommendations, whereas there was a low frequency of recommendations for vocational rehabilitation, resocialization, and related services. The study also showed that 35.5 percent of the patients who returned to the hospital did not use the available aftercare services. Although the discharge rate from mental hospitals has gone up since about 1955, the readmission rate is increasing.

One of the most important factors in aftercare of patients is that they be accepted. The hospital patient on a weekend leave to his home who finds that his room is now used for storage readily gets the idea of what his family thinks of his return. The patient who has been in a mental hospital and adjusted to the institutional life is all too often thrown out into the community and into the hectic affairs of everyday life without the ability to keep up. Unless he and his family receive the assistance they need, the patient will probably very quickly be readmitted. There is no substitute for the home visit to assess the family ecology and interaction. For example, a patient now in his early twenties who has been severely mentally disordered since the age of 12 has a mother who now refuses to talk about her son. In a home visit, the nurse was confronted by his mother who immediately stated, "To be perfectly honest with you, I don't want a thing to do with you and what you are doing with Tom." She became rather upset that the nurse was "delving into the past" of Tom and felt that it was too painful for him. She also stated that "It wouldn't do any good for you to try and find out about Tom's past life; we've been over it many times and it will never do any good." This mother based her criteria for her son's improvement on the time when he would make more friends and socialize more, which was precisely what Tom had not been able to do since he was 12 years old. It is doubtful whether this home will ever be a place to foster the mental health of this patient unless the attitude of the mother changes.

The mental patient returning to the community needs someone to attach himself to. Families also need this kind of person to help them with their special problems. The nurse can be the person to appear when needed and to follow the patient and his family until the need is dissipated.

In the Cassel Hospital, United Kingdom, where whole families are admitted, nurses begin their aftercare *before* the prospective family is admitted (Webster, in Barnes, ed., 1968, p. 176). The work of the nurses in precare can add a new dimension to the treatment plan and also to plans for aftercare. They visit the home beforehand to accomplish at least the following:

To assess adjustment, pressures, and interrelationships around the "sick" member
To find a way to help the family overcome resistances to care
To begin the nurse-family relationship
To offer the family an opportunity to clarify any questions about hospital admission

In preadmission visits, the nurses also determine whether or not it is advisable to separate the patient from the family. Seeing the patient as a part of his particular sociocultural milieu aids the nurse to adjust the assessment of needs accordingly.

Gheel

One situation in which mental patients have been accepted and cared for since the fifteenth century is the colony of Gheel in Belgium. It was originally one of the many shrines dedicated to different saints whose cures were famous in the medieval period. The shrine at Gheel was dedicated to St. Dymphna and mental patients were brought there in large numbers to be cured. From the time of "miracle cures" up to now, mental patients came to Gheel for family treatment. At Gheel the mental patient is accepted. The medical center of the colony of 27,000 inhabitants is a mental hospital for 350 patients with its own staff. Over 2000 patients live in Gheel. The colony is Gheel itself and is split into sections, each with its own psychiatrist and two to three qualified men nurses. The nurses visit patients in their foster homes, talk with the patients and the foster family, see if and how the patients work, look after the bedrooms, clothing, and the food, and give instructions to foster parents. They are responsible for the psychiatric part of the treatment. Each morning there is a conference of all staff involved. Gheel is agricultural and two thirds of the patients live on farms. It is the philosophy of the colony that farm work offers a great variety of activities and that a job can be found for everyone.

Half-way house

In aftercare, diverse services may be used for autistic patients. Transitional services are now on the upswing. Half-way houses provide a sheltered living arrangement for discharged patients. Half-way houses are a kind of dormitory living in the community and accommodate several patients, usually 6 to 15. Patients either have a single room or share a room. Bathrooms and cooking facilities are usually shared and patients expected to maintain their own rooms and laundry. Patients pay rent, plan their own meals, and share the kitchen work. They come and go as they wish. A committee made up of residents and the director plans special events and hears complaints of the residents. Most half-way houses serve only patients with mental disorder, men or women, and get referrals from an agency. Also, most patients who are referred to half-way houses have a potential to adjust to society and to get a job. Most require little supervision and are willing to work toward an early discharge from the house. Half-way houses share certain common functions: (1) residence, (2) transition, (3) socialization and resocialization, (4) vocational assistance, and (5) other ancillary treatment services (Landy and Greenblatt, 1965).

Other transitional services

Transitional services usually provide accessible counseling and socialization. Socially isolated patients have been found to have higher readmission rates than those with some form of social contacts (Dudgeon, 1964). Aiding the discharged patient to socialize is therefore high on the list of priorities in aftercare. The patient who has adjusted himself to institutionalization with staff-planned and staff-directed social activities needs a great deal of help in deciding and planning what to do with his leisure time. Therapeutic social clubs for discharged patients can be used.

The first therapeutic social club was originated by Joshua Bierer in the United Kingdom after his arrival there from Vienna in 1938. The first club of this kind in the United States—Fountain House—originated in 1948. Although there are many psychiatric social clubs now throughout the United States, each one is different. The principal aim of the clubs is rehabilitation. They emerged from the therapeutic community concepts initiated by Main (1946), Jones (1953), and Bierer (1948) in England.

These clubs are for the benefit of individuals who have suffered mental disorder and who have been hospitalized. They are for those who have fragile egos and who are more vulnerable to the stresses and rejections of daily life than most other people and for those who suffer from long-term disturbances. Individuals who use the clubs have few relationships with others. Where relationships occur, closeness is lacking and social isolation is severe. They need to be accepted by others in a milieu in which few demands are placed upon them. Common elements of social clubs are (1) community based, (2) noninstitutional, (3) intrinsically social, (4) democratic emphasis, (5) preference for horizontal merging of staff and volunteer roles, and (5) group activity (Grob, 1968).

The primary aim of the psychiatric social club is to help the discharged mental patient to return to community life and work. The social club is a social-vocational model in that it emphasizes job counseling, personal adjustment counseling, group therapy, and housing services. Mabel Palmer (1966) has written a guide for development of a therapeutic social club.[4]

Senior centers within the community can also be used. Knowledge of the existing community facilities will help you to assist your discharged patient to make use of them. All large cities have many recreational facilities accessible to all age groups.

Patients may also go to foster family homes—homes inspected and approved by professionals where patients live with designated families who are paid for their care. After finding a job, the patient may then move to other accommodations. Availability of industry and other types of housing is a necessary inducement to independent living. Foster family homes have often been located in rural areas where jobs and other types of housing were not easily found. This care is also used for patients who do not require hospitalization but who need some continuous supervision in activities of daily living.

Departments of vocational rehabilitation may assist the patient in getting a job. Counselors attached to community mental health centers are now doing this. A sheltered workshop may be the best place for those patients who require supervision. In California, mental patients no longer lose their professional licenses; therefore, it is easier for people whose work requires a license to go back to work after hospitalization. Nurses, for example, formerly had to take other jobs such as aide work until they could get their license back to practice professional nursing.

---

[4] The reader is referred to F. M. C. Evans: *The Role of the Nurse in Community Mental Health*. New York: The Macmillan Co., 1968, for further discussion of transitional services.

Summary

This chapter concerns itself with withdrawal behavior in persons. Emphasis is placed upon recognition of withdrawal in persons of all ages and ways that nurses may be of aid in case finding, direct care, and referral. Due to the incidence of autistic behavior, attention is focused in this chapter on acceptance of mental disorder in our society and of ways to aid autistic patients and others who are involved in their care.

References

Ackerman, Nathan: *The Psychodynamics of Family Life*. New York: Basic Books, 1958.

American Psychiatric Association: *One Hundred Years of American Psychiatry*. New York: Columbia University Press, 1944.

———— *Diagnostic and Statistical Manual of Mental Disorders, II*. Washington: American Psychiatric Association, 1968.

Barnes, Elizabeth, ed.: *Psychosocial Nursing*. London: Tavistock Publications, 1968.

Bateson, Gregory, Jackson, Donald D.: "Toward a Theory of Schizophrenia," *Behavioral Science*, **1**:4: 251–64, 1956.

Bettelheim, Bruno: *Love Is Not Enough*. New York: The Free Press, 1955.

———— *Truants from Life*. New York: The Free Press, 1955.

———— *The Empty Fortress*. New York: The Free Press, 1968, pp. 233–342.

Bierer, Joshua, ed.: *Therapeutic Social Clubs*. London: H. K. Lewis, 1948.

———— "Great Britain's Therapeutic Social Clubs," *The Journal of Hospital and Community Psychiatry*, **13**: 203ff, April, 1962.

Caplan, Gerald: *Principles of Preventive Psychiatry*. New York: Basic Books, 1964.

Caudill, William, *et al.*: "Social Structure and Interactive Processes on a Psychiatric Ward," *American Journal of Orthopsychiatry*, **22**:314–33, April, 1952.

———— *The Psychiatric Hospital as a Small Society*. Cambridge: Harvard University Press, 1958.

Doane, Leona: *The Therapeutic Termination of Interpersonal Relationships*. Unpublished master's field study, Boston University, 1963.

Dudgeon, Yvonne M.: "The Social Needs of the Discharged Mental Hospital Patient," *The International Journal of Social Psychiatry*, **10**:1:45–54, Winter, 1964.

Evans, F. M. C.: *The Role of the Nurse in Community Mental Health*. New York: The Macmillan Co., 1968.

———— and Esquivel, Piedad: "A Family Study Project: Coordination of Psychiatric and Public Health Nursing for Basic Baccalaureate Students," in *Nursing in Community Mental Health and Retardation Programs*. New York: National League for Nursing, 1965.

Fromm-Reichman, Frieda: *Principles of Intensive Psychotherapy*. Chicago: The University of Chicago Press, 1950, pp. 188–94.

Green, Hannah: *I Never Promised You a Rose Garden*. New York: The New American Library, 1964.

Greenblatt, Milton, Levinson, Daniel J., and Williams, Richard H.: *The Patient and the Mental Hospital*. New York: The Free Press, 1957.

Grob, Samuel: "Psychiatric Social Clubs Come of Age." Hartford, Conn.: The Connecticut Association for Mental Health, 1968.

Jones, Maxwell, Baker, A., Freeman, Thomas, Merry, Julius, Pomryn, B. A., Sandler, Joseph, and Tuxford, Joy: *The Therapeutic Community*. New York: Basic Books, 1953.

———— *Beyond the Therapeutic Community*. New Haven: Yale University Press, 1968.

Kris, Ernst: *Psychoanalytic Explorations in Art*. New York: International Universities Press, Inc., p. 177.

Landy, David, and Greenblatt, Milton: *Half-Way House*. Washington, D.C.: U.S. Department of Health, Education, and Welfare, 1965.

Main, T. F.: "The Hospital as a Therapeutic Institution," *Bulletin of the Menninger Clinic*, **10**:3:66–70, May, 1946.

Merrill, Georgia: "How Fathers Manage When Wives Are Hospitalized for Schizophrenia," *Social Psychiatry*, **4**:1:26–32, 1969.

Modell, Arnold H.: "Hallucinations in Schizophrenia Patients and Their Relation to Psychic Structure," in West, Louis Jolyon, ed.: *Hallucinations*. New York: Grune and Stratton, 1962.

Mosher, Loren R.: "The Center for Studies of Schizophrenia," *Schizophrenia Bulletin*. Washington, D.C.: Government Printing Office, 1969.

Palmer, Mabel: "The Social Club." New York: National Association for Mental Health, 1966.

Rosen, John: *Direct Analysis*. New York: Grune and Stratton, 1953.

Sakel, Manfred: "The Indications of Shock-Therapy Methods," notes taken from presentation at the International Congress of Psychiatry, September 25, 1950, Paris.

Schwing, Gertrud: *A Way to the Soul of the Mentally Ill.* New York: International Universities Press, 1954.
Sechehaye, Marguerite: *Autobiography of a Schizophrenic Girl.* New York: Grune and Stratton, 1951.
———— *Symbolic Realization.* New York: International Universities Press, 1951.
Silverstein, Max: *Psychiatric Aftercare.* Philadelphia: University of Pennsylvania Press, 1968.
Spiegel, John N.: "The Resolution of Role Conflict Within the Family" in Greenblatt, Milton, ed.: *The Patient and the Mental Hospital.* New York: The Free Press, 1957, pp. 545–64.
Stanton, A. H., and Schwartz, M. S.: "Observations on Dissociation as Social Participation," *Psychiatry,* **12**:339–54, 1949.
Sullivan, H. S.: *The Interpersonal Theory of Psychiatry.* New York: W. W. Norton and Co., Inc., 1953.
Tudor, Gwen E.: "A Sociopsychiatric Nursing Approach to Intervention in a Problem of Mutual Withdrawal on a Mental Hospital Ward," *Psychiatry,* May, 1952, pp. 193–217.
Ward, Anita H.: "My Silent Patient," *Perspectives in Psychiatric Care,* **7**:2:87–91, 1969.
Webster, Janice: "Nursing Families," in Barnes, Elizabeth, ed.: *Psychosocial Nursing.* London: Tavistock Publications, 1968, p. 176.
West, Louis Jolyon, ed.: *Hallucinations.* New York: Grune and Stratton, 1962.
Williams, Harold L., Morris, Gary O., and Lubin, Archie: "Illusions, Hallucinations and Sleep Loss," in West, Louis Jolyon, ed.: *Hallucinations.* New York: Grune and Stratton, 1962.
Wilmer, Harry: *Social Psychiatry in Action.* Springfield, Ill.: Charles C Thomas, 1958.

Suggested readings

Aronson, Jason: "Schizophrenia in Transcultural Perspective," notes taken from paper presented at the First International Congress of Social Psychiatry, London, August, 1964.
Bellak, Leopold, and Loeb, Laurence: *The Schizophrenic Syndrome.* New York: Grune and Stratton, 1969.
Berelson, Bernard: *Human Behavior.* New York: Harcourt, Brace and World, 1964.

Bleuler, Eugen: *Dementia Praecox*. Leipzig and Vienna: F. Deuticke, 1911.

Burnham, Donald, Gladstone, Arthur I., and Gibson, Robert W.: *Schizophrenia and the Need-Fear Dilemma*. New York: International Universities Press, Inc., 1969.

Dennehy, Anne: "Nursing Intervention in the Hallucinatory Process," American Nurses' Association, Regional Clinical Conferences, 1965, pp. 22–25.

Deutsch, Albert: *The Mentally Ill in America*. New York: Doubleday Doran and Co., Inc., 1937.

Federn, Paul: "Ego Psychological Aspect of Schizophrenia," in Weiss, Edoardo, ed.: *Ego Psychology and the Psychoses*. New York: Basic Books, 1952, pp. 210–26.

Freeman, H. E., and Simmons, O. G.: "The Social Integration of Former Mental Patients," *International Journal of Social Psychiatry*, **4**:264–71, Spring, 1959.

Freeman, Thomas, *et al.*: *Chronic Schizophrenia*. New York: International Universities Press, 1958.

Fromm-Reichmann, Frieda: "Some Aspects of Psychotherapy with Schizophrenics," in Brody, E. B., and Redlich, F. C., eds.: *Psychotherapy with Schizophrenics*. New York: International Universities Press, 1952, pp. 89–111.

Hewitt, Helon, and Fatka, Nada: "Social Therapeutic Clubs—A Step Toward Rehabilitation," *Perspectives in Psychiatric Care*, **1**:6:31–37, 1963.

Jackson, Don D.: *The Etiology of Schizophrenia*. New York: Basic Books, 1960.

Kris, Ernst: *Psychoanalytic Explorations in Art*. New York: International Universities Press, 1952.

Labreche, Gary, Turner, R. Jay, and Zabo, Lawrence J.: "Social Class and Participation in Outpatient Care by Schizophrenics," *Community Mental Health Journal*, **5**:5:394–402, October, 1969.

Lidz, Theodore, Fleck, Stephen, and Cornielson, Alice R.: *Schizophrenia and the Family*. New York: International Universities Press, 1965.

Melehov, D. E., Grossman, A. V., and Petrunek, A.: "Industrial Rehabilitation of Psychiatric Patients in Open Industry and in Special Workshops," *Social Psychiatry*, **5**:1:12–15, January, 1970.

Mishler, Elliot G., and Waxler, Nancy E.: "Family Interaction Processes and Schizophrenia; a Review of Current Theories," *Merrill-Palmer Quarterly of Behavior and Development*, **11**:4:269–315, 1965.

Moore, Stanley: "A Psychiatric Out-Patient Nursing Service," *Mental Health Bulletin*, Warlingham Park Hospital, United Kingdom, 1961.

Opler, Marvin: *Culture and Mental Health*. New York: The Macmillan Co., 1959.

———— *Culture and Social Psychiatry.* New York: Atherton Press, 1967.

———— "Schizophrenia and Culture," *Scientific American,* **197**:2:103–10, August, 1957.

Pasamanick, Benjamin, Scarpitti, Frank R., and Dinitz, Simon: *Schizophrenics in the Community: An Experimental Study in the Prevention of Hospitalization.* New York: Appleton-Century-Crofts, 1967.

Reuck, A. V. S. de, ed.: *Transcultural Psychiatry.* Boston: Little, Brown and Co., 1965.

Rosenthal, David, and Kety, Seymour S.: *Transmission of Schizophrenia.* Pergamon Press, Inc., 1968.

———— "Problems of Sampling and Diagnosis in the Major Twin Studies of Schizophrenia," *Schizophrenia Bulletin.* Washington, D.C.: U.S. Government Printing Office, 1969, pp. 11–26.

Rubin, Theodore Isaac: *Jordi; Lisa and David.* New York: Ballantine Books, 1962.

Simon, Stanford H., Heggestad, Wayne, and Hopkins, Joseph: "Some Factors Relating to Success and Failure of Male Chronic Schizophrenics on Their First Foster Home Placement," *Community Mental Health Journal,* **4**:4:314–18, August, 1968.

Travelbee, Joyce: *Intervention in Psychiatric Nursing: Process in the One-to-One Relationship.* Philadelphia: F. A. Davis Co., 1969.

Weinberg, S. Kirson: "The Relevance of the Forms of Isolation to Schizophrenia," *International Journal of Social Psychiatry,* **13**:1:33–41, Winter 1966/67.

11   Drug use and drug dependence

The main thesis of this chapter is that drug abuse can apply to any drug. However, the main interest is in drugs that produce changes in mood and behavior since these have the greatest potential for abuse. We live in a society in which drugs are advertised on the mass media as being the answer to many problems. In many cases, the abuse of drugs simply brings on more problems.

Man has known the effect of drugs since antiquity. The drunkenness of Noah is mentioned in the Bible and displayed in sculpture by a fifteenth century artist on a corner of the Doge's Palace in Venice. The Sumerians in Mesopotamia knew about opium, the dried juice of the opium poppy, in 3000 B.C. *Cannabis* and coca leaves seem to have been known since recorded history. Others have appeared on the scene more recently. Almost all drugs have some beneficial use and it is only in drug abuse that something needs to be done. Drug abuse refers to taking drugs to the extent that they result in damage to the individual or to the community by upsetting and disturbing its way of life (World Health Organization, 1967). In psychiatry, tranquilizers were first used on a wide scale in the mid-Fifties. Antidepressants, sleeping pills, coffee, and tobacco also have widespread use in our society. The use of hallucinogenic drugs assumed epidemic proportions in the Sixties. These are three terms that are frequently confused in discussions of drug abuse:

> **Addiction**   *Dependence on a chemical substance to the extent that physiologic dependence is established. The latter manifests itself as withdrawal symptoms (the abstinence syndrome) when the drug is withdrawn.*[1]

> **Habituation**   *a condition, resulting from the repeated consumption of a drug, which involves little or no evidence of tolerance, some psychological dependence, no physical dependence, and a desire (but not a compulsion) to continue taking the drug for the feeling of well-being that it produces.*[2]

---

[1] American Psychiatric Association: *A Psychiatric Glossary*. Washington, D.C., 1969.
[2] Department of Defense: *Drug Abuse: Game Without Winners*. Washington, D.C.: Superintendent of Documents, 1968.

Drug dependence   *Habituation to, abuse of, and/or addiction to a chemical substance. Largely because of psychologic craving, the life of the drug-dependent person revolves about his need for the specific effect of one or more chemical agents on his mood or state of consciousness. The term thus includes not only* addiction *(which emphasizes physiologic dependence), but also drug abuse (where the pathologic craving for drugs seems unrelated to physical dependence).* Alcoholism *is a special type of drug dependence. Other examples are dependence on opiates, synthetic analgesics with morphinelike effects, barbiturates; other hypnotics, sedatives, and tranquilizers; cocaine, marihuana; other psychostimulants; and hallucinogens.*[3]

Recently the World Health Organization has recommended that these terms all be replaced by the term *drug dependence*. The terms *addiction* and *habituation* have international use and probably will not be dropped from the various laws in which they appear. The term *drug dependence* is most likely to be used by those who are medically oriented.

Alcoholism

Alcoholic individuals may be defined as "excessive drinkers, irrespective of the cause, so dependent on alcohol as to be disturbed in physical or mental health or in social activities. The assessment of consumption can only be made in relation to accepted local and national drinking habits."[4]

Etiology

There is no general agreement about the etiology, psychodynamics, and treatment of alcoholism. Four principal theories are (1) *genetic*, (2) *pathophysiological*—dysfunction of the hypophysis-adrenal system or other metabolic dysfunctions, (3) *psychological*—the psychological theories stress seeking security and self-esteem as etiological factors; the psychoanalytic approach emphasizes the presence of strong oral and homosexual

---

[3] American Psychiatric Association: *A Psychiatric Glossary*. Washington, D.C., 1969.
[4] World Health Organization: "WHO and Mental Health, 1949–1961." *WHO Chronicle*, **16**:5:177, May, 1962.

drives in a narcissistic person who uses alcohol to attempt gratification, and (4) *sociocultural*.

The alcoholic is involved in the following circular process: excessive drinking — disapproval — self-recrimination — guilt — rationalization and other defense mechanisms, such as denial and projection — excessive drinking.

The difference between the social drinker and the pathological drinker therefore refers to excessiveness, interference with work and social adjustment, and production of a pathological emotional reaction. The one characteristic common to all alcoholics is that they drink too much. The idea of an alcoholic personality is no longer acceptable. The search for causes for drinking too much has obscured the search for understanding of the mechanism of alcoholism. There are always reasons why people behave the way they do. It is thought that people drink excessively as a defense against anxiety. But there is no clarification as to why alcohol is chosen as a defense against anxiety.

Synonyms for alcohol are ethanol, ethyl alcohol, grain alcohol, and spirit of wine (Taber, 1965). It is readily absorbed from the gastrointestinal tract. Being a central nervous system depressant, it exerts its first action upon the reticular activating system. Alcohol depresses this system and the cortex is released from its integrating control (Goodman and Gilman, 1965, p. 144). Thus the higher centers of judgment, self-criticism, learning, and memory are affected by alcohol. Excitement comes from the resultant lowering of inhibitions. The superego of the individual has been said to be the part of the person that is most soluble in alcohol. Oxidation of alcohol is slow and occurs as follows: alcohol: acetaldehyde: acetic acid: CO_2H_2O. It is thrown off from the body through the breath and the urine.

The hangover results from excessive use of alcohol and is characterized by gastritis, nausea, vomiting, dizziness, headache, malaise, dehydration, and excessive thirst. Himwich (1956, p. 348) cites accumulation of acetaldehyde, retention of potassium, and lactacidemia as possible causes of the hangover. No two hangovers are alike in their emotional pain. It is difficult to adequately describe their affects of despair. Although many "remedies" are suggested for it, the best treatment is probably aspirin, rest, and taking in food.

Alcohol has seven calories per milliliter and is therefore classified by some as a food; others consider it a drug. Ethyl alcohol is made (1) by fermentation of carbohydrates and (2) by the addition of water to ethylene, using sulfuric acid as a catalyst (Grillot, 1964).

Ethyl alcohol has been known since early antiquity. In the human body, alcohol is readily absorbed from the stomach and the small intestine. The rapidity of absorption depends upon the speed of ingestion, concentration of alcohol, volume of alcohol, and the presence and character of other food within the stomach; however, within approximately five minutes after alcohol intake, some of it is in the blood stream. It is almost completely oxidized; in the process, energy is released and carbon dioxide and water are given off.

Although the initial feeling after intake of alcohol is one of expansiveness and euphoria, it is a depressant, not a stimulant. The feeling of well-being is caused by the lowering of inhibitions and the effect of the drug leads the drinker to feel that his performance is improved when, in actuality, it has been impaired. Alcohol taken in moderation stimulates the flow of the digestive juices and thereby aids digestion. Dilation of the blood vessels results in perspiration and heat loss, therefore use of alcohol to keep warm in a cold climate can have disastrous results. Hot toddies for colds and for sleep probably encourage relaxation more than anything else.

Intoxication depends upon the amount of alcohol in the blood stream. A concentration of 0.10 to 0.20 in the blood indicates intoxication whereas 0.50 to 0.90 percent is in the fatal range. Four bottles of beer, four highballs or cocktails will take a 150-pound person up to the 0.10 percent level.[5]

Acute alcoholic intoxication is characterized by euphoria, increased motor activity, clumsiness, incoordination, diplopia, staggering gait, nausea, vomiting, poor control of urination, and finally, loss of consciousness, stupor, and profound coma. Associated with chronic alcoholism are alterations in personality, *delirium tremens*, acute alcoholic hallucinosis, Korsakoff's syndrome, Wernicke's syndrome, cirrhosis of the liver, pellagra, alcoholic polyneuritis, tuberculosis, cardiovascular disease, gastric ulcers, malnutrition, and the various resultant social conditions.

Epidemiology

The number of alcoholics in the United States is unknown. However, estimates are made that there are 5 million (The President's Commission on Law Enforcement and Administration of Justice, 1967). This makes alcoholism the nation's fourth largest health problem. It is also estimated that there are three male alcoholics per each female alcoholic. Alcoholism seems more prevalent within the middle-age group. Seventy-five percent of alcoholics in this country are males between the ages of 35 and 55, and the average age is 42 years. Analysis of the demography of a particular county or metropolitan

[5] The alcohol in a highball or cocktail is based on the use of 1 ounce of 100-proof whiskey or gin (Department of Public Health, San Francisco, 1967).

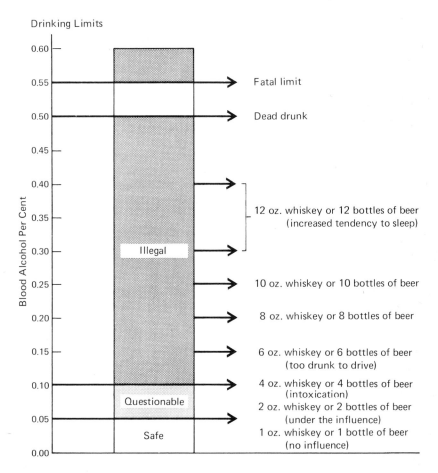

Figure 10   Alcohol intake based on responses of a 150-pound person.

area yields valuable information as to how many alcoholics there actually may be within the area. The incidence of cirrhosis of the liver has formerly been used as an indicator. Cirrhosis of the liver is certainly associated with alcoholism, but there are other causes. Two million arrests in 1965 were for public drunkenness (The President's Commission on Law Enforcement and Administration of Justice, 1967). Repeated arrests for public drunkenness are clearly a sign of alcoholism. An annual expense of $100 million for handling chronic drunkenness is a conservative estimate for the nation. This figure provides no funds for prevention and treatment. Our system of treatment of alcoholics is an abysmal failure (Pittman, 1967). Although the majority of men in Skid Row[6] cannot be defined as alcoholics, the incidence of problem drinking is high (Bogue, 1963). The incidence of arrests is also high, the pattern being arrest, conviction, sentencing, jailing, release, and rearrest within a few days. Although the alcoholic from Skid Row is the one who is most often arrested, only 4 percent of New York's Bowery homeless men were alcoholic (Strauss, 1951).

USERS OF ALCOHOL
Alcohol is available worldwide, although there are areas in which its use is prohibited, for example, in the Moslem countries, India, and "dry" counties in the United States. Its use is associated with tension release and social interaction such as the cocktail party, conventions, picnics, and business luncheons.

WHO IS THE ALCOHOLIC?
Although the people on Skid Row have formerly been thought of as comprising the alcoholic population, these individuals are not all alcoholic and make up only 5 percent of alcoholics (see *Figure 11*). As women move more and more into the world of men, the incidence of alcoholism increases among them or at least is more visible and therefore counted among the statistics; at present, 25 percent are women and 75 percent are men.

Cultural groups, such as Italians and Jews, who use alcohol with meals and serve it to the whole family at ceremonials have lower rates of alcoholism.

Treatment of the alcoholic patient and his family

In his message to the Congress on health, President Lyndon B. Johnson called for a new program in the treatment of alcoholism (1966). He said:[7]

> *The alcoholic suffers from a disease which will yield eventually to scientific research and adequate treatment. Even with the present limited state of our knowledge, much can be done to reduce the untold suffering and uncounted waste caused by this affliction. I have*

---

[6] The term "Skid Row" probably originated in Seattle in the late nineteenth century. Yessler Street was greased to skid logs down the slope into the water. Taverns, hotels, and other places for the loggers lined the street (Pittman, 1967).
[7] Lyndon B. Johnson, Health Message to Congress, 1966.

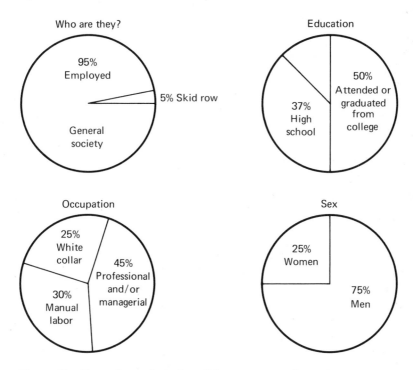

Figure 11 Facts about alcoholics. (13 per cent receive only a grammar school education.)

> *instructed the Secretary of Health, Education, and Welfare to appoint an Advisory Committee on Alcoholism; establish in the Public Health Service a center for research on the cause, prevention, control, and treatment of alcoholism; develop an education program in which to foster public understanding based on scientific fact; and work with public and private agencies on the state and local level to include this disease in comprehensive health programs.*

A coordinating committee at a national level established liaison with representatives of the Veteran's Administration, the Civil Service Commission, the Department of Commerce, the Department of Defense, the Department of Justice, the Department of Labor, and other concerned branches of government. A National Center for Prevention and Control of Alcoholism was then established in the National Institute of Mental Health in 1966. The aims of this new center are (1) to stimulate research, (2) to accelerate communication and application of research findings, (3) to encourage the development of training programs for professional personnel, and (4) to modify public attitudes toward alcoholism by publicizing scientific knowledge through an expanded program of education. The center provides leadership in planning and development of national programs in collaboration with other agencies.

Enabling legislation includes the new Medical Assistance provisions (Title XIX) of the Social Security Act where medical care can be provided in some states for those alcoholics who are medically indigent. The New Comprehensive Health Planning and Public Health Service Amendments of 1966 provide grants to each state to bring health programs in line with needs. Other legislation provides financial support for training manpower and other needs. Alcoholics are apt to have multiple problems and are therefore best treated within their home community, using all possible resources. The provisions of community mental health services by Public Law 88–164 will also aid the alcoholic patient (see *Figure 12*). Vocational rehabilitation is one of the areas in which the alcoholic needs assistance.

DETOXIFICATION CENTERS
In contrast with the punitive approach, the illness approach requires immediate attention to the alcoholic. Detoxification centers can provide the facilities for drying out, thereby replacing jails (Kendis, 1968). This system

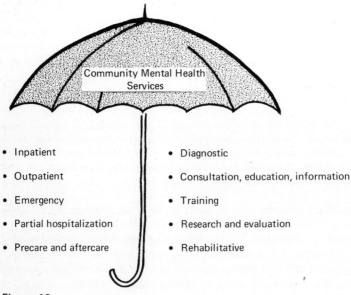

Community Mental Health Services

- Inpatient
- Outpatient
- Emergency
- Partial hospitalization
- Precare and aftercare

- Diagnostic
- Consultation, education, information
- Training
- Research and evaluation
- Rehabilitative

Figure 12

is used successfully in Czechoslovakia. Recently, the U.S. Department of Justice provided funds for two detoxification centers in demonstration projects: in St. Louis and Washington, D.C. The President's Commission on Law Enforcement and Administration of Justice (1967) recommends that *communities should establish detoxification units as part of comprehensive treatment programs.* In the detoxification center, attention is given to a thorough health examination, including a urine test for sugar and acetone. No glucose is given to the acute alcoholic until it is determined whether or not he is diabetic. High protein meals with vitamin and mineral supplements are provided. Twenty-four-hour bed rest and tranquilizers and anti-acids for gastritis are used. Close observation and caring for the alcoholic are necessary to prevent suicide.

Clothing, a bath, laundry facilities, and some recreational activities are provided. Patients are counseled by the staff members; regular lectures, group therapy, films, work projects, vocational rehabilitation, and Alcoholics Anonymous meetings are part of the program. After drying out, referral may be made for further treatment.

ANTABUSE THERAPY

Antabuse (tetraethylthiuram disulfide), first used in Copenhagen in 1948, can be effective in the treatment of alcoholism (Larsen, 1948). A patient may be given a trial reaction in the hospital in which the drug is administered and he is then given his favorite drink. The oxidation of the alcohol is delayed at the acetaldehyde stage and an unpleasant reaction ensues; therefore the patient avoids drinking alcohol to avoid the unpleasant consequences. The success of this treatment depends upon whether the patient takes the medication. Compulsive individuals may be more successful in taking the medication every day than others. Another drug, calcium carbimide (Temposil), has a similar action to Antabuse.

Conditioning and conditioned aversion therapies are being revived once more with some success. The impact of modern learning theory in the behavioral sciences gives impetus to these therapies. An excellent and scholarly review of these treatment approaches from the Thirties up until now is that of Franks (1966). Modeled upon conditioning principles, electro-conditioning therapy of alcoholics sets the sequence, drinking—painful stimulation—no reward, in treatment (Hsu, 1965).

OTHER THERAPIES

Other therapies, individual psychotherapy, family therapy, group psychotherapy, and milieu therapy are also used in different settings for the treatment of the alcoholic patient and his family.

ALCOHOLICS ANONYMOUS

Alcoholics Anonymous is a fellowship group established in 1935 in Akron, Ohio, to help people stop drinking and stay sober. It is conducted by former alcoholics and organized to provide help to alcoholics on a 24-hour basis all over the nation. Every night in the week there is an AA meeting somewhere in every metropolitan area. Every sizable town has its local chapter. It is organized around a religious-social theme and uses many principles of group psychotherapy. A call from an alcoholic at any time of day or night is answered by the members. Group loyalty is high and, in the group, catharsis is experienced and the alcoholic is accepted as he is *except for his drinking behavior*. Anonymity is guarded in AA groups.

Professionals and AA groups now cooperate in their efforts to aid the alcoholic to stop drinking. Alcoholics are helped in the rehabilitation process through the houses run by the AA and in other ways as well. Al-Anon Family Groups are rather new, incorporating in the mid-Fifties. All are self-supporting. Al-Anon is a fellowship group composed of relatives and friends of alcoholics, organized for the following purposes:

To give comfort, hope, and friendship to the families of compulsive drinkers
To learn to grow spiritually through living by the twelve steps adopted from Alcoholics Anonymous
To give understanding and encouragement to the alcoholic [8]

Alateen groups are organized for teen-agers who have a parent who cannot stop drinking. These groups were started in California in 1957 by a boy whose father was an alcoholic. His mother was a member of an Al-Anon Family Group, so he designed Alateen after the Al-Anon group (Al-Anon, 1966).

The role of the nurse

One of the first hurdles for the nurse is self-awareness with regard to one's own attitude toward the alcoholic. If the nurse has a moralistic attitude, the patient will feel it and it will probably further lower his self-esteem. At the other end of the scale, the nurse may think instant reform is possible. An objective attitude is called for in working with the alcoholic patient. When

[8] Al-Anon Family Group Headquarters, Inc., 1969 (P.O. Box 182, Madison Square Station, New York, N.Y. 10010).

diabetic patients go off their diets and have to be regulated, the nurse is not apt to moralize. Is not the chronic alcoholic patient in a similar situation? If the nurse derogates the returning alcoholic patient with the greeting, "What! You again?" his self-esteem is further lowered.

Alcoholic patients are frequently admitted to general hospitals for surgery and for other treatments. While undergoing these procedures, treatment for the alcoholism may be ignored and daily doses of spiritus frumenti ordered by the attending physician. Such situations need to be changed. A health team that heals a surgical wound and ignores the alcohol problem sentences the patient to continued psychic pain. Caring enough about the patient to discuss the alcoholic problem with him may be the catalyst for progress. Admission of alcoholic patients to general hospitals under other diagnoses still occurs and supports continuation of stigma.

Accidents and alcoholism are connected and, unless the accident victim is intoxicated or a very thorough history is taken, the hospitalized alcoholic may go into delirium tremens and die unless preventive measures are instituted. Preventive action would include, for example, a high vitamin, high caloric diet with adequate fluid intake and in-between meal feedings; a box of hard candy by the bedside will assist in the carbohydrate intake. Tranquilizers are now used to assist in relaxation. Vitamin therapy and hypnotics may be ordered by the physician as preventive measures.

Visual hallucinations may be the first sign of impending delirium tremens, as well as nausea and vomiting, and should be reported to the physician at once. The syndrome is also characterized by auditory hallucinations, illusions, disorientation, tremors, fear, restlessness, and insomnia. Recognition of the early signs of delirium tremens will aid in early treatment and recovery of the patient.

The patient with delirium tremens needs someone at his bedside continuously to allay apprehension, and to prevent injury in response to the hallucinations. A light should be kept on in the room to aid orientation, and shadows from its parabola avoided, if possible. The hallucinations are usually very frightening to the patient. They may sometimes *be* pink elephants marching along at the end of the bed. *Restraints should not be used because they tend to further agitate the patient.*

In the treatment of delirium tremens all alcohol and alcohollike medication is stopped. Cough medicines which are made with alcohol should not be given to the patient. Paraldehyde, which is synergistic with alcohol, was once generously used in treatment but is now replaced by other hypnotics and by tranquilizers. When phenothiazines are used, it must be remembered that they potentiate alcohol and that another side effect is orthostatic hypotension. In acute delirium tremens, the first tranquilizer will be given intramuscularly. If the patient cannot tolerate oral liquids, they will be given intravenously.

Orange juice with $\frac{1}{2}$ ounce of dextrimaltose to a 10-ounce glass is given at frequent intervals to replenish glycogen stored in the liver, for vitamin C, sodium chloride, and potassium content. The patient will receive multivitamins and a nonbarbiturate sedative for insomnia. If the patient has status epilepticus, he will be given intravenous barbiturates to control the convulsions. With adequate treatment, the syndrome of delirium tremens is reversible.

Treatment of alcoholics in general hospitals is now gaining impetus. The project at Mt. Zion Hospital, San Francisco, showed that alcoholics can be treated in ordinary general hospital settings in the same room and ward with patients with medical-surgical conditions (Gordon, 1958).

Community nurses who are in the homes of families have an important part to play in the treatment of the alcoholic. They also see people in clinics, schools, industries, and community activities. The community nurse is in a position where high visibility of alcoholism aids identification of cases early in onset. Warning signs of alcoholism should alert the nurse in early recognition of this mental disorder. Some are as follows:

Drinking alone
A feeling of having to have a drink
Missing a day's work due to a hangover
Drinking in the morning
Missing a social engagement due to drinking
Drinking instead of eating
Excessive drinking at meal time

Constructive suggestions to the alcoholic and his family may aid them in seeking help with their problems. For the helping person, knowing one's own limitations in the treatment of the alcoholic person and motivating the alcoholic to accept help are important. Knowing where to get help for the patient is a must whether it be a day treatment center, a community mental health center, a clinic, a psychologist, a physician, psychiatrist, AA, Al-Anon, or Alateen Group. Of equal importance to the nurse is knowing the agencies to approach for consultation and advice such as the local community mental health services.

Specialist community mental health nurses may provide treatment themselves in terms of family therapy, group psychotherapy, and individual psychotherapy. In milieu therapy, the nurse also acts as a role model for the alcoholic patient.

Where the nurse has contact with people in schools, universities, industry, and community activities, an educational program about the use and abuse of alcohol can aid in prevention. In schools, the nurse may set up an educational program for the teachers so that they can better help their students with the question of drinking alcohol.

In one's own life, preventive techniques may be applied, for example, entertaining without the use or overuse of alcohol. I have gone to cocktail parties where the guests were met at the door with a tray of drinks. Pushing drinks onto guests at some parties seems to be taken as generosity of the host, when, in actuality, it may be doing his guests a disservice. If alcohol is served, a wide array of nonalcoholic drinks can also be made available and offered to the guests.

If people must drink, impress upon them the importance of eating. There does seem to be some evidence that early contact with alcohol within the family, at meals and at ceremonials, teaches moderation, the difference between safe and unsafe drinking, and avoidance of a later alcoholic problem. Helping others to have a tolerance for abstaining with complete social acceptance of those who choose to abstain or drink very little is another preventive angle (Plaut, 1966).

Since the greatest impact on alcoholism in the future may come from research rather than from services, nurses have an important role also in this area.

Other drugs

Drug abuse arises from a complex interaction of psychosocial forces, the availability of the drug, the opportunity to take the first dose, and the continuance of its use. Kolb (1968) classifies drug addicts as (1) those seeking pleasure, (2) those seeking reduction of anxiety and tension, and (3) those who have become addicted by receiving drugs throughout long-term illness.

There are many ideas about the cause of the epidemic of drug abuse; the pervasive alienation in our society is one thesis. Certain aspects of our society are relevant to understanding the drug crisis: the drug-saturated society itself, the glorification of drugs by the mass media, the role modeling done by the older generation on drug taking, peer group pressure, over-availability, the interrelatedness of tobacco smoking and cannabis smoking and anxiety (Fort, 1969).

There is some evidence that heroin users are mostly young men, Puerto Rican, Mexican, or Negro who dropped out of high school (Jurgensen, 1967). The highest incidence is among those of low income, poor education, and broken homes, although this picture is rapidly changing. On the other hand, use of hallucinogens is now widespread in middle-class youth, with an upswing also in heroin dependence and dependence on many drugs in the college population (Carey, 1968).

Drug abusers are from every social class, occupation, and walk of life. Young people seem to be the most involved in drug abuse. Children at grade school age are now part of the drug abuse scene. Drug ingestion by children in the home has been a leading problem for years.

The National Institute of Mental Health was reorganized in November, 1968, so that all drug abuse components were in a single division. The Division of Narcotic Addiction and Drug Abuse was formed in recognition of the threat of drug dependence on the mental health of the nation and its impact upon culture.

The enforcement of laws relating to abuse of drugs is in the hands of the Bureau of Narcotics and Dangerous Drugs of the Department of Justice. Research into therapeutic use of drugs is done by the Food and Drug Administration and the Psychopharmacology Research Branch.

The 89th Congress (1966) passed the Narcotic Addict Rehabilitation Act which affords treatment for persons addicted to drugs who are not charged with offense. It also provides for treatment of those addicts who violate federal law. The Narcotic Addict Rehabilitation Branch of the Division of Narcotic Addiction and Drug Abuse is therefore charged with implementation of direct patient care services which were delegated to the Surgeon General and the National Institute of Mental Health. A Center for Studies of Narcotic and Drug Abuse is charged with the task of developing and carrying out a national program of research services and training with regard to the problem of drug abuse. Among others, it is supporting studies of drug abuse behavior among college and high school students, especially in the use of marihuana.

The Alcoholic and Narcotic Addict Rehabilitation Amendments of 1968 (Public Law 90-574) to the Community Mental Health Centers Act (Public Law 88-164) provide matching funds for developing narcotic addict treatment and rehabilitation services and for training personnel.

Since the drugs that affect mood and behavior are most likely the ones that will be abused, some of these are discussed below. They are categorized into *depressants*, *volatile chemicals*, *stimulants*, and *hallucinogens*. Alcohol is the most abused depressant and, because of its epidemiology, has been discussed in the first part of this chapter. Because of their widespread use in psychiatry, some discussion of the nursing care of patients on ataraxic and antidepressive therapy ends this chapter.

Depressants

The depressant effect of a drug is on the central nervous system; it is related to the concentration in the blood. The higher the concentration in the blood, the greater the depressant effect. Tolerance develops with repeated doses.

BARBITURATES

Barbital, the first barbituric acid derivative, was introduced to medicine in the early 1900's; although there are over 2500 barbiturates synthesized since that time, about thirty are now in widespread use. Barbiturates are useful drugs for relief of anxiety and insomnia. They are the most commonly used of the various hypnotics.

It is estimated that there are enough barbiturates manufactured in this country in a year to give every person 250 doses (Carfagni, 1970). They have widespread use as sleeping pills, in suicide attempts (overdose is the leading cause of death by poisoning), and are used now in epidemiologic proportions by children. Illicit traffic in the barbiturates profits many individuals who make trips to Mexico to pick up large supplies, distributed there by the drug companies, return to this country, and resell them (Rice, 1969). Other places where large quantities of barbiturates are obtained illicitly are the supply depots of the armed services. Excess barbiturates can also be obtained through prescriptions.

The abuser administers barbiturates orally, rectally, or intravenously. They are water soluble and can therefore be reduced to liquid. When injected, the user describes an immediate flash which releases tension and spreads throughout the body. It is described as similar to being drunk. The pleasure is the flash and is called the high. There is loss of coordination and emotional control.

The danger of abuse of barbiturates is the development of tolerance, psychological, and physiological dependence. When a person is physiologically dependent, abrupt withdrawal is dangerous and requires medical supervision. After 10 to 12 hours without drugs, there are signs of increasing anxiety, muscle twitching, tremors, weakness, insomnia, nausea, and orthostatic hypotension; changes in the electroencephalogram occur with convulsions. Convulsions may occur within 16 hours or as late as the eighth day in the barbiturate withdrawal syndrome (Department of Defense, 1968). Confusion, agitation, delirium, and hallucinations may also occur.

In addition to the barbiturates, there are other hypnotics that are central nervous system depressants and may cause dependence, for example, glutethimide (Doriden), ethchlorvynol (Placidyl), methyprylon (Noludar), and ethinamate (Valmid) (Schieser, 1968).

Volatile chemicals

Inhaling fumes from glue, gasoline, paint thinner, or lighter fluid produces an effect similar to that of a general anesthetic such as ether (Schieser, 1968).

Glue is squeezed into a rag or bag which is placed over the nose and mouth. Gasoline and paint thinner fumes may be inhaled directly from the container.

The effect of inhalation of these volatile chemicals is excitement and exhilaration, hallucinations, blurring of vision, slurred speech; ringing in the ears and staggering also occur. Further inhalation may lead to unconsciousness of about 1 hour's duration.

Repeated use suggests the development of psychological dependence; other effects are damage to the kidneys, liver, heart, blood, and nervous system. A danger is death by suffocation and the development of psychotic behavior.

Tranquilizers

The phenothiazines are among the most widely used drugs in the practice of medicine. Charpentier synthesized chlorpromazine in 1950. In that year, the French surgeon, Laborit, introduced promethazine as a potentiating agent in general anesthesia (Goodman and Gilman, 1965, p. 163).

Major tranquilizers are used in the treatment of mental disorders and in other ways in general medicine, especially in the control of nausea and vomiting (Goodman and Gilman, 1965, p. 163). These major tranquilizers include the phenothiazine and reserpine-type drugs. Reserpine is also used to treat high blood pressure but is now seldom used in psychiatry. The phenothiazine derivations comprise the large group of tranquilizers. Chlorpromazine may be considered the prototype drug for the phenothiazine group. The phenothiazines not only act upon the central nervous system, they have effects on other organ systems; this is in contrast to the barbiturates and other sedatives.

Chlorpromazine, given in therapeutic doses, diminishes psychomotor activity and results in ataraxia—what one of my patients characterized as "making anxiety peripheral." These drugs do not have the quality of creating euphoria that seems to characterize the drugs that create psychological dependence. Some physiological dependence occurs, and tolerance develops to the sedative effects (Goodman and Gilman, 1965, p. 172). Abuse of the major tranquilizers is rare.

The minor tranquilizers are widely used in relief of anxiety and tension. Many are used as muscle relaxants. Abuses of these drugs are more connected with getting excess drugs on prescription than use in the street. Meprobamate[9] (Equanil, Miltown) and chlordiazepoxide (Librium) are examples of

---

[9] Meprobamate was removed from the *U.S. Pharmacopeia*, May, 1965.

this group. They have been found to cause both psychological and physiological dependence. Abrupt withdrawal may result in symptoms similar to those seen with barbiturates.

Morphinelike narcotics[10] (opiates)

The sticky resin from the capsule of the poppy *Papaver somniferum* is opium. It may be eaten, drunk, or smoked in the crude form. Opium and its derivatives exert a depressant effect upon the central nervous system. They relieve pain and anxiety and comprise one of the most powerful narcotics. Alkaloids of opium—morphine and codeine—are widely used in medicine today. All other pain-relieving drugs are compared with morphine in estimation of their effectiveness. The abuser of morphine takes from 10 to 20 grains per day (Kolb, 1968).

Heroin, a derivative of morphine, is sold as diluted powder in packets called "decks" or "bags" or in capsules. It is prepared and administered intravenously or sniffed. Being a central nervous system depressant, it diminishes hunger, thirst, sexual urges, fear, pain, and relieves anxiety. It produces a sense of well-being and reduces sensitivity to psychological and physical stimuli. Under the influence of the drug, the user is lethargic and indifferent to his personal situation. Heroin produces tolerance and physiological and psychological dependence. Psychological dependence is the more serious because this dependence continues after the drug is discontinued. Tolerance means that more and larger doses are required to achieve the equivalent effect. The pregnant user will continue the drug with full knowledge that the baby will also be addicted and will die after birth unless treated. As the need for the drug increases, the activities of the user are concentrated on how to get a "fix."

Without drugs, withdrawal symptoms develop within 12 to 16 hours and without treatment, the withdrawal syndrome is called "cold turkey." The withdrawal syndrome occurs as follows:

Yawning, lacrimation, rhinorrhea, sneezing, perspiration
Dilated pupils, "gooseflesh," tremor, anorexia

---

[10] The term "narcotic" includes *all* drugs named in the narcotics laws. It is a *legal* term and therefore includes cocaine and marihuana. The medical meaning of the term "narcotic" refers to producing stupor or sleep and relief of pain. Cocaine is a stimulant and marihuana an hallucinogen/sedative but both are, in legal terms, narcotics.

Cramps of the back, abdomen, and legs; uncontrollable muscle twitching; hot and cold flashes
Vomiting and diarrhea
Restlessness, insomnia, increased blood pressure, pulse, temperature, and respiration
Depression and an obsession to get a "fix"

This syndrome reaches its height 48 hours after the last drug and continues for 72 hours, then subsides during the following 5 to 10 days. In contrast with alcoholic and barbiturate withdrawal, this one does not include convulsions. Users know the routine of the different treatment centers and will sometimes turn themselves in to the ones that give the best withdrawal treatment. Detoxification may be done by administration of morphine in diminishing doses or by the use of methadone in diminishing doses or a combination of both drugs. Methadone maintenance programs modeled after Nyswander (1958) are now being developed on an outpatient basis. In these programs, after withdrawal from other addicting drugs, methadone is administered to patients on a long-term basis. They are then able to go about their usual activities such as work and school without spending all their time searching for other drugs. Methadone can be given orally.

Other opium derivatives may be abused, for example, codeine, Dilaudid, and metopon. Demerol, although not chemically related to the opiates, is addicting. One of the dangers of all these drugs is death from overdosage.

Stimulants

Coffee, tea, and colas are stimulants and are widely used in our culture.

NICOTINE
The psychological and physiological dependence of millions of people in this country on tobacco is a form of drug abuse (Fort, 1969). In spite of the relationship between heart disease, cancer, and cigarette smoking, the dependence continues. The Center for Special Problems of the community mental health services of San Francisco treats this problem along with the other problems of drug abuse. In the Soviet Union, the patient takes over his own treatment; for instance, he abstains from smoking for one day, and in the case of relapse, registers each cigarette in writing, giving the reason why he smoked and what was felt while smoking. Various medicinal mixtures are provided for the withdrawal syndrome (Lustig, 1963).

COCAINE

Cocaine is a strong stimulant; legally, it is a narcotic. Cocaine was first used as a local anesthetic but has now been replaced by more suitable ones.

It is called "coke," "C," or "snow" and administered by sniffing, intravenously, or orally. The stimulant effect is excitement, overtalkativeness, euphoria, and a sense of increased physical strength. It dilates the pupils, there is an increase in blood pressure and the pulse, and there is stimulation, followed by depression. Users may have delusions of persecution, agitation, and experience frightening hallucinations after the initial feelings of pleasure. One of the characteristic effects of cocainism is the feeling that there are insects beneath the skin. Withdrawal is not accompanied by the tendency to collapse as seen in the opium derivatives (Kolb, 1968, p. 524). It produces strong psychological dependence, but tolerance does not occur. It does not produce physiological dependence.

AMPHETAMINES

Amphetamines have been in medical use since the 1930's. In medicine today they are used for depressive patients as psychostimulants and also as anorexants for the obese patient. They are also used to counteract drowsiness caused by the sedative drugs. Amphetamines produce an initial increase in blood pressure, palpitations, pallor, dilated pupils, dry mouth, headache, and diarrhea; they also increase alertness and produce euphoria.

Athletes have taken amphetamines to improve performance; they have been given to race horses for the same reason. Truck drivers take them to stay awake and students use them as stimulants to stay up and study. They are called "bennies" (amphetamine), "Christmas tree" (dextroamphetamine and Amytal), "Dexies" (dextroamphetamine), "crystal" and "speed" (methamphetamine). Amphetamines are taken orally or intravenously. Methamphetamine is now one of the most commonly abused drugs of this group.

A subjective description by the user is below:[11]

> The high: after the injection, you experience a flash exploding all over your brain, or waves of heat all over your body. Then you feel a delicious euphoria and a great sense of self-confidence. With large amounts of methamphetamine, the initial flash may be followed by a short period of narcosis similar to that of heroin and soon you are "wired" (stimulated). After several days high on amphetamines, you become very weary and feel weird. You feel completely run down and if you don't shoot some more speed it's a drag. Methamphetamine is a

---

[11] Economic Opportunity Council, Inc. of San Francisco, *Drugs in the Tenderloin*. 1967, p. 44.

psychic energizer as well as a stimulant, and you may feel like you have an IQ of 500. It's almost like you have two bodies. Your inside body is going real fast and your outside body is going so slow you can hardly move.

The user of these drugs takes large doses over a period of 4 or 5 days, without eating or sleeping. The episode can lead to severe weight loss, malnutrition, and psychosis requiring hospitalization.

Tolerance and psychological dependence occur. Most authorities agree that it does not produce physiological dependence or withdrawal syndrome, although depression and fatigue are experienced after withdrawal.

Hallucinogens

Dream images, distortions of perceptions, and hallucinations are characteristic of these drugs. They are also referred to as psychotomimetic[12] or psychedelic. They have no widespread medicinal use, although LSD has been used experimentally with alcoholics and patients with terminal cancer (Pahnke, 1969).

CANNABIS SATIVA

Cannabis is the generic name of Indian hemp (*Cannabis sativa*). *Cannabis sativa* may be divided into two groups: (1) *Cannabis sativa indica* which is grown in India and (2) *Cannabis non-indica*, grown elsewhere. For high potency of the plant, a high temperature and low humidity are necessary (Advisory Committee on Drug Dependence, 1968). Although it was once used in medicine, it is no longer applied. The active ingredients are tetrahydrocannabinols which affect the mind and body in various ways. Although there is controversy over the abuse of *Cannabis sativa*, the World Health Organization Expert Committee on Dependence Producing Drugs states:[13]

There is agreement that Cannabis *produces hilarity, talkativeness, and increased sociability. A sufficiently strong dose will distort perception, particularly of time and space, and impair both judgment and memory.*

---

[12] Psychotomimetic refers to mimicking the psychoses which the hallucinogens were at first thought to be able to do.
[13] World Health Organization, "Drugs, What They Are." *World Health*, July, 1967, p. 8.

There is also a warping of emotional reactions that may take the form of irritability or confusion. For some people, the drug acts as an hallucinogen and lowers the sensory threshold, making paintings seem more vivid and the experience of listening to music more intense. Anxiety and aggressiveness may result from intellectual and sensory confusion. There is no development of physical dependence, nor unequivocal proof that lasting mental disturbances have been produced by Cannabis, *although predisposed people may have temporary psychoses.''*

Pharmacologically it is not a narcotic, although it is controlled under the Marihuana Tax Act of 1937.

LSD

Lysergic acid diethylamide, or LSD, has been known since 1938. This acid is present in ergot, a rye fungus. It is now derived from the chemical laboratory in large quantities for illicit use on a wide scale.

LSD may be obtained in a small white pill, a powder in capsules, or as a tasteless, colorless, or odorless liquid in ampules. It is referred to as acid; it primarily affects the central nervous system. The user of acid may have dilated pupils, tremors, increased temperature and blood pressure, and hyperactive reflexes. The LSD trip involves changes in sight, hearing, touch, body image, time; and sensitivity to sound increases; synesthesia[14] occurs; disorientation and cognitive changes appear. The environment is perceived in an entirely new way. Nausea and vomiting may also occur. The ''bad trip'' refers to perceptual alterations that result in panic where the individual loses control of himself and reacts in ways that are self-destructive. Trivial events take on great significance and any mood may ensue. LSD may create tolerance and psychological dependence may develop, but it is seldom intense; physiological dependence does not occur. Recurrent hallucinations may occur even some months after LSD has been taken.

Other hallucinogens include mescaline from the Mexican cactus (peyote); psilocybin from certain mushrooms found in Mexico; D.M.T. (dimethyltryptamine), now prepared synthetically but a natural constituent of the seeds of certain plants in the West Indies and South America; and S.T.P. (dimethoxymethylamphetamine) (Angrist, 1969). Some morning glory seeds are also known for their hallucinogenic effect.

------

[14] The translation of one sensory phenomenon into another, for example, sounds become visualized.

Treatment of patients with drug dependence

The two federal centers for treatment of drug addicts and clinical research on their condition are located at Lexington, Kentucky, and Fort Worth, Texas. The designation "Clinical Research Center" became effective January 1, 1967, when the National Institute of Mental Health was reorganized as a Bureau of the Public Health Service. The two Clinical Research Centers came under the Division of Narcotic Addiction and Drug Abuse in November, 1968. The two centers are planning to further develop treatment and rehabilitation for their patients. They also offer opportunities for testing new treatments and comparison of established treatment procedures (The Division of Narcotic Addiction and Drug Abuse, 1969).

Nyswander (1958) has shown that outpatient treatment of drug addicts has some success. Methadone maintenance programs are now being established in some urban centers, with New York leading the way. In these programs, methadone is administered to the addict who must come to the clinic for his dose. Methadone blocks the action of heroin and relieves the craving for drugs. The patient is therefore relieved of the need to look for a "fix."

Psychotherapy, both group and individual, and family therapy are used in the treatment of the person who depends on drugs. Although difficult to establish, it should be begun during the withdrawal phase, if possible. In one treatment center, the Connecticut Mental Health Center, New Haven, the head nurse directs the group psychotherapy (Byron, 1969).

Synanon groups have been established by Charles Dederich. In this kind of group, rehabilitation is considered to require several years and people entering it are expected to spend that much time working within Synanon on their problems. Synanon is set up to maintain a permanent community. The principal treatment process is the effect of one person upon the other. People meet people upon a very basic level and there is emphasis upon learning other things besides drugs. The synanon[15] is a group of ten to twelve people, different for each session (to avoid two people's protecting each other), and these groups meet three times per week (Yablonsky, 1965).

The adult needs help with employment and the younger person needs help to complete his education. Synanon may run certain services such as a gas station in which the person can work at a productive job.

---

[15] The small "s" refers to the group and the large "S" (Synanon) to the organization.

Narcotics Anonymous is modeled after Alcoholics Anonymous. There are various other self-help groups such as NARCO (Narcotic Addiction Research and Community Opportunities, New Haven, Connecticut).

The Lower East Side Information and Service Center for Narcotics Addiction is a group in New York City that helps these human beings. Father David Egan, a Roman Catholic priest, known as the "junkie" priest, has given help to young addicts at New York's House of Detention for Women (Jeffee, 1966). The East Harlem Protestant Parish helps addicts to find employment, with family relationships, to use leisure, and also in emergencies by providing help to get food, clothing, and shelter.

Teen Challenge centers its therapy on God; it was founded by David Wilkerson, an evangelist, in 1959. Teen Challenge has headquarters in Brooklyn, New York, and has activities in San Francisco, Boston, Philadelphia, Chicago, Dallas, and Toronto, Canada.

The role of the nurse

A main focus for all helping professionals is to take the myth out of the use of drugs. Young people want to know the facts and telling them only about the bad effects of drugs omits the fact of the initial pleasure. Many youngsters take drugs without knowing what they are and what the results may be. If the group culture is to experiment with drugs, then, in order to be accepted in the group, there will be strong pressure to also experiment. School nurses and other community nurses in public health and community mental health programs are especially in a position to teach people their effects. Teachers need to know about the dangers of drugs and what to do. Young people need to be warned about the social pressure to take drugs and helped to develop other ways to relate. The Office of Communications, National Institute of Mental Health, is using mass media and other activities to disseminate information on drug abuse at the grassroots level. In the community mental health services of San Francisco, Crash Pads have been set up in high schools, manned with professionals from the interdisciplinary mental health team, including nurses. They are actually in the school, on the scene, to be of help to those students who need it. This effort takes the helping person to the scene instead of expecting the young people to come to the community mental health centers for treatment, which they try to avoid.

With regard to the use of barbiturates, the nurse has an important role in teaching moderation of use. Barbiturates are commonly prescribed as sleeping pills in hospitals and given matter-of-factly by the nurse. Sometimes more simple measures to help sleep are superior—a back rub, hot milk, a quiet environment, or a bedtime chat. The same measures can be repeated if the patient awakens in the middle of the night. These measures should especially be provided for patients who are hospitalized for long periods of time, due to the adaptation and adjustment problems that they have. Although the nurse singlehandedly cannot reroute our drug-oriented society, in home visits, families can be taught the fallacy of taking a drug for everything. Helping the parents look at their own modeling to their children and changing it if necessary is another approach. If the nurse is dependent on drugs, nicotine, for example, the patient being taught to quit smoking perceives the hypocrisy and whatever is taught will probably be ignored. Helping people to "turn on" to things other than drugs is another track.

Drug abuse is common in the professions. Among occupational groups, physicians, pharmacists, and nurses have a high rate. Early detection of drug abuse and help at that point or referral may be the deterrent to chronic use. Setting in motion the procedures for dealing with social and emotional problems requires knowing the specific resources of a community.

A nonjudgmental attitude is required in working with people who depend on drugs. Help the individual who has been occupied with the drug culture to communicate about something else; often that is the only thing that he has been able to talk about. The individual may need help with the basic necessities of life and these have to be provided for in some way. New careerists have assisted with some of these needs, finding a place for others to stay, for example.

In withdrawal, the nurse has a central role in the success of the effort. Patients who are being withdrawn will wheedle, cajole, develop myriad symptoms, threaten suicide, and even attempt suicide to try to get their dose of the drug. It takes consistent limit setting to achieve the withdrawal. Even a 10-minute leeway on the time that the next dose is due is pleaded for most strongly. Addicts know how to run up the mercury on a thermometer, put blood in their stools, and various other devices to fake physical illness and therefore be in line for more medication. If the withdrawal is to be successful, the environment has to be controlled so that the patient gets only his prescribed dose. The nurse's observation and reporting of signs and symptoms is an essential part of the treatment process.

Patients who depend on drugs are still admitted to general hospitals without this fact being recorded on their admitting diagnosis. Nursing management problems can sometimes be severe when such facts about the patient are not shared with them. Some orthopedic patients who are immobilized for long periods are subject to drug dependence.

Narcotic orders are written by licensed physicians and no nurse should continue giving narcotics for very long without requesting reassessment by the physician. Some hospitals have a policy that narcotics orders automatically expire within 48 hours. Others require consultation with the supervising nurse before dispensing. The order "q 4 h p.r.n." requires judgment from the nurse as to its administration. Judicious use of narcotics by nurses may prevent addiction. On the other hand, I have seen nurses verbalize fear that their patients would become addicted when, in fact, they were on the brink of death and regular use of the narcotics that were ordered would give relief to suffering.

Nursing care of patients on pharmacotherapy

Discussion of the patients on drug therapy is included here because it is often a part of the treatment of the drug addict during and after withdrawal and also because of its widespread use in the treatment of mental disorders.

Phenothiazines

Chlorpromazine is the prototype drug in the phenothiazine group. The desired effect in therapy is relaxation, relief of hallucinations and delusions, and ataraxia. Side effects include drowsiness, blurred vision, photosensitivity, constipation, overweight, dermatitis, nasal congestion, orthostatic hypotension, and amenorrhea. With heavier doses, salivation, akathisia and dyskinesia, a parkinsonlike syndrome, appear; a tendency to sleep all the time and lowered body temperature may occur.

Chlorpromazine potentiates other drugs, for example, anesthetics, sedatives, and alcohol; therefore the nurse and the patient should be aware of the effect additional drugs may cause. Sunburn can be serious, so precautions against it must be taken. Patients on phenothiazines must be observed closely for jaundice. Reporting all signs and symptoms is an important aspect of treatment, especially with patients who are on long-term pharmacotherapy.

Antidepressants

There are two groups of antidepressant drugs which are used for the treatment of mild or moderate depression and some phobic anxiety states. Group A includes monoamine oxidase inhibitors and group B includes the non-monoamine oxidase inhibitors.

Group A includes isocarboxazide (Marplan), nialamide (Niamid), phenelzine sulfate (Nardil), and tranylcypromine (Parnate). They are mood elevators. Side effects are orthostatic hypotension, dizziness, vertigo, headache, inhibition of ejaculation, weakness, fatigue, dry mouth, blurred vision, skin rashes, and difficulty in urination. Hypertensive crisis is the most serious toxic effect and is associated with the ingestion of cheese (Goodman and Gilman, 1965, p. 197).

Group B includes imipramine (Tofranil) and amitriptyline (Elavil). Their effect is to dull depressive ideation. Orthostatic hypotension is commonly observed; myocardial infarct and congestive heart failure have been reported (Goodman and Gilman, 1965, p. 200).

Side effects are blurred vision, dryness of the mouth, constipation, and urinary retention. Dizziness, tachycardia, excessive perspiration, headache, muscle tremors, and epigastric distress may also occur with the use of antidepressants. There may be severe reactions if these drugs are mixed with group A. There is no evidence of physiological or psychological dependence, but a withdrawal syndrome may occur.

Summary

In this chapter, drug use and abuse have been presented, with particular emphasis upon the epidemiology of alcoholism and other drugs most commonly used. Therapeutic modalities are outlined and the role of the nurse discussed. Discussion of pharmacotherapy with phenothiazines and antidepressants is included. Some special precautions in the administration of the tranquilizing and antidepressant drugs in drug therapy are discussed with reference to the responsibilities of the nurse.

References

Advisory Committee on Drug Dependence: *Cannabis*. London: Her Majesty's Stationery Office, 1968.

Al-Anon: "Youth and the Alcoholic Parent," N.Y., 1968.

———— "Al-Anon Group Impact on Professional Rehabilitation of the Alcoholic," presented by the Public Relations Committee, at the 28th International Congress on Alcohol and Alcoholism, Washington, D.C., September 15–20, 1968.

———— "Purposes of the Al-Anon Family Groups," N.Y., 1969.

American Psychiatric Association: *A Psychiatric Glossary*. Washington, D.C.: American Psychiatric Association, 1969.

Angrist, Burton A.: "Reported Effects of STP—The Unreliability of Hippies as Reporters of Drug Effects," *British Journal of Addiction*, **64**: 231–34, 1969.

Bogue, Donald J.: *Skid Row in American Cities*. Chicago: University of Chicago Press, 1963.

Byron, Christopher M.: "Methadone: The Controversial Method of Treating Drug Addiction," *Yale Alumni Magazine*, pp. 16–23, February, 1969.

Carey, James T.: *The College Drug Scene*. Englewood Cliffs, N.J.: Prentice-Hall, 1968.

Carfagni, Arthur: notes taken from a "Drug Report to the Mental Health Advisory Board of the City and County of San Francisco," January, 1970.

Chein, I., Gerald, D. L., Lee, R. S., and Rosenfeld, E.: *The Road to H*. New York: Basic Books, Inc., 1964.

Department of Defense: *Drug Abuse*. Washington, D.C.: U.S. Government Printing Office, 1968.

Department of Public Health, San Francisco: *Weekly Bulletin*, July 17, 1967.

The Division of Narcotic Addiction and Drug Abuse, National Institute of Mental Health: *Drug Dependence*. Washington, D.C.: U.S. Government Printing Office, 1969.

Economic Opportunity Council, Inc., of San Francisco: *Drugs in the Tenderloin*, 1967.

Fort, Joel: notes taken from lecture on "Sex, Drugs, and Society," San Francisco, August, 1969.

———— *The Pleasure Seekers: The Drug Crisis, Youth and Society*. New York: The Bobbs-Merrill Co., 1969.

Franks, Cyril M.: "Conditioning and Conditioned Aversion Therapies in the Treatment of the Alcoholic," *The International Journal of the Addictions*, 1:2:61–98, June, 1966.

Goodman, Louis S., and Gilman, Alfred: *The Pharmacological Basis of Therapeutics*, 3rd ed. New York: The Macmillan Co., 1965.

Gordon, Jack David, Levy, Robert I., and Perrow, Charles B.: "Open Ward Management of Alcoholism—Experience with a Pilot Program," *California's Medicine*, 89:397–99, December, 1958.

Grillot, Gerald F.: *A Chemical Background to Nursing*. New York: Harper and Row, Publishers, 1964.

Himwich, Harold E.: "Alcohol and Brain Physiology," in Thompson, George N.: *Alcoholism*. Springfield, Ill.: Charles C Thomas, 1956, pp. 291–408.

Hsu, John J.: "Electroconditioning Therapy of Alcoholics," *Quarterly Journal of Studies on Alcohol*, 26:3:449–59, September, 1965.

Jeffee, Saul: *Narcotics—An American Plan*. New York: Paul S. Eriksson, Inc., 1966.

Johnson, President Lyndon B.: "Health Message to Congress," 1966.

Jurgensen, Warren P.: "New Developments at the Lexington Hospital," in Institute on New Developments in the Rehabilitation of the Narcotic Addict: *Rehabilitating the Narcotic Addict*. Washington, D.C.: U.S. Government Printing Office, 1967.

Kendis, Joseph B.: "The Detoxification Center," in Catanzaro, Ronald J., ed.: *Alcoholism: The Total Treatment Approach*. Springfield, Ill.: Charles C Thomas, 1968, pp. 401–406.

Kolb, Lawrence C.: *Noyes' Modern Clinical Psychiatry*. Philadelphia: W. B. Saunders Co., 1968.

Larsen, Valdemar: "The Effect on Experimental Animals of Antabuse (Tetraethylthiuramdisulfide) in Combination with Alcohol," *Acta Pharmacol.*, 4:321–22, 1948.

Lustig, Bruno: *Therapeutic Methods in Soviet Psychiatry*. New York: Fordham University, 1963.

National Institute of Mental Health: *Alcohol and Alcoholism* (Public Health Service Publication No. 1640). Washington, D.C.: U.S. Government Printing Office, 1968.

Nyswander, Marie, *et al.*: "The Treatment of Drug Addicts as Voluntary Outpatients," *American Journal of Orthopsychiatry*, 28:714–27, 1958.

Pahnke, Walter H., Kurland, Albert A., Goodman, Louis E., and Richards, William A.: "LSD-Assisted Psychotherapy with Terminal Cancer Patients," in Hicks, Richard E., and Fink, Paul Jay: *Psychedelic Drugs*. New York: Grune and Stratton, 1969, pp. 33–42.

The Pharmacopoeia of the United States of America, 17th ed. New York: Lippincott, 1965.

Pittman, David J.: "Public Intoxication and the Alcoholic Offender in American Society," in the President's Commission on Law Enforcement and Administration of Justice: *Task Force Report: Drunkenness*. Washington, D.C.: U.S. Government Printing Office, 1967.

Plaut, Thomas F. A.: "Some Major Issues in Developing Community Services for Persons with Drinking Problems" (Background paper prepared for Surgeon General's Conference with the Mental Health Authorities, Washington, D.C., December, 1966), National Center for Prevention and Control of Alcoholism.

——— *Alcohol Problems: A Report to the Nation by the Cooperative Commission on the Study of Alcoholism*. London: Oxford University Press, 1967.

The President's Commission on Law Enforcement and Administration of Justice: *Task Force Report: Drunkenness*. Washington, D.C.: U.S. Government Printing Office, 1967.

Rice, Donald: Testimony to the U.S. House of Representatives, Select Committee on Crime, San Francisco, October 23, 1969.

Schieser, David W., and Cohen, Seymour: "Drugs and Their Effects," *California's Health*, **25**:8:2ff., February, 1968.

Strauss, R., and McCarthy, R. G.: "Nonaddictive Pathological Drinking Patterns of Homeless Men," *Quarterly Journal of Studies in Alcohol*, **12**:601–11, 1951.

Taber, Clarence Wilbur: *Taber's Cyclopedic Medical Dictionary*. Philadelphia: F. A. Davis Co., 1965.

World Health Organization: "WHO and Mental Health, 1949–1961," *WHO Chronicle*, **16**:5:171–81, May, 1962.

——— "Drugs, What They Are." *World Health*, July, 1967.

Yablonsky, Lewis: *The Tunnel Back. Synanon*. New York: The Macmillan Co., 1965.

Suggested readings

Adler, Nathan: "The Antinomian Personality: The Hippie Character Type," *Psychiatry*, **31**:4:325–38, 1968.

Alksne, Harold, Lieberman, Louis, and Brill, Leon: "A Conceptual Model of the Life Cycle of Addiction," *International Journal of Addiction*, **2**:2:221–40, Fall, 1967.

358 Psychosocial nursing

Belden, Ernest: "A Therapeutic Community for Hospitalized Alcoholics," *California's Health*, **20**:12:89–90, December 15, 1962.
Blane, H. T., Hill, M. J., and Brown, Elliot: "Alienation, Self-Esteem and Attitudes Toward Drinking in High School Students," *Quarterly Journal of Studies of Alcohol*, **29**:2:350–54, 1968.
Bloomquist, Edward R.: "Marijuana: Social Benefit or Social Detriment?" *California Medicine*, **106**:5:346–53, 1967.
Byrne, Marcella: "Resocialization of the Chronic Alcoholic," *American Journal of Nursing*, **68**:1:99–100, January, 1968.
Caplan, Gerald, and Grunebaum, Henry: "Perspectives on Primary Prevention," *Archives of General Psychiatry*, **17**:331–46, September, 1967.
Cohen, Sidney: *The Drug Dilemma*. New York: McGraw-Hill Book Co., 1969.
Cooperative Commission on the Study of Alcoholism: *Alcoholic Problems: A Report to the Nation*. London: Oxford University Press, 1967.
Fowler, Grace: "Understanding the Patient Who Uses Alcohol to Solve His Problems," *Nursing Forum*, **4**:4:67, 1965.
Franks, Cyril, ed.: *Conditioning Techniques in Clinical Practice and Research*. New York: Springer, 1964.
Freed, Earl X.: "The Crucial Factor in Alcoholism," *American Journal of Nursing*, **68**:12:2615–16, 1968.
Freud, Sigmund: *Civilization and Its Discontents*. London: Hogarth Press, 1939.
Garb, Solomon: "Narcotic Addiction in Nurses and Doctors," *Nursing Outlook*, **13**:11:30–34, November, 1965.
Gelperin, Abraham, and Gelperin, Eve Arlin: "The Inebriate in the Emergency Room," *American Journal of Nursing*, **70**:7:1494–97, July, 1970.
Giordano, Henry L.: "The Dangers of Marihuana . . . Facts You Should Know," Bureau of Narcotics and Dangerous Drugs, Washington, D.C.: U.S. Government Printing Office, 1968.
Glatt, M. M.: "Rehabilitation of the Addict," *British Journal of Addictions*, **64**:165–82, 1969.
Godber, Sir George E.: "Smoking Disease: A Self-Inflicted Injury," *American Journal of Public Health*, **60**:2:235–42, February, 1970.
Goode, Erich, ed.: *Marijuana*. New York: Atherton Press, 1969.
Grinspoon, Lester: "Marihuana," *Scientific American*, **221**:6:17–26, December, 1969.
Haberman, Paul W., and Sheinberg, Jill: "Public Attitudes Toward Alcoholism as an Illness," *American Journal of Public Health*, **59**:7:1209–16, July, 1969.
Halleck, Seymour L.: "Psychiatric Treatment for the Alienated College Student," *American Journal of Psychiatry*, **124**:5:642–50, 1967.

Hollander, Charles, ed.: *Background Papers on Student Drug Involvement.* Washington, D.C.: United States National Student Association, 1967.

Huessy, Hans, Marshall, Carlton D., Lincoln, Elizabeth K., and Finan, John L.: "The Indigenous Nurse as Crisis Counselor and Intervenor," *American Journal of Public Health,* **59**:11:2022—29, November, 1969.

Kalinowsky, Lothar B., and Hippius, Hanns: *Pharmacological, Convulsive and Other Somatic Treatments in Psychiatry.* New York: Grune and Stratton, 1969.

Kalkman, Marion E.: *Psychiatric Nursing.* New York: McGraw-Hill Book Co., 1967, pp. 161—77.

Kendall, Lillian: "The Role of the Nurse in the Treatment of the Alcoholic Patient," in Fox, Ruth, ed.: *Alcoholism: Behavioral Research, Therapeutic Approaches.* New York: Springer Publishing Co., Inc., 1967, pp. 285—92.

Keniston, Kenneth: *The Uncommitted; Alienated Youth in American Society.* New York: Harcourt, Brace and World, Inc., 1965.

———— "The Sources of Student Dissent," *Journal of Social Issues,* **23**:3:108—37, 1967.

Krause, Merton S., Ransohoff, Daniel J., and Cohen, Pauline: "Promoting Possible Alcoholism Referrals," *Community Mental Health Journal,* **4**:1:13—16, February, 1968.

Krieg, Margaret B.: *Green Medicine.* Skokie, Ill.: Rand McNally and Co., 1966.

Layton, Sister Mary Michele: "Behavior Therapy and Its Implications for Psychiatric Nursing," *Perspectives in Psychiatric Care,* **4**:2:38—52, 1966.

Leonard, B. E.: "*Cannabis*: A Short Review of Its Effects and the Possible Dangers of Its Use," *British Journal of Addictions,* **64**:121—30, 1969.

Lester, David, *et al.*: "Driving Under the Influence of Alcohol," *Quarterly Journal of Studies on Alcohol,* **14**:4:614—19, 1953.

Lewis, Garland K.: "Communication: A Factor in Meeting Emotional Crises," *Nursing Outlook,* **13**:8:36—39, August, 1965.

McNatt, Juanita, and Sahler, Sandra: "Alcoholism: Caring for the Alcoholic on a Medical Unit," *American Journal of Nursing,* **65**:3:114—16, March, 1965.

Manheimer, Dean I., and Mellinger, Glen D.: "The Use of Psychotherapeutic Drugs Among Adults in California," *California's Health,* **26**:8:3—6, February, 1969.

National Institute of Mental Health: *Thinking About Drinking* (Public Health Service Publication No. 1683). Washington, D.C.: U.S. Government Printing Office, 1968.

Nelson, Bryce: "Alcoholism: The Small Beginnings of a Significant Federal Program," *Science,* **158**:475—77, October 27, 1967.

Otto, Herbert: "The Human Potential of Nurses and Patients," *Nursing Outlook*, **13**:8:32—35, August, 1965.

Parry, Allen A.: "Alcoholism," *American Journal of Nursing*, **65**:3:111—14, March, 1965.

Pazdur, Helen C.: "Innovation: The School Nurse as a Mental Health Specialist," *Mental Health Digest*, **1**:12:28—30, December, 1969.

Price, Gladys: "Alcoholism—A Family, Community and Nursing Problem," *American Journal of Nursing*, **67**:5:1022—26, May, 1967.

Proceedings of a Nurse's Conference on Alcoholism: *Nurse's Role in the Problem of Alcoholism*. New Orleans: November 18—20, 1964.

Rosenberg, Bernard: *Analyses of Contemporary Society: I.* New York: Thomas Y. Crowell Co., 1966.

San Francisco Council on Alcoholism: "The Community's Response to Substance Misuse," *International Journal of the Addictions*, **1**:2:99—105, 1966.

Schoenfeld, Eugene: *Dear Doctor Hippocrates*. New York: Grove Press, Inc., 1968.

Skinner, B. F.: *Science and Human Behavior*. New York: The Macmillan Co., 1953.

Smith, Jean Paul: "LSD: The False Illusion," *FDA Papers*. Washington, D.C.: U.S. Government Printing Office, July-August, 1967.

Ujhely, Gertrud B.: "Nursing Intervention with the Acutely Ill Psychiatric Patient," *Nursing Forum*, **8**:3:311—25, 1969.

United Nations: *International Control of Narcotic Drugs*. New York, 1965.

U.S. Department of Health, Education, and Welfare: *Social Welfare and Alcoholism, Conference Proceedings*. Washington, D.C.: U.S. Government Printing Office, 1968.

Way, Leong E., and Adler, T. K.: *The Biological Disposition of Morphine and Its Surrogates*. Geneva: World Health Organization, 1962.

Willmar State Hospital: *The Manual for the Alcoholic*. Willmar, Minn.: Willmar State Hospital, 1964.

——— *The Therapist's Manual*. Willmar, Minn.: Willmar State Hospital, 1964.

Wolff, Ilse S.: "The Role of the Public Health Nurse in the Treatment of the Alcoholic," in Fox, Ruth, ed.: *Alcoholism: Behavioral Research, Therapeutic Approaches*. New York: Springer Publishing Co., Inc., 1967, pp. 293—98.

World Health Organization: "Neurophysiology and Behavioral Science in Psychiatry," *WHO Chronicle*, **22**:5:204—207, May, 1968.

Appendix A Developmental tasks from infancy through later maturity[1]

Infancy and early childhood (birth to 6 years)
1. Learning to walk
2. Learning to take solid foods
3. Learning to talk
4. Learning to control the elimination of body wastes
5. Learning sex differences and sexual modesty
6. Achieving physiological stability
7. Forming simple concepts of social and physical reality
8. Learning to relate oneself emotionally to parents, siblings, and other people
9. Learning to distinguish right and wrong and developing a conscience

Middle childhood (6 to 12 years)
1. Learning physical skills necessary for ordinary games
2. Building wholesome attitudes toward oneself as a growing organism
3. Learning to get along with age-mates
4. Learning an appropriate masculine or feminine social role
5. Developing fundamental skills in reading, writing, and calculating
6. Developing concepts necessary for everyday living
7. Developing conscience, morality, and a scale of values
8. Achieving personal independence
9. Developing attitudes toward social groups and institutions

Adolescence (12 to 18 years)
1. Achieving new and more mature relations with age-mates of both sexes
2. Achieving a masculine or feminine social role
3. Accepting one's physique and using the body effectively
4. Achieving emotional independence of parents and other adults
5. Achieving assurance of economic independence
6. Selecting and preparing for an occupation
7. Preparing for marriage and family life

---

[1] Robert J. Havighurst: *Human Development and Education*. New York: Longmans, Green and Co., Inc., 1953, by permission, New York, David McKay Co., Inc. These tasks represent a maturity-expectancy score for the given periods.

8. Developing intellectual skills and concepts necessary for civic competence
9. Desiring and achieving socially responsible behavior
10. Acquiring a set of values and an ethical system as a guide to behavior

Early adulthood (18 to 35 years)
1. Selecting a mate
2. Learning to live with a marriage partner
3. Starting a family
4. Rearing children
5. Managing a home
6. Getting started in an occupation
7. Taking on civic responsibility
8. Finding a congenial social group

Middle age (35 to 60 years)
1. Achieving adult civic and social responsibility
2. Establishing and maintaining an economic standard of living
3. Assisting teen-age children to become responsible and happy adults
4. Developing adult leisure-time activities
5. Relating oneself to one's spouse as a person
6. Accepting and adjusting to the physiological changes of middle age
7. Adjusting to ageing parents

Later maturity (60 and older)
1. Adjusting to decreasing physical strength and health
2. Adjusting to retirement and reduced income
3. Adjusting to death of spouse
4. Establishing an explicit affiliation with one's age group
5. Meeting social and civic obligation
6. Establishing satisfactory physical living arrangements

Appendix B   Classification of mental disorders: the diagnostic nomenclature [1]

LIST OF MENTAL DISORDERS AND THEIR CODE NUMBERS
I. Mental retardation
Mental retardation (310–315)
  310   Borderline mental retardation
  311   Mild mental retardation
  312   Moderate mental retardation
  313   Severe mental retardation
  314   Profound mental retardation
  315   Unspecified mental retardation

The fourth-digit subdivisions cited below should be used with each of the above categories. The associated physical condition should be specified as an additional diagnosis when known.

  .0   Following infection or intoxication
  .1   Following trauma or physical agent
  .2   With disorders of metabolism, growth, or nutrition
  .3   Associated with gross brain disease (postnatal)
  .4   Associated with diseases and conditions due to (unknown) prenatal influence
  .5   With chromosomal abnormality
  .6   Associated with prematurity
  .7   Following major psychiatric disorder
  .8   With psychosocial (environmental) deprivation
  .9   With other [and unspecified] [2] condition

II. Organic brain syndromes
(Disorders Caused by or Associated with Impairment of Brain Tissue Function) In the categories under IIA and IIB the associated physical condition should be specified when known.

---

[1] From the American Psychiatric Association: *Diagnostic and Statistical Manual of Mental Disorders. II*. Washington, D.C., 1968, Section 2, pp. 5–13.
[2] The brackets used in this list indicate categories in *The International Classification of Diseases*, Eighth Revision, World Health Organization, 1968, that are to be avoided in the United States or used by record librarians only.

IIA. Psychoses associated with organic brain syndromes (290–294)

290   Senile and presenile dementia
 .0   Senile dementia
 .1   Presenile dementia
291   Alcoholic psychosis
 .0   Delirium tremens
 .1   Korsakov's psychosis (alcoholic)
 .2   Other alcoholic hallucinosis
 .3   Alcohol paranoid state
 .4* Acute alcohol intoxication* [3]
 .5* Alcoholic deterioration*
 .6* Pathological intoxication*
 .9   Other [and unspecified] alcoholic psychosis
292   Psychosis associated with intracranial infection
 .0   Psychosis with general paralysis
 .1   Psychosis with other syphilis of central nervous system
 .2   Psychosis with epidemic encephalitis
 .3   Psychosis with other and unspecified encephalitis
 .9   Psychosis with other [and unspecified] intracranial infection
293   Psychosis associated with other cerebral condition
 .0   Psychosis with cerebral arteriosclerosis
 .1   Psychosis with other cerebrovascular disturbance
 .2   Psychosis with epilepsy
 .3   Psychosis with intracranial neoplasm
 .4   Psychosis with degenerative disease of the central nervous system
 .5   Psychosis with brain trauma
 .9   Psychosis with other [and unspecified] cerebral condition
294   Psychosis associated with other physical condition
 .0   Psychosis with endocrine disorder
 .1   Psychosis with metabolic or nutritional disorder
 .2   Psychosis with systemic infection
 .3   Psychosis with drug or poison intoxication (other than alcohol)
 .4   Psychosis with childbirth
 .8   Psychosis with other and undiagnosed physical condition
 [.9 Psychosis with unspecified physical condition]

IIB Nonpsychotic organic brain syndromes (309)

309   Nonpsychotic organic brain syndromes (mental disorders not specified as psychotic associated with physical conditions)

---

[3] The asterisks used in this list indicate categories added to the ICD-8 for use in the United States only.

.0   Nonpsychotic OBS with intracranial infection

[.1   Nonpsychotic OBS with drug, poison, or systemic intoxication]

.13* Nonpsychotic OBS with alcohol* (simple drunkenness)

.14* Nonpsychotic OBS with other drug, poison, or systemic intoxication*

.2   Nonpsychotic OBS with brain trauma

.3   Nonpsychotic OBS with circulatory disturbance

.4   Nonpsychotic OBS with epilepsy

.5   Nonpsychotic OBS with disturbance of metabolism, growth, or nutrition

.6   Nonpsychotic OBS with senile or presenile brain disease

.7   Nonpsychotic OBS with intracranial neoplasm

.8   Nonpsychotic OBS with degenerative disease of central nervous system

.9   Nonpsychotic OBS with other [and unspecified] physical condition

[.91* Acute brain syndrome, not otherwise specified*]

[.92* Chronic brain syndrome, not otherwise specified*]

III Psychoses not attributed to physical condition listed previously (295–298)

295   Schizophrenia

.0   Schizophrenia, simple type

.1   Schizophrenia, hebephrenic type

.2   Schizophrenia, catatonic type

.23* Schizophrenia, catatonic type, excited*

.24* Schizophrenia, catatonic type, withdrawn*

.3   Schizophrenia, paranoid type

.4   Acute schizophrenic episode

.5   Schizophrenia, latent type

.6   Schizophrenia, residual type

.7   Schizophrenia, schizo-affective type

.73* Schizophrenia, schizo-affective type, excited*

.74* Schizophrenia, schizo-affective type, depressed*

.8*   Schizophrenia, childhood type*

.90* Schizophrenia, chronic undifferentiated type*

.99* Schizophrenia, other [and unspecified] types*

296   Major affective disorders

.0   Involutional melancholia

.1   Manic-depressive illness, manic type

.2   Manic-depressive illness, depressed type

.3   Manic-depressive illness, circular type

.33* Manic-depressive illness, circular type, manic*
.34* Manic-depressive illness, circular type, depressed*
.8   Other major affective disorder
[.9   Unspecified major affective disorder]
      [Affective disorder not otherwise specified]
      [Manic-depressive illness not otherwise specified]
297   Paranoid states
.0   Paranoia
.1   Involutional paranoid state
.9   Other paranoid state
298   Other psychoses
.0   Psychotic depressive reaction
[.1   Reactive excitation]
[.2   Reactive confusion]
      [Acute or subacute confusional state]
[.3   Acute paranoid reaction]
[.9   Reactive psychosis, unspecified]
[299   Unspecified psychosis]
      [Dementia, insanity, or psychosis not otherwise specified]

IV Neuroses (300)
300   Neuroses
.0   Anxiety neurosis
.1   Hysterical neurosis
.13* Hysterical neurosis, conversion type*
.14* Hysterical neurosis, dissociative type*
.2   Phobic neurosis
.3   Obsessive compulsive neurosis
.4   Depressive neurosis
.5   Neurasthenic neurosis
.6   Depersonalization neurosis
.7   Hypochondriacal neurosis
.8   Other neurosis
[.9   Unspecified neurosis]

V Personality disorders and certain other nonpsychotic mental disorders (301–304)
301   Personality disorders
.0   Paranoid personality
.1   Cyclothymic personality
.2   Schizoid personality

.3 Explosive personality
.4 Obsessive compulsive personality
.5 Hysterical personality
.6 Asthenic personality
.7 Antisocial personality
.81* Passive-aggressive personality*
.82* Inadequate personality*
.89* Other personality disorders of specified types*
[.9 Unspecified personality disorder]
302 Sexual deviations
.0 Homosexuality
.1 Fetishism
.2 Pedophilia
.3 Transvestism
.4 Exhibitionism
.5* Voyeurism*
.6* Sadism*
.7* Masochism*
.8 Other sexual deviation
[.9 Unspecified sexual deviation]
303 Alcoholism
.0 Episodic excessive drinking
.1 Habitual excessive drinking
.2 Alcohol addiction
.9 Other [and unspecified] alcoholism
304 Drug dependence
.0 Drug dependence, opium, opium alkaloids, and their derivatives
.1 Drug dependence, synthetic analgesics with morphinelike effects
.2 Drug dependence, barbiturates
.3 Drug dependence, other hypnotics and sedatives or "tranquilizers"
.4 Drug dependence, cocaine
.5 Drug dependence, *Cannabis sativa* (hashish, marihuana)
.6 Drug dependence, other psychostimulants
.7 Drug dependence, hallucinogens
.8 Other drug dependence
[.9 Unspecified drug dependence]

VI Psychophysiologic disorders (305)
305 Psychophysiologic disorders
.0 Psychophysiologic skin disorder
.1 Psychophysiologic musculoskeletal disorder

.2   Psychophysiologic respiratory disorder
.3   Psychophysiologic cardiovascular disorder
.4   Psychophysiologic hemic and lymphatic disorder
.5   Psychophysiologic gastrointestinal disorder
.6   Psychophysiologic genitourinary disorder
.7   Psychophysiologic endocrine disorder
.8   Psychophysiologic disorder of organ of special sense
.9   Psychophysiologic disorder of other type

VII Special symptoms (306)

306   Special symptoms not elsewhere classified
.0   Speech disturbance
.1   Specific learning disturbance
.2   Tic
.3   Other psychomotor disorder
.4   Disorders of sleep
.5   Feeding disturbance
.6   Enuresis
.7   Encopresis
.8   Cephalalgia
.9   Other special symptom

VIII Transient situational disturbances (307)

307*   Transient situational disturbances
.0* Adjustment reaction of infancy*
.1* Adjustment reaction of childhood*
.2* Adjustment reaction of adolescence*
.3* Adjustment reaction of adult life*
.4* Adjustment reaction of late life*

IX Behavior disorders of childhood and adolescence (308)

308   Behavior disorders of childhood and adolescence
.0* Hyperkinetic reaction of childhood (or adolescence)*
.1* Withdrawing reaction of childhood (or adolescence)*
.2* Overanxious reaction of childhood (or adolescence)*
.3* Runaway reaction of childhood (or adolescence)*
.4* Unsocialized aggressive reaction of childhood (or adolescence)*
.5* Group delinquent reaction of childhood (or adolescence)*
.9* Other reaction of childhood (or adolescence)*

X Conditions without manifest psychiatric disorder and nonspecific conditions (316*–318*) [4]

316*   Social maladjustments without manifest psychiatric disorder

.0* Marital maladjustment*

.1* Social maladjustment*

.2* Occupational maladjustment*

.3* Dyssocial behavior*

.9* Other social maladjustment*

317*   Nonspecific conditions*

318*   No mental disorder*

XI Nondiagnostic terms for administrative use (319*)

319*   Nondiagnostic terms for administrative use*

.0* Diagnosis deferred*

.1* Boarder*

.2* Experiment only*

.9* Other*

---

[4] The terms included in this category would normally be listed in that section of ICD-8 that deals with "Special conditions and examinations without sickness."

Appendix C Major drugs used for mind alteration*

Morphine (an opium derivative)

Pharmacologic classification   Central nervous system depressant
Controls   Narcotic (per Harrison Act, 1914)
Medical use   To relieve pain
Potential for physical dependence   Yes
Potential for psychological dependence   Yes
Tolerance   Yes
Possible effects when abused   Drowsiness or stupor, pinpoint pupils
How taken when abused   Orally or by injection
Comments   Morphine is the standard against which other narcotic analgesics are compared. Legally available on prescription only.

Heroin (a morphine derivative)

Pharmacologic classification   Depressant
Controls   Narcotic (per Harrison Act, 1914)
Medical use   To relieve pain
Potential for physical dependence   Yes
Potential for psychological dependence   Yes
Tolerance   Yes
Possible effects when abused   Same as morphine
How taken when abused   Sniffed or by injection
Comments   Not legally available in United States. Used medically in some countries for relief of pain.

Codeine (an opium derivative)

Pharmacologic classification   Depressant
Controls   Narcotic (per Harrison Act, 1914)
Medical use   To relieve pain and coughing
Potential for physical dependence   Yes
Potential for psychological dependence   Yes
Tolerance   Yes
Possible effects when abused   Drowsiness, pinpoint pupils

---

* Dept. of Defense, U.S. Government Printing Office. *Drug Abuse; Game Without Winners*, 1968.

371

How taken when abused   Orally (usually as cough syrup)

Comments   Preparations containing specified minimal amounts of codeine are classified as "exempt" narcotics and can be obtained without prescription in some states.

Paregoric (preparation containing opium)

Pharmacologic classification   Depressant

Controls   Narcotic (per Harrison Act, 1914)

Medical use   For sedation and to counteract diarrhea

Potential for physical dependence   Yes

Potential for psychological dependence   Yes

Tolerance   Yes

Possible effects when abused   Same as morphine

How taken when abused   Orally or by injection

Comments   Paregoric is often boiled to concentrate narcotic content prior to injection. Classified as an exempt narcotic. In some states may be obtained without prescription.

Merperidine (synthetic morphinelike drug)

Pharmacologic classification   Depressant

Controls   Narcotic (brought under Harrison Act in 1944)

Medical use   To relieve pain

Potential for physical dependence   Yes

Potential for psychological dependence   Yes

Tolerance   Yes

Possible effects when abused   Similar to morphine, except that at higher doses, excitation, tremors, and convulsions occur

How taken when abused   Orally or by injection

Comments   Shorter acting than morphine. Frequent dosing required. Withdrawal symptoms appear quickly. Prescription only.

Methadone (synthetic morphinelike drug)

Pharmacologic classification   Depressant

Controls   Narcotic (a 1953 amendment to the Harrison Act brought drugs like methadone under control)

Medical use   To relieve pain

Potential for physical dependence   Yes

Potential for psychological dependence   Yes

Tolerance   Yes

Possible effects when abused   Same as morphine

How taken when abused   Orally or by injection

Comments   Longer acting than morphine. Withdrawal symptoms develop more slowly, are less intense and more prolonged. Prescription only.

Cocaine
Pharmacologic classification   Central nervous system stimulant
Controls   Narcotic (per Harrison Act, 1914)
Medical use   Local anesthetic
Potential for physical dependence   No
Potential for psychological dependence   Yes
Tolerance   No
Possible effects when abused   Extreme excitation, tremors, hallucinations
How taken when abused   Sniffed or by injection
Comments   Although cocaine does not have the narcotic properties of morphine, it has been classified as a narcotic by law because its abuse potential necessitates the same stringent control measures.

Marihuana
Pharmacologic classification   Hallucinogen
Controls   Narcotic (per Marihuana Tax Act, 1937, plus subsequent restrictive legislation which covered marihuana and narcotics together)
Medical use   None
Potential for physical dependence   No
Potential for psychological dependence   Yes
Tolerance   No
Possible effects when abused   Drowsiness or excitability, dilated pupils, talkativeness, laughter, hallucinations
How taken when abused   Smoked or orally
Comments   From a legal control standpoint, marihuana is treated as a narcotic. It is almost never legally available in the United States.

Barbiturates (e.g., amobarbital, pentobarbital, secobarbital)
Pharmacologic classification   Depressant
Controls   Controlled drug products (per Drug Abuse Control Amendments, 1965)
Medical use   For sedation, sleep-producing, epilepsy, high blood pressure
Potential for physical dependence   Yes
Potential for psychological dependence   Yes

Tolerance   Yes

Possible effects when abused   Drowsiness, staggering, slurred speech

How taken when abused   Orally or by injection

Comments   Prescription only. Original prescription expires after 6 months. Only 5 refills permitted within this period. Dependence generally occurs only with the use of high doses for a protracted period of time.

Amphetamine drugs (e.g., amphetamine, dextroamphetamine, methamphetamine—also known as desoxyephedrine)

Pharmacologic classification   Stimulant

Controls   Controlled drug products (per Drug Abuse Control Amendments, 1965. Methamphetamine added to list of controlled drugs in May, 1966.)

Medical use   For mild depression, anti-appetite, narcolepsy

Potential for physical dependence   No

Potential for psychological dependence   Yes

Tolerance   Yes

Possible effects when abused   Excitation, dilated pupils, tremors, talkativeness, hallucinations

How taken when abused   Orally or by injection

Comments   Prescription only. Original prescription expires after 6 months. Only 5 refills permitted within this period.

LSD (also mescaline [peyote], psilocybin, DMT)

Pharmacologic classification   Hallucinogen

Controls   (Brought under Drug Abuse Control Amendments in September, 1966)

Medical use   (Medical research only)

Potential for physical dependence   No

Potential for psychological dependence   Yes

Tolerance   Yes

Possible effects when abused   Excitation, hallucinations, rambling speech

How taken when abused   Orally or by injection

Comments   In 1966, LSD was brought under the control of Drug Abuse Control Amendments of 1965. Control under one of the International Narcotics Conventions is being considered. Not legally available except for medical research.

Glue (also paint thinner, lighter fluid)
> *Pharmacologic classification*   Depressant
> *Controls*   No federal controls. Glue sales restricted in some states.
> *Medical use*   None
> *Potential for physical dependence*   Unknown
> *Potential for psychological dependence*   Yes
> *Tolerance*   Yes
> *Possible effects when abused*   Staggering, drowsiness, slurred speech, stupor
> *How taken when abused*   Inhaled
> *Comments*   Freely available as commercial products, except that some states have laws forbidding the sale of glue to persons under 18.

Index